Breastfeeding and Lactation Care

Breastfeeding and Lactation Care

Editor: Emily Belcher

AMERICAN
MEDICAL PUBLISHERS
www.americanmedicalpublishers.com

AMERICAN
MEDICAL PUBLISHERS
www.americanmedicalpublishers.com

Cataloging-in-Publication Data

Breastfeeding and lactation care / edited by Emily Belcher.
p. cm.
Includes bibliographical references and index.
ISBN 978-1-63927-607-3
1. Breastfeeding. 2. Lactation. 3. Infants--Nutrition. 4. Lactation--Nutritional aspects.
5. Breastfeeding--Physiological aspects. I. Belcher, Emily.
RJ216 .B74 2023
649.33--dc23

American Medical Publishers,
41 Flatbush Avenue,
1st Floor, New York,
NY 11217, USA

ISBN 978-1-63927-607-3 (Hardback)

Contents

Preface

Lactation is a process which involves the secretion of milk through the mammary glands. It also describes the period in which a mother lactates to feed her new born child. The procedure normally occurs in all sexually mature female mammals. The process of feeding a child with breast milk is called breastfeeding or nursing. Breast milk can be fed directly from the breast, or it can be pumped to be given to the child later. Breastfeeding starts a few hours after the birth of a baby and can be continued as long as the baby needs it. The infants cannot be fed with any foods or drinks till they turn six months old. New-born babies are prescribed vitamin D for ensuring that they are able to absorb calcium and phosphorus. After completing six months, the baby can be fed foods advised by the doctors, but breastfeeding should continue till one or two years of age. This book explores all the important aspects of breastfeeding and lactation care in the present day scenario. The topics included herein are of utmost significance and bound to provide incredible insights to readers. This book will serve as a reference to a broad spectrum of readers.

The information shared in this book is based on empirical researches made by veterans in this field of study. The elaborative information provided in this book will help the readers further their scope of knowledge leading to advancements in this field.

Finally, I would like to thank my fellow researchers who gave constructive feedback and my family members who supported me at every step of my research.

Editor

1

Is there an Association between Breastfeeding and Dental Caries among Three-Year-Old Australian Aboriginal Children?

Dandara G. Haag [1,2], Lisa M. Jamieson [1], Joanne Hedges [1] and Lisa G. Smithers [2,*]

1 Indigenous Oral Health Unit, Australian Research Centre for Population Oral Health, The University of Adelaide, Adelaide, SA 5005, Australia; dandara.haag@adelaide.edu.au (D.G.H.); lisa.jamieson@adelaide.edu.au (L.M.J.); joanne.hedges@adelaide.edu.au (J.H.)

2 School of Public Health, The University of Adelaide, Adelaide, SA 5005, Australia

* Correspondence: lisa.smithers@adelaide.edu.au

Abstract: An unresolved question about breastfeeding is its effect on caries, in particular, early childhood caries (ECC). In secondary analyses of data from an ECC intervention, we describe breastfeeding among Aboriginal children and associations between breastfeeding and ECC. Breastfeeding (duration and exclusivity to six months) was grouped into mutually exclusive categories. ECC was observed by a calibrated dental professional. Outcomes were prevalence of ECC (% decayed, missing, and filled teeth in the primary dentition (% dmft>0)) and caries severity (mean number of decayed, missing, and filled surfaces (mean dmfs)) in children aged three years. Analyses were adjusted for confounding. Multiple imputation was undertaken for missing information. Of 307 participants, 29.3% were never breastfed, 17.9% exclusively breastfed to six months, and 9.3% breastfed >24 months. Breastfeeding >24 months was associated with higher caries prevalence (adjusted prevalence ratio (PR_a) 2.06 (95%CI 1.35, 3.13, *p*-value = 0.001) and mean dmfs (5.22 (95% CI 2.06, 8.38, *p*-value = 0.001), compared with children never breastfed. Exclusive breastfeeding to six months with breastfeeding <24 months was associated with 1.45 higher caries prevalence (95% CI –0.92, 2.30, *p*-value = 0.114) and mean dmfs 2.04 (−0.62, 4.71, *p*-value = 0.132), compared with never breastfeeding. The findings are similar to observational studies on breastfeeding and caries but not with randomized controlled trials of breastfeeding interventions. Despite attending to potential biases, inconsistencies with trial evidence raises concerns about the ability to identify causal effects of breastfeeding in observational research.

Keywords: breastfeeding; caries; childhood; Aboriginal

---

1. Introduction

Breastfeeding has many well-established benefits for both mother and baby, and is recommended by governments, scientific, and health institutions all over the world. The World Health Organization (WHO) recommends that infants are exclusively breastfed to age six months, and that breastfeeding continues to two years of age [1]. Individual countries may vary slightly in their recommendations, for example, the Australian government recommends exclusive breastfeeding to six months and continued breastfeeding to up to and beyond one year [2]. Despite these recommendations, there is little recent evidence on adherence to these guidelines by marginalized communities, such as Aboriginal and Torres Strait Islander peoples. Breastfeeding is culturally supported by Aboriginal and Torres Strait Islanders and is encouraged by local Aboriginal Community Controlled Health Service workers and midwifes.

An unresolved question about breastfeeding is its effect on caries, in particular, early childhood caries (ECC). ECC is defined as the presence of one or more decayed (cavitated or not), missing (due to dental caries), or filled tooth surfaces in any primary tooth among children aged <6 years old [3]. In recent years, there have been a number of systematic reviews reporting the effect of breastfeeding on ECC that have arrived at slightly differing conclusions. One of the first systematic reviews published by Tham et al. [4] included 63 papers published up until 2014. Tham et al. concluded that breastfeeding protected against ECC but breastfeeding beyond 12 months of age increased the risk of ECC. Cui et al. suggested similar findings from a search up to 2015 that included 35 studies but called for more studies to strengthen the evidence [5]. While it seems that breastfeeding in the early postnatal period is protective, the time at which the association reverses and breastfeeding becomes a risk factor for ECC is unclear. Earlier this year, Moynihan et al. published a systematic review that investigated this further [6], where they examined studies that compared the effects of breastfeeding ≥12 months compared to <12 months on ECC, and studies of breastfeeding ≥24 months compared to <24 months. For the 21 studies comparing breastfeeding <12 vs. ≥12 months, a null association was observed. The evidence from the eight studies comparing breastfeeding ≥24 months compared to <24 months varied widely, with some studies reporting strong positive associations with ECC, but studies were too small to generate a precise effect estimate and a null association was inferred.

We previously collected breastfeeding and ECC information from Australian Aboriginal children and their families who participated in a randomized controlled trial of an early childhood caries intervention. In Australia, oral health inequalities between Aboriginal and non-Aboriginal people start to emerge in childhood. According to the Australian National Child Oral Health Study (NCOHS) conducted between 2012 and 2014, the prevalence of untreated dental caries in the primary dentition among Indigenous children aged 5–10 years old was 44% compared to 26% among their non-Indigenous counterparts [7]. This difference represents a 70% increase in the prevalence of untreated dental caries, and it was larger than the inequalities observed according to other important sociodemographic factors, such as household income, parental education, and residential location. Furthermore, not only the prevalence of untreated dental caries is higher among Indigenous children, but they also have more severe disease. Indigenous Australian children aged 5 to 10 years old have, on average, almost three times the mean number of decayed tooth surfaces observed among their non-Indigenous counterparts (3.4 vs. 1.2). This means that Indigenous children are more likely to be exposed to the consequences of dental caries, such as dental pain, treatment under general anesthesia, poorer concentration in a classroom setting, and higher school absenteeism. Therefore, understanding potential drivers of dental caries at an early age in this population is the first step to developing culturally appropriate interventions to manage dental disease in its early stages, and to instituting effective preventive measures to improve oral health in adulthood. Here, we conduct a secondary (observational) analyses of these data with two aims: (1) To describe patterns of breastfeeding among Australian Aboriginal children, and (2) to examine the association between different categories of breastfeeding on three-year-old ECC outcomes.

2. Materials and Methods

2.1. Participants and Study Design

The current study comprises a secondary analysis using data from an early childhood caries intervention that involved 448 women who identified as being pregnant with an Aboriginal and/or Torres Strait Islander child between February 2010 and May 2011 [8].

Recruitment was mainly through the antenatal clinics at South Australian hospitals and through Aboriginal Community Controlled Health Organizations. The study was a 2-arm parallel, outcome assessor-blinded, randomized controlled trial that aimed to assess if an intervention involving dental care to mothers during pregnancy, application of fluoride varnish to the teeth of children, anticipatory guidance, and motivational interviewing reduced prevalence of dental disease among Aboriginal children in South Australia at follow-up ages of 24 and 36 months [9,10]. The intervention took place during pregnancy and when children were aged 6, 12, and 18 months for the early intervention group, and when children were aged 24, 30, and 36 months for the delayed intervention group. Three-year follow-up data were collected from November 2014 to February 2016. All information was collected at participants' households or at their ACCHO. Children with any information collected at baseline, 2,- and 3-year-old follow-up were included in the study (n = 307).

All participants provided written informed consent. Both the original trial and the follow-up studies were conducted in accordance with the Declaration of Helsinki, and the protocol was approved by the Ethics Committee of The University of Adelaide Human Research Ethics Committee (Project code: H-057-2010), the Aboriginal Health Council of South Australia (Project code: 04-09-362), the South Australian Department for Health, including the human research ethics committees of participating South Australian hospitals (Flinders Medical Centre (Project code: 435-10), Lyell McEwin Hospital (Project code: 2010-160), and Women's and Children's Hospital (Project code: REC2322/11/13)).

2.2. *Breastfeeding (Exposure)*

Breastfeeding information was collected when children were aged 24 months by asking mothers the duration of breastfeeding and the period of exclusive breastfeeding. Patterns of breastfeeding were categorized according to two definitions based on previous studies examining the effect of breastfeeding on dental caries (definition A) [4,6] and following the WHO recommendations (definition B) [1]. Definition A allows us to compare the risks of ECC for breastfeeding over 12 months with other durations of breastfeeding, whereas definition B aligns with the WHO's international breastfeeding recommendations. Definition A consisted of four categories including children who were never breastfed, breastfed for <12 months, breastfed for 12–23 months, and breastfed for 24 months or longer. Definition B consisted of the following four categories of breastfeeding; never breastfed, breastfed for <24 months with exclusive breastfeeding until 6 months, breastfed for <24 months with no exclusive breastfeeding until 6 months, and breastfed for 24 months or longer.

2.3. *Oral Health (Outcomes)*

The primary outcome was the prevalence of ECC, which is the proportion of children with ≥1 decayed teeth (with or without a break in the tooth surface), ≥1 missing teeth due to dental caries, and ≥1 filled teeth) at 3 years of age (% dmft>0). The primary dentition comprises 20 teeth, which normally erupt in the oral cavity between 6 and 24 months of age. Dental decay was considered since its initial stages, which consists of white areas on the surface of the tooth. We also examined the severity of ECC by assessing the mean number of tooth surfaces with decayed, missing, and filled surfaces (mean dmfs). Oral examinations were conducted by calibrated and masked examiners following a standardized protocol to record dental disease experience. Children were examined in the knee-to-knee position on their mother's lap, as is considered appropriate for this age group. Teeth were dried with cotton pads before examination. The light source was a fiber-optic light and standard infection control procedures were followed. Only visual criteria were used to assess diagnoses. Any children identified as having untreated dental decay were referred to the South Australian Dental Service (SADS).

2.4. *Confounding*

Confounding factors included a range of variables that share a causal association with both exposures and outcomes and were assessed at baseline. These included smoking and alcohol consumption in pregnancy (yes/no), child sex, main source of household income (job vs. government social welfare support), maternal education (secondary school or less vs. trade/technical and university), parity (first time mother vs. others), maternal age (continuous), maternal ethnicity (Aboriginal vs. non-Aboriginal), and a national indicator of socioeconomic position calculated from residential postcode (the index of relative socioeconomic advantage and disadvantage (IRSAD) [11]. Additionally, we adjusted for randomization group because breastfeeding occurred during the intervention, even though there were no differences in breastfeeding duration between the treatment groups.

2.5. Statistical Analysis

In order to address potential bias due to missing data, we undertook multiple imputation by chained equations under the assumption that data were missing at random conditional on the observed data [12]. Twenty imputed datasets were generated from imputation models containing all the variables included in the final regression analyses. Imputed values were generated for smoking in pregnancy (missing $n = 1$), alcohol consumption in pregnancy (missing $n = 1$), main source of household income at baseline (missing $n = 1$), IRSAD (missing $n = 3$), breastfeeding duration (missing $n = 3$), exclusive breastfeeding duration (missing $n = 9$), and mean number of tooth surfaces with dental caries (missing $n = 1$). All other variables were fully observed. Analyses were conducted by combining all imputed datasets following Robin's rules on a final sample of $n = 307$ children who had some information collected at baseline, 2-, and 3-year-old follow-up.

Descriptive statistics were computed for the response sample, complete cases, and imputed sample, and included the distribution of participants according to exposures (breastfeeding), confounding factors (listed above), and outcomes (prevalence of ECC and mean dmfs). Generalized linear models with a log-Poisson link function and robust standard errors were used to estimate the prevalence ratios [13] and their 95% confidence intervals (CI) of dental caries according to breastfeeding patterns (definitions A and B). Next, adjusted PRs and their respective 95% CIs were assessed after the inclusion of the abovementioned confounding variables in the models. Unadjusted and adjusted and linear regressions were used to estimate the association between breastfeeding patterns and mean dmfs.

Analyses were carried out using STATA 15.0.

3. Results

The sample consisted of 307 children who had some information collected at baseline, 2-, and 3-year-old follow-up. Sample characteristics are shown in Table 1. Most children were born to mothers who identified as Aboriginal (82.7%). On average, mothers were 24.7 years old at baseline. Just over half of the children (52.1%) were boys and 39.4% were the first child. Four in five children (82.4%) lived in households where government support was the main source of income and over two-thirds of mothers (71.7%) had high school or less educational attainment. Over half of the children (55.3%) lived in the most disadvantaged IRSAD quintile. Smoking in pregnancy was observed among half of the sample, whereas 10.8% of mothers reported alcohol consumption during pregnancy. One in three children were never breastfed (29.2%), whereas half of the sample (49.9%) were breastfed for less than 12 months. The proportion of children breastfed for 12–23 months and 24 or more months was 11.5% and 9.3%, respectively. One in four children were exclusively breastfed until six months (23.8%) (data not shown). At three years of age, one-third had experienced dental caries, and the mean number of decayed, missed, or filled tooth surfaces was 3.2 (Table 1).

Table 1. Characteristics of the study sample.

	Response Sample %	Complete Cases % (n = 292)	Imputed Sample % (n = 307)
Exposure: Breastfeeding patterns			
Breastfeeding pattern A			
Never breastfed	29.3	29.8	29.2
Breastfed for <12 months	49.8	51.7	49.9
Breastfed for 12 to 23 months	11.4	11.3	11.5
Breastfed for 24 months or more	9.5	7.2	9.3
Breastfeeding pattern B (WHO recommendations)			
Never breastfed	29.3	29.8	29.2
Breastfed for <24 months, exclusively until 6	17.9	18.5	18.2
Breastfed for <24 months, not exclusively until 6	43.3	44.5	43.2
Breastfed for 24 months or more	9.5	7.2	9.3
Outcomes at child age 3 years			
Any decayed, missed or filled tooth (% dmft>0)	32.0	31.9	32.1
Mean number of decayed, missed or filled tooth surfaces (mean dmfs)	3.1	3.2	3.2
Potential confounding factors			
Child sex (male)	52.1	52.1	52.1
Mean maternal age at childbirth	24.7	24.6	24.7
Main household income source			
Job	17.6	18.2	17.6
Government support	82.4	81.9	82.4
Maternal education at birth			
High school or less	71.7	71.2	71.7
TAFE or university	28.3	28.8	28.3
Index of Relative Socioeconomic Advantage and Disadvantage			
1st quintile (most disadvantaged)	55.4	55.1	55.3
2nd quintile	17.3	16.8	17.4
3rd quintile	21.1	23.6	21.0
4th quintile	2.6	2.7	2.6
5th quintile (most advantaged)	1.6	1.7	1.6
Alcohol consumption in pregnancy (yes)	10.8	10.6	10.8
Smoking in pregnancy (yes)	50.1	50.7	50.0
Parity (first child)	39.4	40.1	39.4
Maternal Ethnicity (Aboriginal and/or Torres Strait Islander)	82.7	82.5	82.7
Child received the intervention (early)	49.5	49.0	49.5

WHO: World Health Organization.

Figure 1 displays the prevalence of dental caries experience (% dmft>0) and mean dmfs according to breastfeeding patterns (definition A). In comparison with children who were never breastfed, the prevalence of ECC was lower among those who were breastfed <12 months (33.1% vs. 25.7%), although both groups exhibited a similar mean dmfs (2.3 vs. 3.0). Over two-thirds of the children breastfed for 12 to 23 months had dental caries (37.0%). The highest prevalence (56.4%) and severity (6.6 mean dmfs) of disease was observed among children breastfed for 24 months.

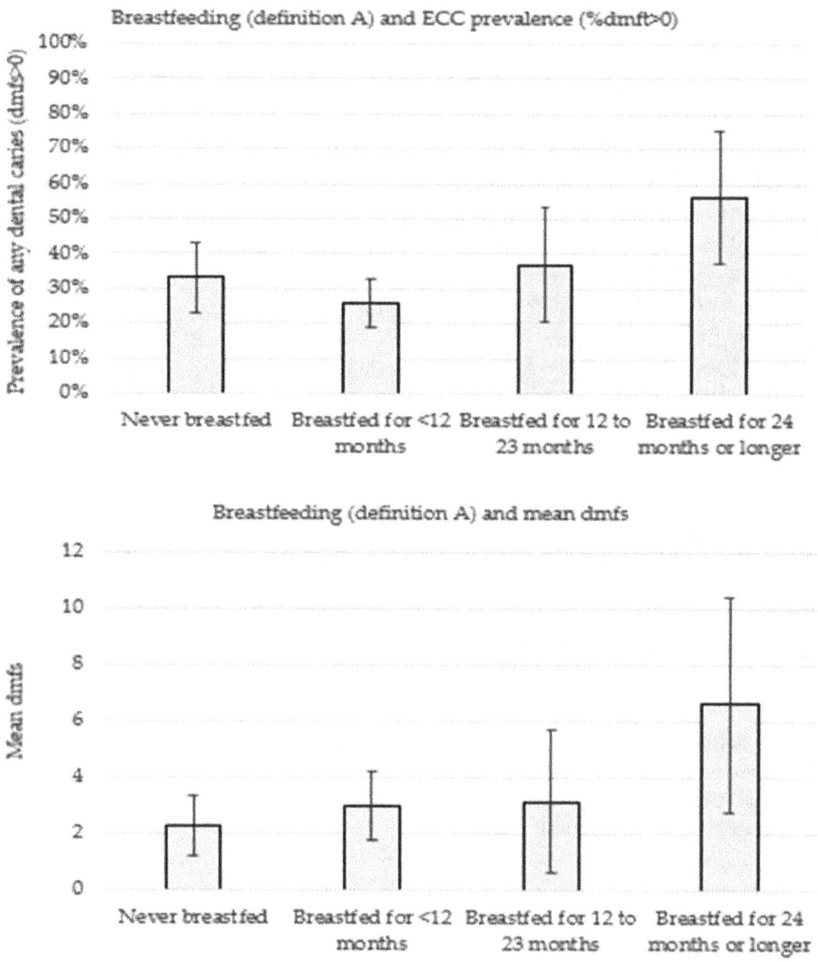

Figure 1. Prevalence of early childhood caries (ECC) and mean number of decayed, missing, and filled teeth (mean dmfs) according to breastfeeding patterns (definition A).

Figure 2 displays the prevalence of dental caries experience (% dmft>0) and mean dmfs according to breastfeeding patterns (definition B). While a higher prevalence of dental caries was observed among children breastfed for less than 24 months with exclusive breastfeeding until six months (33.1%) in comparison with those breastfed for the same duration but without exclusive breastfeeding (25.7%), both groups exhibited a similar mean dmfs (3.0 vs. 3.1).

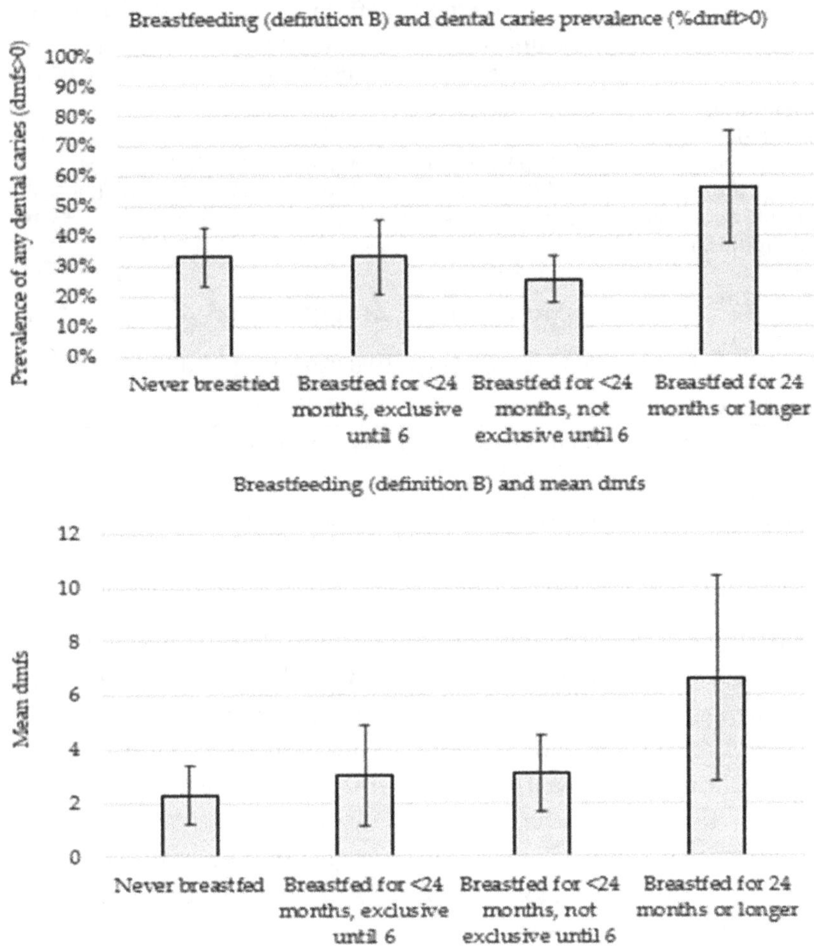

Figure 2. Prevalence of early childhood caries (ECC) and mean number of decayed, missing, and filled teeth (mean dmfs) according to breastfeeding patterns (definition B).

Table 2 displays the unadjusted and adjusted associations between breastfeeding patterns (definitions A and B) with % dmft>0 and mean dmfs. For definition A, the point estimate for prevalence of % dmft>0 was 6% lower among children who were breastfeeding <12 months compared with no breastfeeding (PR = 0.94 (95%CI 0.63; 1.41)). Breastfeeding for 12 to 23 months and breastfeeding for two years or more were associated with a 47% (PR = 1.47 (95%CI 0.85; 2.54)) and two-fold higher ECC prevalence (PR = 2.06 (95%CI 1.35; 3.13)), respectively. In comparison with children who were never breastfed, adjusted models for the mean dmfs showed higher dmfs among children breastfed for less than 12 months (β = 1.31 (95%CI-0.66; 3.30)), those breastfed for 12 to 13 months (β = 2.24 (95%CI –0.74; 5.24)), and among those breastfed for 24 months or longer (β = 5.22 (95%CI 2.06; 8.39). For definition B, breastfeeding up to 23 months and exclusively until six months was associated with a 45% (PR = 1.45 (95%CI 0.92; 2.30)) higher ECC prevalence and a higher dmfs (β = 2.04 (95%CI –0.62; 4.71)).

Table 2. Associations between breastfeeding patterns with dental caries prevalence and severity.

	Any Decayed, Missed or Filled Tooth (% dmft>0)		Number of Decayed, Missed or Filled Tooth Surfaces (Mean dmfs)	
	Unadjusted PR (95%CI)	**Adjusted PR (95%CI)**	**Unadjusted β (95%CI)**	**Adjusted β (95%CI)**
Breastfeeding (definition A)				
Never breastfed	Ref	Ref	Ref	Ref
Breastfed for <12 months	0.77 (0.52; 1.17)	0.94 (0.63; 1.41)	0.72 (−1.02; 2.65)	1.31 (−0.66; 3.30)
Breastfed for 12 to 23 months	1.11 (0.66; 1.89)	1.47 (0.85; 2.54)	0.88 (−2.00; 3.76)	2.24 (−0.74; 5.24)
Breastfed for 24 months or longer	1.70 (1.09; 2.64)	2.06 (1.35; 3.13)	4.31 (1.19; 7.43)	5.22 (2.06; 8.39)
Breastfeeding (definition B)				
Never breastfed	Ref	Ref	Ref	Ref
Breastfed for <24 months, exclusively until 6	1.00 (0.52; 1.17)	1.45 (0.92; 2.30)	0.70 (−1.85; 3.24)	2.04 (−0.62; 4.71)
Breastfed for <24 months, not exclusively until 6	0.77 (0.66; 1.89)	0.90 (0.59; 1.36)	0.77 (−1.23; 2.77)	1.26 (−0.79; 3.31)
Breastfed for 24 months or longer	1.70 (1.09; 2.64)	2.06 (1.35; 3.13)	4.31 (1.19; 7.43)	5.22 (2.05; 8.39)

Prevalence ratios obtained from Poisson regressions. Beta coefficients obtained from linear regressions. Models adjusted for child: Child sex, household main income source, maternal education at childbirth, index of relative socioeconomic advantage and disadvantage, alcohol consumption in pregnancy, smoking in pregnancy, parity, maternal ethnicity, and whether the child received the intervention (early, delayed).

4. Discussion

The results presented here are secondary, observational analyses from a sample of Aboriginal families in South Australia who were enrolled in an early childhood caries intervention. They show that that around one-third of children are never breastfed, half are breastfed for less than 12 months, and one-fifth are breastfed for longer than 12 months (breastfeeding definition A). Applying the WHO breastfeeding recommendations in breastfeeding definition B shows that almost one-fifth of children are breastfed exclusively for six months. For our aim of investigating observational associations between breastfeeding and oral health, these results suggest that breastfeeding for 24 months or longer is associated with twice the prevalence of ECC and four-fold higher severity of caries (indicated by mean dmfs). Both duration and exclusivity of breastfeeding may be important, but evidence from the current study is stronger for the duration of breastfeeding. Evidence for duration comes from the breastfeeding pattern A results, where the adjusted point estimates suggest monotonically increasing risks of both % dmft>0 and dmfs from 12–23 and then ≥24 months of breastfeeding. Breastfeeding pattern B provides some suggestive observational evidence of an increased risk of caries with exclusive breastfeeding to six months, although there are major challenges with disentangling duration and exclusivity (discussed further below). Additionally, the modest sample size has likely contributed to imprecision in estimating these effects. Notably, this sample has poor oral health with 25% prevalence of ECC even though children were only three years old, which has contributed to why we have been able to detect these associations at such a young age.

It is important to emphasize that any potential effects of breastfeeding on caries can be mitigated by better oral hygiene and access to oral healthcare, and these should be the targets of public policy, particularly since oral health is a major cause of problems (such as hospitalizations, extractions) in children. Maternal-child health nurses encourage breastfeeding and with appropriate training they might present an opportunity for teaching caregivers to begin clean deciduous teeth as soon as they erupt. The promotion of wide-spread water fluoridation is also important in reducing oral health inequalities, particularly between Indigenous and non-Indigenous Australian children [7].

Compared with Australian national statistics on breastfeeding the prevalence, data reported here appear lower. For example, national data indicate that around 80% of Aboriginal children were ever breastfed [14], whereas 70% of children in the current study were reportedly ever breastfed. The national data were collected in 2014–2015, at a similar time to our study, so temporal shifts in breastfeeding cannot explain this discrepancy. This is probably not due to selection bias as, compared with birth registry data, we enrolled around half of all eligible Aboriginal children born in the state over the recruitment period, and families who were not enrolled or dropped out are likely to be more marginalized. While it is difficult to pinpoint exactly why we found lower breastfeeding outcomes compared with national averages, we speculate that this may be because our participants are more disadvantaged than families included in the national data. The high level of disadvantage is indicated in Table 1, where half of the participants in our study are in the most disadvantaged quintile for socioeconomic position (on a national scale), half smoked during pregnancy, and about 80% received government income support. The state of South Australia has a more disadvantaged socioeconomic profile than other mainland Australian states. However, many other (non-socioeconomic) issues around breastfeeding should also be considered. Such factors might include mothers being very time-poor, impediments to breastfeeding due to mental health problems (postnatal depression, anxiety), low self-confidence in their ability to breastfeed, and lack of partner support. Taking a strengths-based view, since only one-third of women did not breastfeed, this indicates this is an area of cultural strength. Contributors to breastfeeding success are other key women involved in perinatal care and social networks of new mothers', which may improve self-confidence in their ability to successfully initiate and maintain breastfeeding for longer. Social context and culturally safe birthing programs are important influences on breastfeeding among Aboriginal women [15,16].

The debate about whether breastfeeding has a causal role in ECC remains, with discussions on the evidence from the three systematic reviews on this topic vary. Our results appear to confirm concepts raised in previous systematic reviews that the risk of ECC increases with breastfeeding beyond 12 months and possibly with exclusive breastfeeding [4,6]. We were surprised to find suggestive evidence that exclusive breastfeeding to six months (among children breastfed for less than 24 months) was linked to higher caries, as first teeth only erupt around six months. It is possible that the exclusive breastfeeding to six months is an indicator of other related factors, such as mothers being more committed to breastfeeding and more likely to breastfeed for longer. Support for this idea comes from the fact that the duration of breastfeeding among children exclusively breastfed to six months was 2.5 times longer than the duration observed among children who were not exclusively breastfed to six months (10 vs. 4 months). It is clearly difficult to separate out effects of exclusive breastfeeding from the effect of duration of breastfeeding in observational research, and for this reason we look to the literature for evidence from specific breastfeeding randomized controlled trials (RCTs). The standout in this field is the large Promotion of Breastfeeding Intervention Trial (PROBIT), trial which is a cluster-RCT where intervention hospitals implemented the baby-friendly hospital initiative, and this resulted in increased breastfeeding duration and exclusivity [13]. Follow up of caries data in the PROBIT participants indicated no differences in caries outcomes between the groups, despite having more women in the intervention group breastfeeding for longer durations and higher proportions of women exclusively breastfeeding to six months of age [17]. Another cluster RCT of an intervention that increased exclusive breastfeeding to six months conducted in Uganda also indicated no effect of caries outcomes at five years of age [18]. Observational research on breastfeeding is notoriously confounded and one way forward might be to apply different study designs that can help overcome such problems, as has been done for the effects of breastfeeding on intelligence quotient and obesity [19].

We approached this study with causal inference in mind. With respect to study validity, we tried to minimize confounding by adjusting for multiple variables that were identified through content knowledge and literature. One issue relevant to this field is whether to adjust for confounding by other aspects of the child's diet such as sugary foods and beverages. In causal inference theory, confounding is considered to be a common cause of the exposure and outcome [20]. While there is no doubt that the sugar content of the diet has a direct effect on caries, it is not a direct cause of initiating breastfeeding. Any reduction in breastfeeding will lead to consumption of other foods and therefore sugary foods may be a mediator on the breastfeeding → diet → caries pathway. Factors further back in the causal chain, such as parental education, influence breastfeeding and diet, a phenomenon occasionally referred to as M-bias in the epidemiological literature. Our approach was to adjust for many of these more distal factors to block the influence of these cofounders. It is also worth noting that the participants were involved in a health promotion trial and therefore their breastfeeding behaviors may have been different had they not been involved in the trial. We used multiple imputation to address bias due to missing information, which is uncommon in this field [4,6]. Some effect estimates have wide confidence intervals which is likely due to the sample size, which was limited to the original trial. Increasing the sample size was not possible because the study is estimated to have enrolled around half of the local Aboriginal and Torres Strait Islander children in the state of South Australia at the time of recruitment.

5. Conclusions

There is room to improve breastfeeding prevalence, duration, and exclusivity among mothers of Aboriginal children in South Australia, and this could have flow on effects of improving other health outcomes. Regarding ECC, the observational analyses presented here suggest that breastfeeding for longer and more exclusively may be linked to poorer outcomes. Despite attempting to address sources of bias, doubt is raised about interpreting this observational research as causal.

Author Contributions: Conceptualization, D.G.H. and L.G.S.; data curation, L.M.J., J.H., and L.G.S.; formal analysis, D.G.H.; funding acquisition, L.M.J. and J.H.; methodology, D.G.H. and L.G.S.; project administration, L.M.J.; supervision, L.G.S.; writing—original draft, D.G.H. and L.G.S.; writing—review and editing, D.G.H., L.M.J., J.H., and L.G.S..

Acknowledgments: The authors acknowledge the support of the Baby Teeth Talk study participants and staff including the Aboriginal Reference Group (Chaired by Cathy Leane); support of staff from the South Australian Aboriginal Community-Controlled Health Organisations. We thank Colgate Palmolive for donations of toothpaste, toothbrushes, dental floss and disclosing tables that were offered as part of a 'thank you' package to participants and their families.

References

1. World Health Organization. Breastfeeding. Available online: https://www.who.int/topics/breastfeeding/en/ (accessed on 27 September 2019).
2. National Health and Medical Research Council. *Infant Feeding Guidelines*; National Health and Medical Research Council: Canberra, Australia, 2013.
3. Wyne, A.H. Early childhood caries: Nomenclature and case definition. *Community Dent. Oral Epidemiol.* **1999**, *27*, 313–315. [CrossRef] [PubMed]
4. Tham, R.; Bowatte, G.; Dharmage, S.C.; Tan, D.J.; Lau, M.X.; Dai, X.; Allen, K.J.; Lodge, C.J. Breastfeeding and the risk of dental caries: A systematic review and meta-analysis. *Acta Paediatr.* **2015**, *104*, 62–84. [CrossRef] [PubMed]
5. Cui, L.; Li, X.; Tian, Y.; Bao, J.; Wang, L.; Xu, D.; Zhao, B.; Li, W. Breastfeeding and early childhood caries: A meta-analysis of observational studies. *Asia Pac. J. Clin. Nutr.* **2017**, *26*, 867–880. [CrossRef] [PubMed]
6. Moynihan, P.; Tanner, L.M.; Holmes, R.D.; Hillier-Brown, F.; Mashayekhi, A.; Kelly, S.A.M.; Craig, D. Systematic Review of Evidence Pertaining to Factors That Modify Risk of Early Childhood Caries. *JDR Clin. Transl. Res.* **2019**, *4*, 202–216. [CrossRef] [PubMed]
7. Do, L.G.; Ha, D.H.; Roberts-Thomson, K.F.; Jamieson, L.; Peres, M.A.; Spencer, A.J. Race- and income-related inequalities in oral health in Australian children by fluoridation status. *JDR Clin. Trans. Res.* **2018**, *3*, 170–179. [CrossRef] [PubMed]
8. Merrick, J.; Chong, A.; Parker, E.; Roberts-Thomson, K.; Misan, G.; Spencer, J.; Broughton, J.; Lawrence, H.; Jamieson, L. Reducing disease burden and health inequalities arising from chronic disease among Indigenous children: An early childhood caries intervention. *BMC Public Health* **2012**, *12*, 323. [CrossRef] [PubMed]
9. Jamieson, L.; Smithers, L.; Hedges, J.; Parker, E.; Mills, H.; Kapellas, K.; Lawrence, H.P.; Broughton, J.R.; Ju, X. Dental Disease Outcomes Following a 2-Year Oral Health Promotion Program for Australian Aboriginal Children and Their Families: A 2-Arm Parallel, Single-blind, Randomised Controlled Trial. *E Clin. Med.* **2018**, *1*, 43–50. [CrossRef] [PubMed]
10. Jamieson, L.M.; Smithers, L.G.; Hedges, J.; Aldis, J.; Mills, H.; Kapellas, K.; Lawrence, H.P.; Broughton, J.R.; Ju, X. Follow-up of an Intervention to Reduce Dental Caries in Indigenous Australian Children: A Secondary Analysis of a Randomized Clinical Trial. *JAMA Netw. Open* **2019**, *2*, e190648. [CrossRef] [PubMed]

11. Australian Bureau of Statistics. Information Paper: An Introduction to Socio-Economic Indexes for Areas (SEIFA). 2006. Available online: http://www.ausstats.abs.gov.au/Ausstats/subscriber.nsf/0/D729075E079F9FDECA2574170011B088/$File/20390_2006.pdf (accessed on 27 September 2019).
12. Bhaskaran, K.; Smeeth, L. What is the difference between missing completely at random and missing at random? *Int. J. Epidemiol.* **2014**, *43*, 1336–1339. [CrossRef] [PubMed]
13. Kramer, M.S.; Chalmers, B.; Hodnett, E.D.; Sevkovskaya, Z.; Dzikovich, I.; Shapiro, S.; Collet, J.-P.; Vanilovich, I.; Mezen, I.; Ducruet, T.; et al. Promotion of Breastfeeding Intervention Trial (PROBIT): A Randomized Trial in the Republic of Belarus. *J. Am. Med. Assoc.* **2001**, *285*, 413–420. [CrossRef] [PubMed]
14. Australian Government Department of Health. *Australian National Brestfeeding Strategy 2018 and Beyond: Draft for Public Consultation*; Australian Government Department of Health: Canberra, Australia, 2018; pp. 1–47.
15. Hartz, D.L.; Blain, J.; Caplice, S.; Allende, T.; Anderson, S.; Hall, B.; McGrath, L.; Williams, K.; Jarman, H.; Tracy, S.K. Evaluation of an Australian Aboriginal model of maternity care: The Malabar Community Midwifery Link Service. *Women Birth* **2019**, *32*, 427–436. [CrossRef] [PubMed]
16. Brown, S.; Stuart-Butler, D.; Leane, C.; Glover, K.; Mitchell, A.; Deverix, J.; Francis, T.; Ah Kit, J.; Weetra, D.; Gartland, D.; et al. Initiation and duration of breastfeeding of Aboriginal infants in South Australia. *Women Birth* **2019**, *32*, e315–e322. [CrossRef] [PubMed]
17. Kramer, M.S.; Vanilovich, I.; Matush, L.; Bogdanovich, N.; Zhang, X.; Shishko, G.; Muller-Bolla, M.; Platt, R.W. The effect of prolonged and exclusive breast-feeding on dental caries in early school-age children. New evidence from a large randomized trial. *Caries Res.* **2007**, *41*, 484–488. [CrossRef] [PubMed]
18. Birungi, N.; Fadnes, L.T.; Okullo, I.; Kasangaki, A.; Nankabirwa, V.; Ndeezi, G.; Tumwine, J.K.; Tylleskar, T.; Lie, S.A.; Astrom, A.N. Effect of Breastfeeding Promotion on Early Childhood Caries and Breastfeeding Duration among 5 Year Old Children in Eastern Uganda: A Cluster Randomized Trial. *PLoS ONE* **2015**, *10*, e0125352. [CrossRef] [PubMed]
19. Smithers, L.G.; Kramer, M.S.; Lynch, J.W. Effect of breastfeeding on obesity and intelligence: Causal insights from different study designs. *JAMA Pediatrics* **2015**, *169*, 707–708. [CrossRef] [PubMed]
20. Glymour, M.M.; Greenland, S. Causal diagrams. In *Modern Epidemiology*, 3rd ed.; Rothman, K.J., Greenland, S., Lash, T.L., Eds.; Lippincott Williams & Wilkins: Philadelphia, PA, USA, 2008; pp. 183–209.

2

Relationships between Breastfeeding Patterns and Maternal and Infant Body Composition over the First 12 Months of Lactation

Zoya Gridneva [1,*], Alethea Rea [2], Anna R. Hepworth [1], Leigh C. Ward [3], Ching T. Lai [1], Peter E. Hartmann [1] and Donna T. Geddes [1]

[1] School of Molecular Sciences, M310, The University of Western Australia, Crawley, Perth, WA 6009, Australia; arhepworth@westnet.com.au (A.R.H.); ching-tat.lai@uwa.edu.au (C.T.L.); peter.hartmann@uwa.edu.au (P.E.H.); donna.geddes@uwa.edu.au (D.T.G.)

[2] Centre for Applied Statistics, The University of Western Australia, Crawley, Perth, WA 6009, Australia; alethea.rea@uwa.edu.au

[3] School of Chemistry and Molecular Biosciences, The University of Queensland, St. Lucia, Brisbane, QLD 4072, Australia; l.ward@uq.edu.au

[*] Correspondence: zoya.gridneva@uwa.edu.au

Abstract: Breastfeeding has been implicated in the establishment of infant appetite regulation, feeding patterns and body composition (BC). A holistic approach is required to elucidate relationships between infant and maternal BC and contributing factors, such as breastfeeding parameters. Associations between maternal and breastfed term infant BC (n = 20) and feeding parameters during first 12 months of lactation were investigated. BC was measured at 2, 5, 9 and/or 12 months postpartum with ultrasound skinfolds (US; infants only) and bioimpedance spectroscopy (infants and mothers). 24-h milk intake (MI) and feeding frequency (FFQ) were measured. Higher FFQ was associated with larger 24-h MI ($p \leq 0.003$). Higher 24-h MI was associated with larger infant fat mass (FM) (US: $p \leq 0.002$), greater percentage FM (US: $p \leq 0.008$), greater FM index (FMI) (US: $p \leq 0.001$) and lower fat-free mass index (FFMI) (US: $p = 0.015$). Lower FFQ was associated with both larger FFM (US: $p \leq 0.001$) and FFMI (US: $p < 0.001$). Greater maternal adiposity was associated with smaller infant FFM measured with US (BMI: $p < 0.010$; %FM: $p = 0.004$; FMI: $p < 0.011$). Maternal BC was not associated with FFQ or 24-h MI. These results reinforce that early life is a critical window for infant programming and that breastfeeding may influence risk of later disease via modulation of BC.

Keywords: human milk; breastfed infants; body composition; anthropometrics; milk intake; bioelectrical impedance spectroscopy; ultrasound skinfolds; maternal factors

---

1. Introduction

The importance of lactocrine programming has been highlighted recently, with breastfeeding identified as one of the most economical preventative measures for non-communicable diseases (NCD) including obesity later in life [1–5]. The development of body composition (BC) in early life is known to play an important role in the programming of these health outcomes [6]. This reduction in risk may be a result of multiple mechanisms associated not only with composition of human milk (HM) but also with infant breastfeeding patterns and behavior [7–9], all of which may influence the growth and development of breastfed infants. Differences in the weight and BC between breastfed and formula-fed infants have been attributed to the stark compositional differences of HM and formula [10,11]. Despite the evidence that volume of HM is a main driver of growth [11–13], a major focus of at present limited research on infant growth and BC development has been on the composition of HM and maternal pre-pregnancy body mass index (BMI), and to a lesser extent on the effect of the volume of HM and maternal adiposity. Although these findings suggest a dose-dependent effect of breastfeeding on development of infant BC, the pathways of this effect are not fully understood.

Indeed, in utero maternal influences are apparent in obese women who generally deliver heavier infants with greater adiposity [14] thus maternal weight is a major predictor of infant birth weight (BW) [15,16]. However, recent studies have shown the infant BW is not associated with increased maternal BMI in women with BMI above 24 kg/m^2 [17]. To further complicate our understanding, overweight women deliver infants with higher adiposity [18] but not fat-free mass (FFM) [19,20]. Unfortunately, the majority of the studies have analyzed maternal pre-pregnancy BMI or gestational weight gain (parameters that are often self-reported and potentially misleading) as measures of adiposity. Considering that HM composition is influenced by the current maternal BC [21] rather than pre-pregnancy BMI, longitudinal studies with multiple measures of both maternal and breastfed infant BC are necessary [22] to elucidate the positive mechanistic effects of breastfeeding.

In a few recent studies, maternal BC was measured during pregnancy and a positive association between maternal BC and infant BW was found [23–26], showing maternal FFM or total body water, but not fat mass (FM) are the strongest predictors. Interestingly, longer duration of breastfeeding is shown to attenuate the adverse effects of BW and early weight gain on infant FM gain [27]. Further, the majority of participants are either newborns or children between 2 and 11 years of age, and infant adiposity (fat mass (FM) and percentage FM (%FM)) has been measured rather than FFM, yet the metabolic rate is largely determined by the FFM [28,29]. Furthermore, despite 24-h milk intake (MI) having a strong positive relationship with infant weight gain [12,13,30], there has been no investigation of the effect of either 24-h MI or feeding frequency (FFQ) on infant BC, yet these factors are highly variable between infants [31]. Our recent research of gastric emptying in term breastfed infants indicated that shorter, smaller and leaner infants fed more frequently (maternal self-report) [32], highlighting the need to connect not only maternal and infant BC, but also contributing factors, such as milk production and composition, infant MI and FFQ and, in turn, the development of the breastfed infant BC (Figure 1).

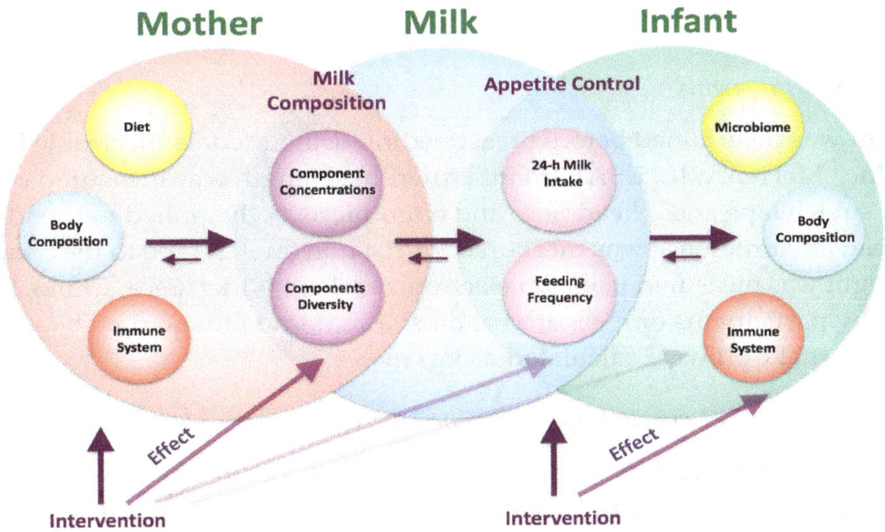

Figure 1. Framework for possible interconnecting pathways of lactocrine programming of the infant, and points of intervention for potential improvement of infant growth, development and health, based on available research.

It is important to understand the mechanisms by which maternal BC, breastfeeding and HM components may influence infant BC, as this will allow for more targeted interventions that may potentially reduce both infant and adult overweight and obesity. Therefore, the aim of this longitudinal study was to investigate relationships between maternal and infant BC during the first 12 months of lactation. Further, exploration of relationships of infant 24-h MI and FFQ with maternal and infant BC was carried out.

2. Materials and Methods

2.1. Study Participants

Breastfed infants (n = 20; 10 males, 10 females) of English-speaking, predominantly Caucasian, mothers of higher social-economic status from a developed country were recruited from the community, primarily from the West Australian branch of the Australian Breastfeeding Association. Inclusion criteria were: healthy singletons, gestational age ≥37 weeks, exclusively breastfed [33] at 2 and 5 months, and maternal intention to breastfeed until 12 months. Exclusion criteria were: infant factors that could potentially influence growth and development of BC, maternal smoking, and low milk supply. All mothers provided written informed consent to participate in the study, which was approved by The University of Western Australia Human Research Ethics Committee (RA/1/4253, RA/4/1/2639) and registered with the Australian New Zealand Clinical Trials Registry (ACTRN12616000368437).

2.2. Study Session

Measurements were made when the infants were 2 and/or 5, 9 and 12 months of age. Participants visited our laboratory at King Edward Memorial Hospital for Women (Subiaco, Perth, WA, Australia) for up to four monitored breastfeeding sessions between March 2013 and September 2015. At each study session, the infant was weighed pre-feed, and then the mother breastfed her infant. Infant bioelectrical impedance spectroscopy (BIS) measurements were made pre-feed, unless impractical, then they were made post-feed [34]. Ultrasound skinfold (US) and anthropometric measurements were made post-feed. This combination of methods for measuring infant BC was used to ensure safe, non-invasive and accurate assessment, and to avoid the inherent limitations of a singular technique [35]. Clothing was removed for the measurements except for a dry diaper and a singlet.

Maternal weight, height and BIS measurements were recorded. Current FFQ of the infants was self-reported by mothers.

2.3. Anthropometric Measurements

Infants weight was determined before breastfeeding using Medela Electronic Baby Weigh Scales (±2.0 g; Medela Inc., McHenry, IL, USA). Infant crown-heel length was measured once to the nearest 0.1 cm using non-stretch tape and a headpiece and a footpiece, both applied perpendicularly to a hard surface. Infant head circumference was measured with a non-stretch tape to the nearest 0.1 cm.

Maternal weight was measured using an electronic scale (±0.1 kg; Seca, Chino, CA, USA). Height was self-reported by participants or measured against a calibrated marked wall (accuracy ± 0.1 cm).

Infant and maternal BMI were calculated as kg/m^2.

2.4. Body Composition with Bioelectrical Impedance Spectroscopy

Whole body bioimpedance (wrist to ankle) of infants and mothers was measured using the Impedimed SFB7 bioelectrical impedance analyzer (ImpediMed, Brisbane, QLD, Australia) according to the manufacturer's instructions.

Mothers were measured in supine position on a non-conductive surface. A series of ten consecutive measurements (fat mass (FM), percentage fat mass (%FM) and fat-free mass (FFM)) were taken within 1–2 min and averaged for data analysis. The within participant coefficient of variation (CV) for maternal %FM was 0.21% [21].

Infants were measured by applying an adult protocol as used previously in infants but with data analyzed using settings customized for infants [35,36]. Resistance (ohm) at 50 kHz (R_{50}) was determined from the curve of best fit, averaged for analysis purposes and used in the Lingwood et al. [36]

age-matched (3 and 4.5 month-old infants) BIS equations for FFM of 2 and 5 month-old infants respectively, and Bocage [37] total body water (TBW) equations for 9 and 12 month-old infants:

$$\text{TBW} = (0.418 \times \text{Weight (kg)} + 1936/\text{R}_{50} + 0.8649) \times \text{Length (cm)}/100 \quad (1)$$

FFM was further determined using sex and age-appropriate hydration factors (HF) calculated from Butte et al. [38]:

$$\text{FFM} = \text{TBW}/\text{HF}. \quad (2)$$

%FM was calculated as follows:

$$\%\text{FM} = 100 \times (\text{Weight (kg)} - \text{FFM (kg)})/\text{Weight (kg)}. \quad (3)$$

Within participant CV for infant R_{50} was 1.5% [34].

2.5. Ultrasound Skinfold Measurements

Infant skinfolds were measured using the Aplio XG (Toshiba, Tokyo, Japan) US machine with a 14–8 MHz transducer (PLT-1204BX) and sterile water-based ultrasonic gel (Parker Laboratories Inc., Fairfield, NJ, USA) as described previously [35]. Single US scans of four anatomical sites (biceps, subscapular, suprailiac and triceps) were performed on the left side of the body with minimal compression. Subcutaneous tissue thickness (skin thickness and the skin-fat interface to fat-muscle interface distance) was measured directly from images on the screen using electronic calipers. One experienced sonographer with good interrater reliability [39] performed all of the measurements. US measurements were doubled [40] for use in skinfold equations developed for subcutaneous tissue thickness measurement with skinfold calipers. At all time points, infant %FM with 2-skinfolds (US 2SF: triceps, subscapular; Slaughter et al. [41]) and density (d; kg/L) with 4-skinfolds (US 4SF: biceps, subscapular, suprailiac and triceps; Brook [42]) were calculated with %FM further determined using Lohman equation [43]:

$$\%\text{FM} = 100 \times (5.28/d - 4.89). \quad (4)$$

2.6. Body Composition Indices

The indices of height-normalized BC were calculated for mothers and infants: fat mass index (FMI) was calculated as FM/length^2, and fat-free mass index (FFMI) was calculated as FFM/length^2; both expressed as kg/m^2 [44].

2.7. 24-H Milk Intake and Feeding Frequency

Infant MI was measured by mothers using the 24-h milk production (MP) protocol, weighing infants at home with the Medela Electronic Baby Weigh Scales pre- and post each breastfeed during a 24-h period plus one breastfeeding, and recording amounts of HM (g) consumed by the infant (including expressed HM if any) [45]. 24-h MI was determined as previously described with potential underestimation of 3–10% [45] and FFQ (meals per day) was recorded [31]. 24-h MI was measured at three time points: between 2 and 5 (4.0 $\pm$ 1.3) months, when MI is shown to be stable [31], and within two weeks of 9 (9.4 $\pm$ 0.3) and 12 (12.2 $\pm$ 0.4) months. Given that measuring 24-h MI is not always practical, particularly at the later stages of lactation, mothers were also asked how frequently the infant fed, and self-reported the typical time between the feeds (e.g., each 2 h) during the week prior to the study session as a proxy measure of FFQ.

2.8. Statistical Analyses

Statistical analysis was performed in R 3.1.2 for Mac OSX [46]. Additional packages were used for linear mixed effects models (nlme, lme4 and car) [47–49], intra-class correlations (irr) [50], Tukey's all pair comparisons (multcomp) [51] and graphics (ggplot2) [52]. Descriptive statistics are reported as mean ± standard deviation (SD) (range); model parameters as estimate ± SE (standard error).

During this longitudinal study infants were measured at four time points (2 and/or 5, 9 and 12 months). An approximate sample size was calculated using the 'F tests–Linear multiple regression: Fixed model: R^2 increase' option in G*Power [53] as if this was a cross-sectional study with equal numbers at each time. Allowing four predictors (3 for age comparisons), $\alpha = 0.05$ and 14 participants (56 sample points = 14 participants × 4 time points) gave the study power of 0.80 to detect an effect size of 0.15. This approach was selected, as there is no closed form expression suitable for the calculation of sample sizes for this research design [54], with the consideration that longitudinal study design is more powerful. Recruitment of participants at the 5 months point was introduced, as many mothers would not commit to a study that required breastfeeding to 12 months, when approached at 2 months ($n = 8$). As a result, required number of participants was increased to 20 in order to maintain predicted power; this also addressed issues relating to missed visits. Missing data was dealt with using available case analysis.

Maternal BC was analysed using an intercept only linear mixed effects model for the calculation of CV for maternal %FM measurements ($n = 10$, 10 measurements each).

Infant BC was analysed using linear mixed effects models with random intercept per participant to determine whether BC measurements (%FM, FM, FMI, FFM and FFMI) differed systematically by age, measurement method (US 2SF, US 4SF and BIS) and infant sex. As interactions between sex and methods were non-significant ($p > 0.52$), reported associations are for pooled data. Months after birth were accounted for in all models; results reported account for this, regardless of significance.

Survey responses relating to FFQ were analysed using a one-way intra-class correlation for agreement of single measures.

The analyses for systematic differences in all measured parameters (maternal characteristics, infant characteristics and breastfeeding characteristics) at different months after birth and between different measurement methods used general linear hypothesis tests (Tukey's all pair comparisons).

Relationships between infant BW and maternal and infant BC at four time points after birth were analysed using linear regression models accounting for gestational age and sex, which were identified as significant covariates using a stepwise regression analysis. Since major postpartum weight/adiposity loss happens during the first 4 to 6 months in women of high social-economic status [55,56], maternal BC at 5, 9 and 12 months was considered instead of unavailable pre-pregnancy BMI.

Relationships between: (a) infant BC and breastfeeding characteristics; (b) breastfeeding characteristics and maternal BC; and (c) infant and maternal BC were analysed using linear mixed effects models. Each breastfeeding characteristic or infant BC measure/index was considered separately as the response variable, and each model contained fixed effects of infant age (months), a predictor (breastfeeding measure or maternal BC measure/index) and an interaction between infant age and predictor, as well as a random intercept per participant.

Owing to the large number of comparisons, a false discovery rate adjustment [57] was performed on associated subgroupings of results. p-values were considered to be significant below 0.018 for associations between infant BW and maternal BC; below 0.047 for associations between infant BW and infant BC; below 0.018 for associations between infant FFM and maternal BC; below 0.038 for associations between infant FFMI and maternal BC; below 0.029 for associations between infant BC and MI; below 0.040 for associations between infant BC and self-reported FFQ; below 0.05 for associations between infant BC and 24-h MP FFQ; below 0.0004 for associations between infant BC changes between the time points and 24-h MI; below 0.001 for associations between infant BC changes between the time points and self-reported FFQ; below 0.004 for associations between infant BC changes between the time points and 24-h MP FFQ; below 0.009 for associations between maternal BC changes between time points and 24-h MI; below 0.014 for associations between maternal BC changes between time points and self-reported FFQ; and below 0.05 for associations between maternal BC changes between time points and 24-h MP FFQ. The significance was set at the 5% level otherwise.

3. Results

3.1. Subjects

Twenty-two infants were recruited; 2 infants (1 male, 1 female) were excluded from the study after the 2-month visit (starting supplementation with formula; personal circumstances). One female infant started supplementation with formula/weaning at 6 months and was excluded from further analysis. Nineteen remaining infants were breastfed at 2, 5 and 9 months. Seventeen infants (94%) continued to breastfeed at 12 months, but one male was too sick to attend the last session. Out of 18 infants measured at 12 months 16 infants (89%) still continued to breastfeed. One male infant ceased breastfeeding 2 weeks before the 12-month appointment and one female infant stopped at 10 months after birth. Both infants and their mothers were measured at 12 months.

Some sessions were not attended by some participants leading to incomplete data. Five infants did not start at 2 months, two did not attend at 9 months and two at 12 months. Overall 80 measures were expected, however some were missing, specifically: infant weight ($n = 9$); infant %FM, FM, FMI, FFM and FFMI measured with US 2SF, and maternal age, weight, height, BMI, %FM, FM, FMI, FFM and FFMI ($n = 10$); infant head circumference ($n = 11$); infant length, BMI and %FM, FM, FMI, FFM and FFMI measured with US 4SF ($n = 12$); infant %FM, FM, FMI, FFM and FFMI measured with BIS ($n = 13$); self-reported FFQ ($n = 20$). Missing data also occurred due to difficulties with conducting 24-h MI measurements at later stages of lactation. The following measurements from the 60 expected were missing: FFQ from 24-h MP ($n = 26$) and 24-h MI ($n = 27$). Missing data were spread across the time points (Table 1).

Breastfeeding characteristics, infant and maternal demographics and anthropometrics as well as maternal BC measures at the four study sessions are presented in Table 1. Mean maternal age at the start of the study was 33.3 ± 4.7 (24–44) years, mean height was 167.4 ± 7.4 (150–181) cm and mean parity was 2.3 ± 0.9 (1–4). Infant male/female ratio was 10/10, mean BW was 3.486 ± 0.498 (2.660–4.455) kg and mean gestational age was 39.4 (37.6–43) weeks. After accounting for infant age males were heavier (0.85 [0.12, 1.57], $p = 0.025$) and had larger head circumferences than females (1.89 [0.81, 2.96], $p = 0.002$), while no significant difference between sexes was seen for either length (1.68 [−0.24, 3.59], $p = 0.083$) or BMI (1.09 [−0.15, 2.32], $p = 0.081$).

Table 1. Participant anthropometric and breastfeeding characteristics.

Characteristic	2 Months [a]	5 Months [b]	9 Months [c]	12 Months [d]
	Mean ± SD	Mean ± SD	Mean ± SD	Mean ± SD
	(Range)	(Range)	(Range)	(Range)
Mothers				
Weight (kg)	78.8 ± 19.3	70.1 ± 17.8	63.0 ± 10.0	64.2 ± 17.3
	(57.5–116.2)	(53.7–115.3)	(50.4–121.9)	(51.4–121.9)
BMI (kg/m^2)	27.2 ± 5.5	24.8 ± 5.0	22.7 ± 3.9	23.9 ± 5.9
	(20.4–35.5)	(19.0–35.2)	(17.9–37.2)	(18.2–37.2)
Fat-free Mass [e] (kg)	49.5 ± 8.2	45.4 ± 6.6	44.1 ± 4.1	45.4 ± 6.7
	(38.2–66.2)	(37.4–60.9)	(35.1–68.5)	(35.9–67.7)
Fat Mass [e] (kg)	29.3 ± 11.8	24.6 ± 12.0	18.9 ± 7.4	18.8 ± 11.0
	(15.2–50.0)	(13.9–54.4)	(11.4–53.4)	(10.0–54.3)
Fat Mass [e] (%)	36.0 ± 6.4	33.8 ± 7.0	29.2 ± 6.7	27.7 ± 7.9
	(25.7–44.7)	(23.2–47.2)	(20.0–44.3)	(19.4–44.5)
FFMI [e] (kg/m^2)	16.8 ± 2.1	16.2 ± 1.9	16.1 ± 2.3	16.4 ± 2.4
	(13.7–20.2)	(13.2–20.0)	(12.4–20.9)	(12.7–20.7)

Table 1. *Cont.*

Characteristic	2 Months [a] Mean ± SD (Range)	5 Months [b] Mean ± SD (Range)	9 Months [c] Mean ± SD (Range)	12 Months [d] Mean ± SD (Range)
Mothers				
FMI [e] (kg/m^2)	9.5 ± 3.3 (6.2–15.3)	8.4 ± 3.3 (4.8–16.6)	7.9 ± 3.5 (3.9–16.3)	7.5 ± 3.5 (3.6–16.6)
Infants				
Sex (M/F)	9M/6F	10M/10F	10M/9F	9M/9F
Age (months)	2.04 ± 0.14 (1.87–2.33)	5.16 ± 0.22 (4.77–5.47)	9.22 ± 0.27 (8.83–9.77)	12.26 ± 0.28 (11.63–12.67)
Length (cm)	58.1 ± 1.9 (54.2–60.0)	64.8 ± 2.3 (60.5–69.5)	71.7 ± 1.9 (66.0–74.0)	73.6 ± 3.2 (69.0–78.5)
Weight (kg)	5.630 ± 0.660 (4.420–7.400)	7.431 ± 1.134 (5.808–9.510)	8.836 ± 0.975 (6.675–10.095)	9.650 ± 0.618 (7.165–11.085)
BMI (kg/m^2)	16.6 ± 1.2 (14.5–18.1)	17.6 ± 1.9 (14.9–20.4)	17.7 ± 1.7 (14.2–20.2)	17.8 ± 0.9 (13.7–19.2)
Head circumference (cm)	39.7 ± 1.6 (37.0–42.0)	42.1 ± 1.5 (40.0–45.9)	45.6 ± 1.7 (43.0–48.5)	46.6 ± 1.7 (44.2–49.5)
Breastfeeding characteristics				
24-h milk intake (g)	n/a [f]	818.8 ± 204.9 (498–1185)	502.3 ± 157.8 (300–775)	445.5 ± 200.4 (255–795)
24-h feeding frequency (MP)	n/a [f]	8.1 ± 1.4 (6–11)	5.4 ± 1.2 (4–7)	4.4 ± 1.9 (2–8)
Feeding frequency (SR)	2.3 ± 0.4 [g] (1.5–3.0)	2.8 ± 0.8 (1.5–4.0)	3.7 ± 1.2 (2.0–6.0)	5.4 ± 2.9 (2.2–12.0)

Data are mean ± SD and ranges. [a] n = 15; [b] n = 20; [c] n = 19; [d] n = 18. [e] Maternal body composition as measured with bioelectrical impedance spectroscopy. [f] Milk intake and feeding frequency as meals per 24-h was determined from 24-h milk production (MP) measured between 2 and 5 months (presented at 5 months here, n = 17) and within 2 weeks of 9 (n = 8) and 12 months (n = 9 for feeding frequency, n = 8 for milk intake). [g] Maternal self-report (SR) of feeding frequency at the time of the visit as a typical time between feeds (e.g., each 2 h) (n = 11, n = 19, n = 17, n = 13 at 2, 5, 9 and 12 months respectively). BMI—body mass index; FFMI—fat-free mass index; FMI—fat mass index, n/a—not applicable.

3.2. Maternal Body Composition

Maternal BC is presented in Table 1. At the session attended at 5 months postpartum none of the participants were classified as being underweight (BMI < 18.5; %FM < 21). They were classified as: normal weight (BMI 18.5–24.9, 65%, n = 13; %FM 21–32.9, 55%, n = 11), overweight (BMI 25–29.9, 20%, n = 4; %FM 33–38.9, 30%, n = 6) or obese (BMI > 30, 15%, n = 3; %FM > 39, 15%, n = 3) [58].

3.3. Infant Body Composition

Infant BC measured with three measurement techniques (BIS, US 2SF and US 4SF) is presented in Table S1.

Male infants were compared to female infants using all three measurement techniques. FFM was significantly greater in males overall (0.66 [0.19, 1.14] kg, p = 0.009) and when the methods were considered separately (US 2SF: 0.55 [0.07, 1.03] kg, p = 0.027; US 4SF: 0.70 [0.20, 1.20] kg, p = 0.009; BIS: 0.74 [0.25, 1.22] kg, p = 0.005). FFMI was significantly higher in males overall (0.95 [0.21, 1.69] kg,

$p = 0.015$) and when determined with US 4SF and BIS (US 4SF: 1.01 [0.29, 1.73] kg, $p = 0.009$; BIS: 1.09 [0.37, 1.81] kg, $p = 0.005$) but not with US 2SF (0.70 [−0.12, 1.52] kg, $p = 0.089$).

Differences were not seen for %FM, FM and FMI overall (males %FM: −0.38 [−3.02, 2.26] %, $p = 0.77$; FM: 0.19 [−0.17, 0.55] kg, $p = 0.27$; FMI: 0.16 [−0.52, 0.85] kg/m^2, $p = 0.62$) or when the methods were considered separately (%FM: $p \geq 0.30$; FM: $p \geq 0.095$; FMI: $p \geq 0.25$).

A comparison of measurement methods showed no difference for %FM ($p \geq 0.074$), FM ($p \geq 0.11$), FMI ($p \geq 0.077$) and FFM ($p \geq 0.15$). Overall FFMI determined with BIS was significantly higher compared with US 2SF (0.24 ± 0.10, $p > 0.039$) with no further differences between the methods ($p \geq 0.24$).

3.4. Infant Birth Weight and Maternal and Infant Body Composition

After accounting for infant sex and gestational age no significant associations between BW and any maternal BC parameter were seen at any time point after birth after adjusting for the false discovery rate ($p \geq 0.018$) (the raw p-values for negative associations between maternal adiposity/BC indices at 5, 9 and 12 months postpartum and infant BW before the adjustment were: %FM (5 months: −0.03 ± 0.01, $p = 0.026$; 9 months: −0.03 ± 0.01, $p = 0.021$; 12 months: −0.03 ± 0.01, $p = 0.018$), BMI (5 months: −0.04 ± 0.02, $p = 0.024$; 9 months: −0.03 ± 0.02, $p = 0.046$; 12 months: −0.04 ± 0.02, $p = 0.019$), FMI (5 months: −0.06 ± 0.02, $p = 0.032$; 9 months: −0.05 ± 0.02, $p = 0.038$; 12 months: −0.06 ± 0.02, $p = 0.023$), and FFMI (5 months: −0.10 ± 0.04, $p = 0.042$; 12 months: −0.09 ± 0.04, $p = 0.032$)).

After accounting for infant sex and gestational age and adjusting for the false discovery rate ($p \geq 0.047$) larger BW was associated with larger infant FFM measured at all-time points and with all three methods (2 months: US 2SF, 0.81 ± 0.17, $p = 0.001$; US 4SF, 0.95 ± 0.23, $p = 0.004$; BIS, 0.75 ± 0.22, $p = 0.010$; 5 months: US 2SF, 1.03 ± 0.30, $p = 0.004$; US 4SF, 1.24 ± 0.29, $p < 0.001$; BIS, 0.87 ± 0.17, $p < 0.001$; 9 months: US 2SF, 1.20 ± 0.32, $p = 0.002$; US 4SF, 1.17 ± 0.33, $p = 0.004$; BIS, 1.37 ± 0.39, $p = 0.004$; 12 months: US 2SF, 1.46 ± 0.32, $p < 0.001$; US 4SF, 1.55 ± 0.32, $p < 0.001$; BIS, 1.42 ± 0.42, $p = 0.006$). Also, larger BW was associated with larger FM only at 5 months and only when measured with BIS (0.70 ± 0.25, $p = 0.014$).

3.5. 24-H Milk Intake and Feeding Frequency

A moderate level of agreement (ICC = 0.602 [0.339, 0.779], $p < 0.001$) was seen between FFQ measured with 24-h MP as meals per 24-h and FFQ self-reported by mothers as hours between meals. Short intervals between feeds were associated with higher self-reported values than 24-h MP values; this effect was not seen with longer intervals between feeds.

FFQ and 24-h MI did not differ by infant sex ($p \geq 0.54$). Greater FFQ was associated with larger 24-h MI (24-h MP FFQ: 81.1 ± 18.5, $p < 0.001$; self-reported FFQ: −50.6 ± 13.3, $p = 0.003$).

3.6. Longitudinal Changes in Maternal, Breastfeeding and Infant Characteristics

Maternal weight, BMI, %FM, FM and FMI decreased significantly between 2 and 12 months (Table S2), while FFM and FFMI did not differ (FFM: $p = 0.10$; FFMI: $p = 0.076$). Over the first year of lactation, maternal adiposity decreased (Figure 2) (%FM: −2.03% ± 0.59, $p = 0.001$, month of lactation: $p < 0.001$; BMI: −0.78 ± 0.24, $p = 0.002$, month of lactation: $p < 0.001$; FMI: −0.64 ± 0.18, $p < 0.001$, month of lactation: $p = 0.001$), after accounting for the month of lactation as a factor.

FFQ and 24-h MI decreased significantly across the lactation (Table S2).

Infant anthropometrics and both FM and FFM measured with all methods increased significantly as age increased (Table S3). BMI, FFMI determined with US 4SF, FMI determined with US 2SF and FM determined with BIS initially increased and then plateaued, while %FM and FMI measured with BIS initially increased and then decreased (Figure 3). %FM measured with US skinfolds and FFMI determined with US 2 SF did not differ significantly (%FM US 2SF: $p = 0.56$; %FM US 4 SF: $p = 0.11$; FFMI US 2SF: $p = 0.13$).

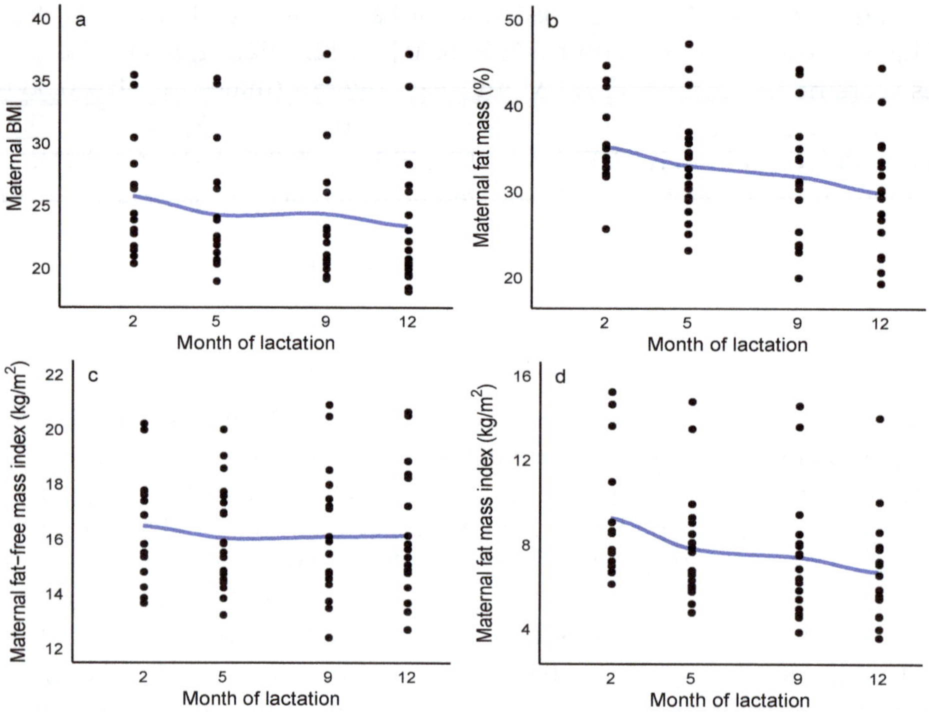

Figure 2. Longitudinal changes in: (**a**) maternal body mass index (BMI); (**b**) maternal percentage fat mass, (**c**) fat-free mass index and (**d**) fat mass index measured with bioelectrical impedance spectroscopy from 2 to 12 months of lactation. Blue line represents local regression smoother (LOESS), grey areas represent ± confidence interval, ($n = 14$, $n = 20$, $n = 18$, $n = 18$ at 2, 5, 9 and 12 months respectively).

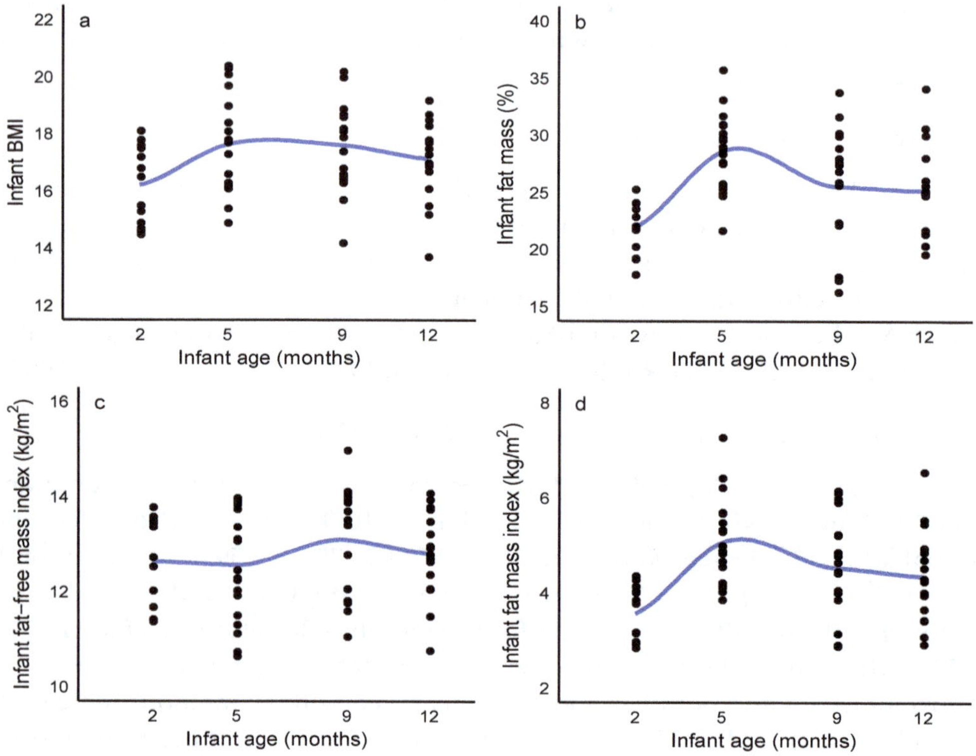

Figure 3. Longitudinal changes in: (**a**) infant body mass index (BMI); (**b**) percentage fat mass, (**c**) infant fat-free mass index and (**d**) infant fat mass index from 2 to 12 months after birth measured with bioelectrical impedance spectroscopy. Blue line represents local regression smoother (LOESS), grey areas represent ± confidence interval, ($n = 14$, $n = 20$, $n = 18$, $n = 18$ at 2, 5, 9 and 12 months respectively).

3.7. Relationships between Infant and Maternal Body Composition

Significant negative associations between infant FFM and maternal adiposity were seen after accounting for month after birth and interaction between month after birth and maternal characteristic (Table A1). After adjusting for the false discovery rate, higher maternal BMI was associated with smaller infant FFM measured with both US 2SF ($p = 0.007$) and US 4SF ($p = 0.010$) (Figure 4a); greater maternal FM was associated with smaller infant FFM measured with US 2SF ($p = 0.004$) (Figure 4b); and greater maternal FMI was associated with smaller infant FFM measured with both US 2SF ($p = 0.005$) and US 4SF ($p = 0.011$). There were no other significant associations between the measured maternal and infant BC parameters. No significant interactions between month after birth and maternal predictors were seen.

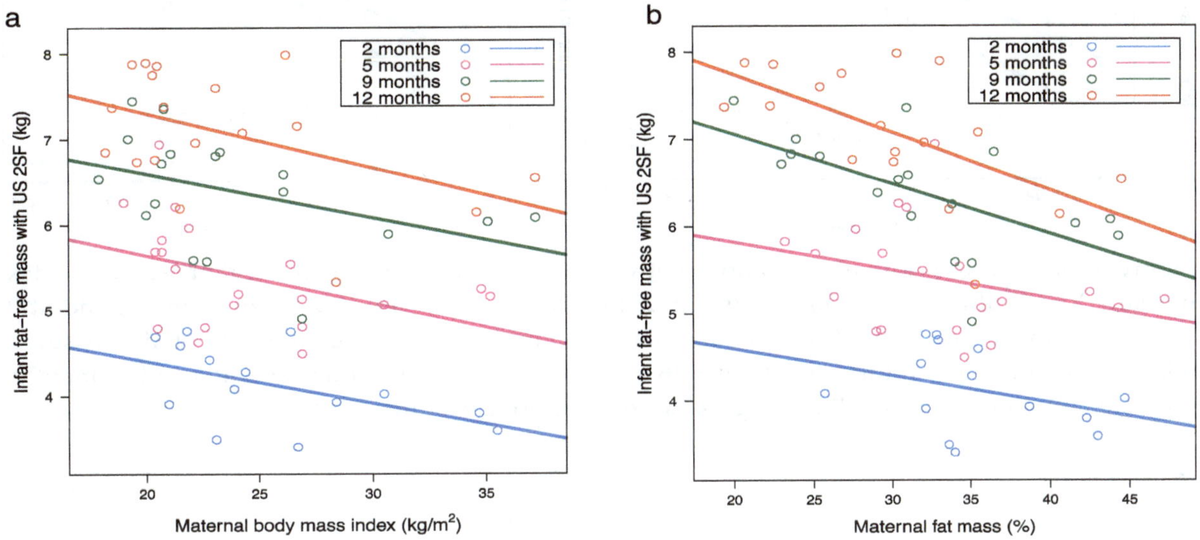

Figure 4. Significant negative associations between: (**a**) maternal body mass index and infant fat-free mass measured with ultrasound (2 skinfolds; US 2SF); (**b**) maternal percentage fat mass (%FM) and infant fat-free mass measured with US 2SF. Lines represent linear regression, one line for each time point ($n = 14$, $n = 20$, $n = 18$, $n = 18$ at 2, 5, 9 and 12 months respectively).

3.8. Infant Body Composition and Breastfeeding Parameters

Significant associations between infant BC and feeding parameters (FFQ, 24-h MI) were seen after accounting for the month after birth and interaction between month after birth and feeding parameters (Table A2).

After adjusting for false discovery rate, higher 24-h MI was associated with greater infant FM measured with both US 2SF ($p = 0.004$) and US 4SF ($p = 0.002$), greater %FM measured with both US 2SF ($p = 0.008$) and US 4SF ($p < 0.001$), greater FMI measured with US 2SF ($p = 0.001$) and US 4SF ($p < 0.001$) and lower FFMI measured with US 4SF ($p = 0.015$) (Table A2, Figure 5).

After adjusting for false discovery rate, longer intervals between feeds (self-reported FFQ) were associated with larger infant FFM (US 2SF: $p = 0.001$; US 4SF: $p < 0.001$; BIS: $p = 0.019$) and FFMI (US 2SF: $p = 0.013$; US 4SF: $p < 0.001$; BIS: $p = 0.017$) (Table A2, Figure 6). No significant associations were seen for 24-h MP FFQ (meals per 24 h).

Significant interactions between breastfeeding parameters and the month after birth were seen for infant BC characteristics (Table A2). 24-h MI and the month after birth: the slope for infant BMI changes from positive (5 months) to flat (9 months) and then negative (12 months) ($p = 0.018$) indicating that associations between 24-h MI and infant BMI weakens over the first 12 months of lactation; the slope for infant FFMI measured with US 4SF changes from flat (5 and 9 months) to negative (12 months) ($p = 0.024$) indicating that associations between 24-h MI and infant FFMI strengthens over the first 12 months of lactation. 24-h MP FFQ and the month after birth: the slope for infant FM measured with

US 2 SF changes from negative (5 months) to positive (9 and 12 months) ($p = 0.014$) indicating that associations between FFQ and infant FM strengthens over the first 12 months of lactation.

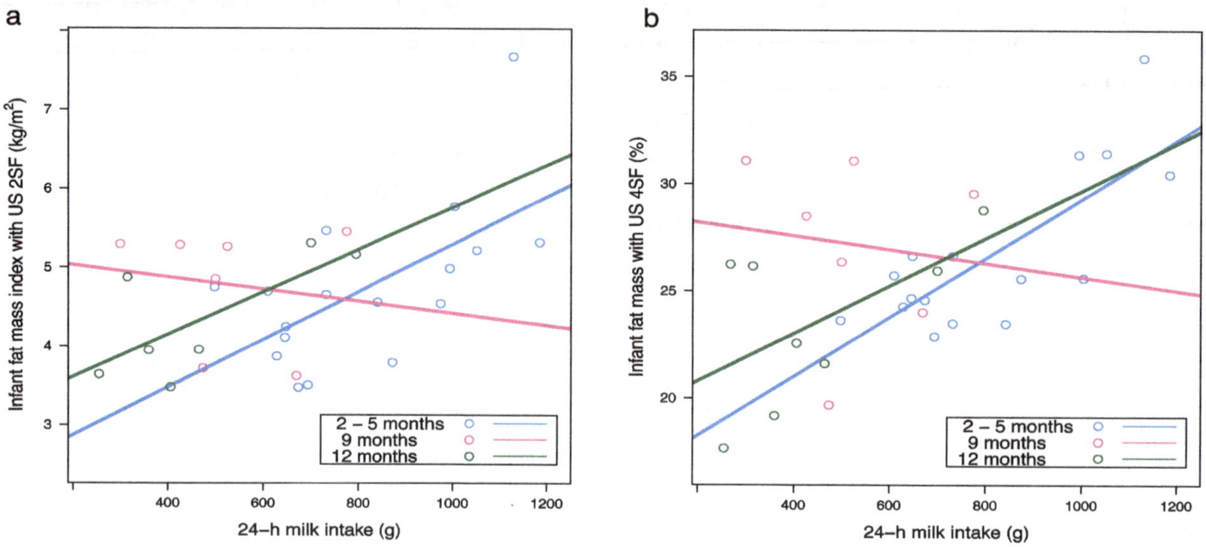

Figure 5. Significant positive associations between: (**a**) 24-h milk intake and infant fat mass index measured with ultrasound (2 skinfolds; US 2SF) (n = 17, n = 7, n = 7 between 2 and 5, and at 9 and 12 months respectively); (**b**) 24-h milk intake and infant percentage fat mass (%FM) measured with ultrasound (4 skinfolds; US 4SF) (n = 16, n = 7, n = 7 between 2 and 5, and at 9 and 12 months respectively). Lines represent linear regression, one line for each time point.

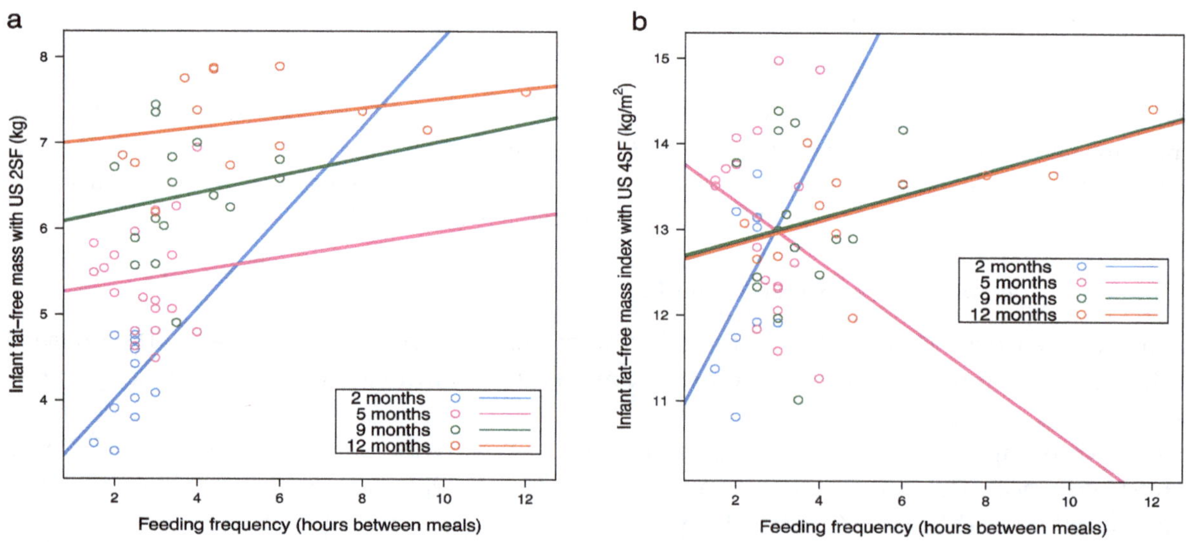

Figure 6. Significant positive associations between: (**a**) self-reported feeding frequency (hours between feeds) and infant fat-free mass measured with ultrasound (2 skinfolds; US 2SF) (n = 11, n = 19, n = 16, n = 13 at 2, 5, 9 and 12 months respectively); (**b**) self-reported feeding frequency and infant fat-free mass index measured with ultrasound (4 skinfolds; US 4SF) (n = 10, n = 18, n = 16, n = 12 at 2, 5, 9 and 12 months respectively). Lines represent linear regression, one line for each time point.

After adjusting for false discovery rate, no associations were seen between changes in infant BC and either 24-h MI ($p \geq 0.0004$) or FFQ ($p \geq 0.001$ for self-reported FFQ, and $p \geq 0.004$ for 24-h MP FFQ) at any practical time points (Tables A3 and A4).

3.9. *Maternal Body Composition and Breastfeeding Parameters*

No associations were seen between maternal BC and 24-h MI and both FFQ (24-h MP and self-reported) (BMI: $p \geq 0.45$; FFM: $p \geq 0.51$; FFMI: $p \geq 0.13$; FM: $p \geq 0.82$; FMI: $p \geq 0.69$; %FM: $p \geq 0.67$) after accounting for the month after birth ($p < 0.001$ for all) and interaction between month after birth and maternal characteristics.

Significant interaction was seen between maternal BMI and the month after birth (2 months: reference; 5 months: -0.03 ± 0.07; 9 months: 0.01 ± 0.07; 12 months: 0.76 ± 0.17, $p < 0.001$; month after birth: $p < 0.001$) and maternal FFMI and the month after birth (2 months: reference; 5 months: -0.13 ± 0.16; 9 months: 0.11 ± 0.16; 12 months: 1.18 ± 0.22, $p < 0.001$; month after birth: $p < 0.001$) for self-reported FFQ indicating that the association between both, BMI and FFMI, and self-reported FFQ (hours between feeds) strengthens over the first 12 months of lactation. No significant interaction with month after birth was seen for other maternal characteristics.

After adjusting for the false discovery rate, no associations were seen between decrease in maternal BMI, FFM, FFMI, FM, %FM and FMI and either 24-h MI ($p \geq 0.009$) or FFQ (self-reported FFQ: $p \geq 0.014$; 24-h MP FFQ: $p \geq 0.068$) at any practical time points (Table A5).

4. Discussion

The life period spanning from pre-conception to early life is a critical period when appetite control and BC are programmed and is the greatest window of opportunity for intervention to significantly improve infant outcome. This period is influenced by the maternal factors and early nutrition [5] and breastfeeding can have long-term beneficial health effects at both the individual and population levels [4]. Furthermore, longer duration of breastfeeding is shown to reduce risk for rapid growth patterns in early childhood [59] and attenuate the adverse effects of BW and early weight gain on infant FM gain [27], suggesting dose-dependent effect of breastfeeding on development of infant BC, but the mechanisms of this effect are not fully understood. Our study expands previous research, identifies specific risk factors and critical periods and sheds new light on the mechanisms by which breastfeeding influences infant BC. FFQ and 24-h MI are implicated in development of infant FM while maternal BC is associated with infant FFM, all of these emphasizing the critical role of breastfeeding in programming growth in the first 12 months of life (Figure 7).

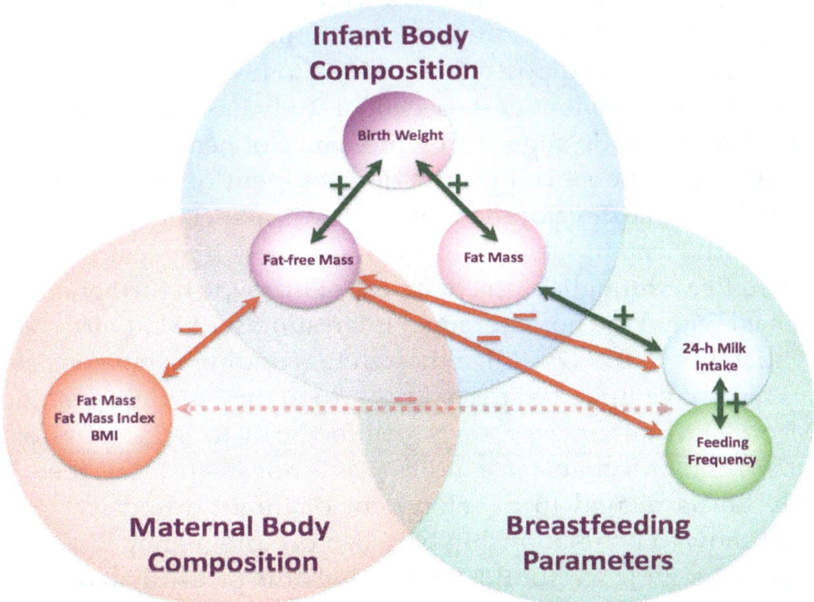

Figure 7. Interconnecting pathways of lactocrine programming of the infant as researched. Green arrows indicate positive associations between measured parameters; red arrows indicate negative associations; red dotted arrow indicates significant interaction terms (negative). BMI—body mass index.

Milk intake is a major driver of infant growth and here we show a link between infant breastfeeding behavior, as in FFQ, where more frequent feeders consumed more milk and subsequently had greater adiposity (FM, %FM, FMI) and less lean mass (FFM, FFMI) over the first 12 months of life. This supports a study, in which 24-h MI had no associations with infant weight, but was positively associated with both weight-for-length and weight-for-age [60], suggesting infant BC rather than weight drives this relationship [61]. The lack of association between FFQ and infant 24h-MI in previous studies of the exclusive breastfeeding period is likely due to no consensus on definitions of a breastfeed or meal and non-compliance to demand feeding [31,62]. One cross-sectional study has reported a positive association between FFQ and 24-h MI, however, not all mothers exclusively breastfed for 6 months and study did not account for FFQ in early life [63], which is known to reduce in established lactation [64]. In our study, the association between FFQ and infant adiposity strengthened with duration of lactation, similar to the study, which found that the later breastfeeding was discontinued the more infant %FM was observed at 6 months [65], further highlighting the importance of breastfeeding in the weaning period during the gradual introduction of food.

It is not fully understood what influences infant FFQ, which generally declines with the duration of lactation [62,64]. We have previously reported that smaller, shorter and leaner (less %FM), but not younger infants fed more frequently in a cohort of 2 and 5 month-old fully breastfed infants [32] and we have now extended this relationship to FFM, although it is not clear which comes first: are smaller infants in greater demand for nutrients, or is higher FFQ/MI provide more HM components that may regulate/slow down the growth? The results of this study were not uniform between self-reported FFQ and 24-h MP FFQ. This could be explained by the fact that both methods of measuring FFQ have some limitations: self-reported FFQ was shown to be biased towards reporting higher numbers of feeds in frequent feeders compared with 24-h MP FFQ, which itself is limited to one measure at the time point of data collection. Nevertheless, the associations between infant BC and both FFQ and 24-h MI indicate that, with more comprehensive investigation, these provide a window for adjustment of infant growth rate, during both, exclusive breastfeeding period and specifically from 9 to 12 months, where HM could potentially make a greater contribution to optimal infant growth rate and adiposity (Figure 1).

Previous studies based on maternal BMI [14,15] or BC measured during pregnancy [23–26,66] reported a positive relationship with infant BW. Our study showed no relationship of BW with either maternal BMI or BC, although none of our mothers were categorised as underweight and only 15% were obese, and correction for multiple comparisons eliminated statistical significance. However, we did find that increased maternal adiposity was related to lower infant FFM over the course of the first year of life whereas only one previous cross-sectional study has found this at 5 to 35 days of life [67]. Therefore, this sustained relationship suggests maintenance of healthy maternal pre-pregnancy and possibly lactational adiposity is beneficial for the development of infant lean body mass. Optimal lean body mass is desirable, since development of obesity is associated with increased FFM [68] and compositional changes of the lean tissue [69]. Further, we show in breastfed infants increased BW is associated with increased FFM throughout the first year of life, which further emphasizes the necessity for maternal BC to remain within the normal range. Interestingly, FFM at birth has also been shown to explain most of the variability in BW [70–72], although this finding is not consistent [19,73].

Previous studies also have linked maternal pre-pregnancy BMI or gestational weight gain to increased infant FM or %FM either very early in life (birth to 4 months) or later in childhood (2–11 years) [19,20,67,74,75]. Mechanistic studies have not been attempted to understand how breastfeeding in early life is related to development of infant adiposity. Similar to one recent longitudinal study that showed no relationship between pre-pregnancy BMI and infant postpartum %FM during first 6 months [76], we found no relationship of estimated pre-pregnancy/current maternal BC and infant FM, leading us to speculate that breastfeeding may modulate infant FM development, contributing in part to protection against obesity. Further, other studies have not measured breastfeeding parameters and have included formula-fed infants, this combined with the historic cohorts including mothers with BMI significantly lower than current cohorts [77] may have influenced their findings.

BW is not a reliable predictor of newborn adiposity [78]. We found no association between BW and infant FM during the first 12 months of life, with the exception of a positive association at 5 months, when measured with BIS only. Similarly, Chomtho et al. have reported positive association between BW and infant FM measured with stable isotope at 3 months [73]. The emergence of positive associations of BW with infant FM only at 3 months [73] and 5 months (our study) in the first year of life might be explained by relative proximity of the measures to the peaking of infant adiposity at around 6–7 months [38,79] and a reduction in the adverse effect of BW and early infant weight gain on FM later in infancy with increased duration of breastfeeding [27,80]. Our findings therefore point to maternal BC being implicated in lean tissue development rather than fat accrual in the infant post birth, while breastfeeding parameters appear to be involved in development of adipose tissue.

Higher FM in infants is usually considered as a negative result [81], however some studies observed %FM to be consistently higher due to lower FFM in breastfed infants compared to formula-fed [82] which may be related to the neurodevelopmental and cognitive differences between these two groups [83]. Curiously, duration of breastfeeding has been found to associate positively with infant subcutaneous but not visceral fat [76], indicating that breastfeeding may ensure a beneficial adipose phenotype, associated with a reduced risk of NCD and obesity [76,84]. It will be necessary to study the development of visceral fat in breastfed infants over time, since it cannot be extrapolated to %FM [76].

Infant BC also influenced by the infant sex. In our recent cross-sectional study of 2, 5, 9 and 12 months old infants we showed that %FM was lower in males than in females [35]. Similar to some longitudinal studies [85,86] and contrary to others [38,87,88], we have seen no difference in adiposity between sexes in this study, although, as expected, we observed that lean mass in males was greater (FFM and FFMI). Larger sample sizes will allow for more robust findings with respect to sex and BC of breastfeeding infants.

Given the evidence confirming that obese mothers experience greater physical difficulties in breastfeeding as well as being at higher risk of not producing adequate volumes of milk [60,61,89–91], one might expect maternal BC to influence breastfeeding parameters. Our study, however, did not find any associations between maternal BC or indicators of milk production (24-h MI) and breastfeeding behaviour (FFQ). This may be because all of our mothers produced enough milk for their infants [31] and that only 15% of our mothers were obese. Furthermore, infants in our study displayed appropriate patterns of growth according to WHO growth standards [92], with 18 out of 20 infants residing between 15th and 97th weight-for-age centiles over the first year of life, and only three infants crossing two major centiles in downward and one in upward trend from birth to 12 months. Before correction for multiple comparisons however, we found that the reduction in maternal adiposity was associated with higher 24-h MI in the later stages of lactation, these findings are further supported by significant interaction between maternal BMI and the month after birth, which indicated the strengthening of the association between BMI and FFQ at the later stages of lactation. It is biologically plausible that higher FFQ and MI at the later stages of lactation/during weaning may contribute to greater reduction in maternal adiposity due to the energetic demand of lactation. Indeed, exclusive breastfeeding promotes greater maternal %FM loss than mixed feeding during the early postpartum period [93], and at the later stages of lactation [56,94], with more frequent feeding associating with greater fat reduction at 6 months postpartum [94]. One must be cautious, as FFQ is also related to 24-h MI. These findings support the limited data that suggests that duration of lactation is associated with protection against incidence of obesity, CVD, type 2 diabetes and prevalence of the metabolic syndrome [95], enabled by the mobilization of the stored fat and persisting beyond weaning.

The strength of this proof-of-concept study is the wide variation of adiposity levels among the mothers and that measurements were performed on breastfeeding dyads feeding on demand over a wide period of lactation, from 2 to 12 months. The limitations are the small number of 24-h MP at the later stages of lactation and the modest number of participants as a result of time constraints associated with multiple measurement time points. Our population was predominantly Caucasian term healthy fully breastfed singletons from mothers of higher social-economic status therefore, the results may not be applicable to dyads from other backgrounds. Further analysis including a holistic approach is required to understand multiple levels of breastfeeding programing and regulatory effects. Elucidation of the effect of maternal BC on infant BC via both composition and the quantity of HM will help to understand the intergenerational nature of obesity allowing for the possibility of interventions. These interventions would include maintaining/achieving healthy maternal BC pre-conception and during pregnancy and lactation, as well as supporting breastfeeding from 9 to 12 months and beyond, as outlined in the NHMRC [96] and WHO infant feeding guidelines [97], to improve the outcomes for breastfeeding dyads. An example of an 'intervention' is Norway's promotion of breastfeeding (and extended breastfeeding), which is deployed by overweight/obese mothers as a weight loss strategy, since Norwegian women with greater pre-pregnancy weight concerns are more likely to initiate breastfeeding and breastfeed for longer [98].

5. Conclusions

This study found that infant BC was associated with both maternal adiposity and breastfeeding patterns over the first 12 months of lactation. These results confirm that the first year of life is a critical window of infant developmental programming that has the potential for intervention to improve outcomes for the infant, and emphasise the importance of including quantitative measures in order to elucidate the mechanisms by which breastfeeding affects infant BC (Figure 1).

Acknowledgments: All authors critically reviewed and approved the final manuscript. This study was supported by an unrestricted research grant from Medela AG (Switzerland). Zoya Gridneva was supported by an Australian Postgraduate Award from The University of Western Australia (Australia). Many thanks are extended to all mothers who participated in this study.

Author Contributions: Zoya Gridneva designed the study, collected the data, conducted data analysis and interpreted results, and wrote the manuscript; Alethea Rea conducted data analysis and interpreted results; Anna R. Hepworth provided consultation for research design and conducted data analysis and interpretation; Ching T. Lai provided technical and analytical support; Leigh C. Ward contributed to the design of the study and provided technical and educational support; Peter E. Hartmann substantially contributed to the conception and design of the study and contributed reagents/materials/analysis tools for research; Donna T. Geddes designed the study, collected the data and interpreted results.

Appendix A

Table A1. Significant associations between infant body composition and maternal body composition.

Predictor	2 Months		5 Months		9 Months		12 Months		p-Value		
	Intercept (SE)	Slope (SE)	Intercept (SE)	Slope (SE)	Intercept (SE)	Slope (SE)	Intercept (SE)	Slope (SE)	Predictor	Infant Age (Months)	Interaction
Infant fat-free mass with ultrasound 2 skinfolds (kg)											
Maternal BMI [d] (kg/m^2)	5.62 (0.79) [a]	−0.06 (0.03)	6.81 (0.69)	−0.06 (0.03)	7.78 (0.61)	−0.06 (0.03)	8.55 (0.60)	−0.06 (0.03)	**0.007** [b]	**<0.001** [c]	0.99 [c]
Maternal FM [d] (%)	5.30 (0.84)	−0.03 (0.02)	6.22 (0.63)	−0.03 (0.02)	7.87 (0.57)	−0.05 (0.02)	8.68 (0.55)	−0.05 (0.02)	**0.004**	**<0.001**	0.40
Maternal FM (kg)	4.79 (0.40)	−0.03 (0.02)	5.81 (0.32)	−0.02 (0.01)	6.99 (0.31)	−0.03 (0.01)	7.72 (0.29)	−0.03 (0.01)	0.018	**<0.001**	0.62
Maternal FMI [d] (kg/m^2)	4.91 (0.43)	−0.09 (0.05)	5.98 (0.35)	−0.07 (0.04)	7.15 (0.32)	−0.09 (0.04)	7.87 (0.31)	−0.11 (0.04)	**0.005**	**<0.001**	0.72
Infant fat-free mass with ultrasound 4 skinfolds (kg)											
Maternal BMI	5.90 (0.84)	−0.07 (0.03)	7.05 (0.74)	−0.07 (0.03)	7.82 (0.66)	−0.06 (0.03)	8.84 (0.65)	−0.07 (0.03)	**0.010**	**<0.001**	0.93
Maternal FM (%)	5.01 (0.88)	−0.03 (0.03)	6.06 (0.67)	−0.02 (0.02)	7.75 (0.63)	−0.04 (0.02)	8.74 (0.60)	−0.05 (0.02)	0.024	**<0.001**	0.29
Maternal FM (kg)	4.82 (0.43)	−0.03 (0.02)	5.86 (0.35)	−0.02 (0.01)	7.01 (0.33)	−0.02 (0.01)	7.90 (0.32)	−0.03 (0.01)	0.033	**<0.001**	0.54
Maternal FMI [d] (kg/m^2)	4.93 (0.46)	−0.09 (0.05)	6.03 (0.38)	−0.07 (0.04)	7.17 (0.35)	−0.09 (0.04)	8.05 (0.33)	−0.11 (0.04)	**0.011**	**<0.001**	0.71
Infant fat-free mass with bioelectrical impedance spectroscopy (kg)											
Maternal BMI	5.76 (0.89)	−0.06 (0.03)	6.54 (0.76)	−0.05 (0.03)	7.85 (0.68)	−0.06 (0.03)	8.32 (0.68)	−0.05 (0.03)	0.030	**<0.001**	0.99
Maternal FMI [d] (kg/m^2)	4.93 (0.48)	−0.07 (0.05)	5.73 (0.39)	−0.05 (0.04)	7.16 (0.36)	−0.09 (0.04)	7.72 (0.36)	−0.08 (0.04)	0.037	**<0.001**	0.79
Infant fat-free mass index with ultrasound 2 skinfolds (kg/m^2)											
Maternal FM [d] (%)	13.90 (1.56)	−0.04 (0.05)	14.10 (1.14)	−0.04 (0.03)	15.10 (1.04)	−0.07 (0.03)	14.50 (1.00)	−0.06 (0.03)	0.038	0.12	0.85

[a] Data are parameter estimate ± SE; effects of predictors taken from linear mixed effects models that accounted for infant age and an interaction between infant age and predictor. [b] Results are presented only for predictors with $p < 0.05$; after the false discovery rate adjustment, the predictor p-values were considered to be significant at <0.018 for infant fat-free mass measures (indicated by the bold text) and at <0.038 for fat-free mass index (none are significant). [c] Significant results for month after birth and the interaction between predictor and month after birth ($p < 0.05$, indicated by the bold text). [d] BMI—body mass index; FM—fat mass; FMI—fat mass index; %FM—percentage fat mass.

Table A2. Significant associations between infant body composition and feeding characteristics.

Predictor	2 Months		5 Months		9 Months		12 Months		p-Value		
	Intercept (SE)	Slope (SE)	Intercept (SE)	Slope (SE)	Intercept (SE)	Slope (SE)	Intercept (SE)	Slope (SE)	Predictor	Infant Age (Months)	Interaction
Infant body mass index (kg/m^2)											
24-h milk intake (g) [c]	n/a [c]	n/a [c]	15.20 (1.16) [a]	0.003 (0.001)	17.7 (1.25)	0.001 (0.002)	18.90 (0.90)	−0.003 (0.002)	0.40 [b]	0.61	**0.018** [b]
Infant fat mass with ultrasound 2 skinfolds (%)											
24-h milk intake (g)	n/a	n/a	17.20 (3.45) [a]	0.01 (0.004)	29.5 (4.72)	−0.005 (0.01)	21.50 (3.03)	0.01 (0.006)	**0.008**	0.30	0.20
Infant fat mass with ultrasound 4 skinfolds (%)											
Feeding frequency SR [d]	18.40 (5.71)	3.06 (2.42)	25.40 (2.91)	0.32 (1.01)	30.50 (2.73)	−1.21 (1.01)	27.00 (2.01)	−0.64 (0.32)	0.040	0.34	0.26
Feeding frequency MP	n/a	n/a	24.30 (5.49)	0.29 (0.66)	18.9 (6.50)	1.53 (1.17)	16.60 (3.17)	1.52 (0.69)	0.029	0.16	0.38
24-h milk intake (g)	n/a	n/a	15.20 (3.30)	0.01 (0.004)	28.2 (4.46)	−0.002 (0.01)	18.90 (2.87)	0.01 (0.006)	**<0.001**	**0.043**	0.20
Infant fat mass with ultrasound 2 skinfolds (kg)											
24-h milk intake (g)	n/a	n/a	0.93 (0.37)	0.001 (0.0004)	2.53 (0.43)	−0.0002 (0.001)	2.10 (0.28)	0.001 (0.001)	**0.004**	**<0.001**	0.18
Feeding frequency MP	n/a	n/a	2.89 (0.57)	−0.11 (0.07)	2.00 (0.56)	0.08 (0.10)	1.94 (0.30)	0.12 (0.06)	0.63	**0.036**	**0.014**
Infant fat mass with ultrasound 4 skinfolds (kg)											
24-h milk intake (g)	n/a	n/a	0.81 (0.37)	0.001 (0.0004)	2.37 (0.45)	0.0001 (0.001)	1.88 (0.29)	0.001 (0.001)	**0.002**	**<0.001**	0.28
Infant fat mass with bioelectrical impedance spectroscopy (kg)											
24-h milk intake (g)	n/a	n/a	1.20 (0.44)	0.001 (0.001)	1.79 (0.57)	0.001 (0.001)	2.22 (0.41)	0.0004 (0.001)	0.045	**0.030**	0.65
Infant fat mass index with ultrasound 2 skinfolds (kg/m^2)											
24-h milk intake (g)	n/a	n/a	2.17 (0.79)	0.003 (0.001)	4.88 (1.0)	0.0001 (0.002)	3.57 (0.72)	0.002 (0.001)	**0.001**	0.060	0.25
Feeding frequency MP	n/a	n/a	4.39 (1.28)	0.04 (0.16)	2.90 (1.57)	0.35 (0.28)	2.55 (0.82)	0.37 (0.17)	0.046	0.42	0.32
Infant fat mass index with ultrasound 4 skinfolds (kg/m^2)											
Feeding frequency MP	n/a	n/a	3.81 (1.34)	0.12 (0.16)	2.82 (1.58)	0.39 (0.28)	2.36 (0.82)	0.36 (0.17)	0.025	0.14	0.52
24-h milk intake (g)	n/a	n/a	1.78 (0.77)	0.004 (0.001)	4.76 (1.03)	0.0003 (0.002)	2.91 (0.74)	0.002 (0.002)	**<0.001**	**0.022**	0.23

Table A2. *Cont.*

Predictor	2 Months		5 Months		9 Months		12 Months		p-Value		
	Intercept (SE)	Slope (SE)	Intercept (SE)	Slope (SE)	Intercept (SE)	Slope (SE)	Intercept (SE)	Slope (SE)	Predictor	Infant Age (Months)	Interaction
Infant fat mas index with bioelectrical impedance spectroscopy (kg/m²)											
24-h milk intake (g)	n/a	n/a	2.71 (0.92)	0.003 (0.001)	3.56 (1.18)	0.001 (0.002)	4.37 (0.85)	0.00003 (0.002)	0.029	0.75	0.31
Infant fat-free mass with ultrasound 2 skinfolds (kg)											
Feeding frequency SR	4.41 (0.61)	−0.09 (0.25)	4.94 (0.32)	0.17 (0.11)	5.82 (0.31)	0.16 (0.11)	6.58 (0.24)	0.10 (0.03)	**0.001**	**<0.001**	0.67
Infant fat-free mass with ultrasound 4 skinfolds (kg)											
Feeding frequency SR	4.14 (0.51)	0.04 (0.21)	5.19 (0.28)	0.09 (0.09)	5.56 (0.27)	0.24 (0.09)	6.58 (0.22)	0.13 (0.03)	**<0.001**	**<0.001**	0.25
Infant fat-free mass with bioelectrical impedance spectroscopy (kg)											
Feeding frequency SR	4.37 (0.75)	−0.001 (0.32)	5.14 (0.41)	0.06 (0.14)	5.69 (0.37)	0.22 (0.14)	6.74 (0.29)	0.08 (0.04)	**0.019**	**<0.001**	0.48
Infant fat-free mass index with ultrasound 2 skinfolds (kg/m²)											
Feeding frequency SR	12.10 (1.26)	0.19 (0.53)	13.10 (0.67)	−0.07 (0.23)	12.80 (0.61)	0.08 (0.23)	11.90 (0.46)	0.19 (0.07)	**0.013**	0.20	0.68
Infant fat-free mass index with ultrasound 4 skinfolds (kg/m²)											
Feeding frequency SR	11.50 (1.01)	0.44 (0.43)	13.40 (0.57)	−0.13 (0.19)	12.20 (0.51)	0.26 (0.19)	11.90 (0.39)	0.25 (0.06)	**<0.001**	**0.031**	0.25
24-h milk intake (g)	n/a	n/a	13.60 (0.80)	−0.001 (0.001)	13.30 (0.82)	−0.001 (0.002)	15.40 (0.60)	−0.004 (0.001)	**0.015**	0.057	**0.024**
Infant fat-free mass index with bioelectrical impedance spectroscopy (kg/m²)											
Feeding frequency SR	12.20 (1.15)	0.30 (0.49)	13.10 (0.62)	−0.15 (0.21)	12.40 (0.57)	0.21 (0.21)	12.20 (0.44)	0.15 (0.06)	**0.017**	0.16	0.49

[a] Data are parameter estimate ± SE; effects of predictors taken from linear mixed effects models that accounted for infant age and an interaction between infant age and predictor. [b] Results are presented only for interactions (indicated by the bold text) or predictors with $p < 0.05$; after the false discovery rate adjustment, the predictor p-values were considered to be significant at <0.029 for 24-h milk intake, at <0.040 for self-reported feeding frequency (indicated by the bold text) and at <0.05 for 24-h milk production feeding frequency (none are significant). [c] 24-h milk intake and feeding frequency as meals per 24-h (MP) were measured between 2 and 5 months ($n = 17$; presented here at 5 months) and within 2 weeks of 9 ($n = 8$) and 12 months ($n = 9$ for feeding frequency, $n = 8$ for milk intake). [d] Feeding frequency was self-reported by mothers (SR) at the time of the visit as a typical time between feeds (e.g., each 2 h) ($n = 11$, $n = 19$, $n = 17$, $n = 13$ at 2, 5, 9 and 12 months respectively). n/a—not applicable.

Table A3. Associations between 24-h milk intake at given time points and infant body composition changes between time points.

Changes in Infant Characteristic	Months after Birth					
	5 and 2	9 and 2	12 and 2	9 and 5	12 and 5	12 and 9
	24-h milk intake between 2 and 5 months [e]					
BMI [d] (kg/m^2)	**0.014** [a,c] **0.003 ± 0.001** [b]	0.54 0.001 ± 0.002	0.94 0.0002 ± 0.002	0.55 −0.001 ± 0.001	0.29 −0.002 ± 0.002	0.35 −0.001 ± 0.001
Fat-free mass US 2SF [d] (kg)	0.65 −0.004 ± 0.001	**0.013** **0.002 ± 0.001**	0.10 0.002 ± 0.001	0.56 0.004 ± 0.001	0.56 0.004 ± 0.001	0.88 0.0 ± 0.0
Fat-free mass US 4SF [d] (kg)	0.35 0.001 ± 0.001	**0.004** **0.003 ± 0.001**	**0.007** **0.003 ± 0.001**	0.38 0.001 ± 0.001	0.29 0.001 ± 0.001	0.26 0.0004 ± 0.003
Fat-free mass BIS [d] (kg)	0.096 0.001 ± 0.0003	0.14 0.002 ± 0.001	**0.009** **0.003 ± 0.001**	0.46 0.001 ± 0.001	0.20 0.001 ± 0.001	0.23 0.001 ± 0.001
Fat-free mass index US 4SF (kg/m^2)	0.068 0.003 ± 0.001	0.092 0.003 ± 0.001	**0.035** **0.005 ± 0.002**	0.63 0.001 ± 0.001	0.84 0.0003 ± 0.001	0.91 0.0001 ± 0.001
Fat-free mass index BIS (kg/m^2)	**0.031** **0.002 ± 0.001**	0.47 0.001 ± 0.002	0.37 0.002 ± 0.002	0.68 0.001 ± 0.001	0.92 0.0001 ± 0.001	0.68 0.001 ± 0.001
Fat mass US 2SF (kg)	**0.037** **0.002 ± 0.001**	0.46 0.001 ± 0.001	0.47 0.001 ± 0.001	0.77 −0.0002 ± 0.001	0.60 −0.0003 ± 0.001	0.97 0.0 ± 0.0
Fat mass index US 2SF (kg/m^2)	**0.033** **0.004 ± 0.002**	0.98 0.0 ± 0.0	0.87 −0.0004 ± 0.002	0.50 −0.001 ± 0.001	0.25 −0.002 ± 0.001	0.39 −0.001 ± 0.001
Fat mass index US 4SF (kg/m^2)	0.47 0.001 ± 0.001	0.23 −0.003 ± 0.002	0.19 −0.004 ± 0.003	0.38 −0.001 ± 0.001	0.074 −0.002 ± 0.001	**0.047** **−0.001 ± 0.001**
Fat mass index BIS (kg/m^2)	0.065 0.002 ± 0.001	0.97 0.0 ± 0.0	0.46 −0.001 ± 0.001	0.37 −0.001 ± 0.001	**0.034** **−0.003 ± 0.001**	0.21 −0.002 ± 0.001
	24-h milk intake at 12 months [e]					
Fat-free mass index US 2SF (kg/m^2)	n/a [f]	n/a [f]	0.14 −0.005 ± 0.002	n/a [f]	**0.003** **−0.006 ± 0.001**	0.064 −0.003 ± 0.001
Fat-free mass index US 4SF (kg/m^2)	n/a	n/a	0.31 −0.005 ± 0.004	n/a	**0.0004** **−0.005 ± 0.0004**	0.18 −0.003 ± 0.002
Fat mass US 2SF (kg)	n/a	n/a	**0.023** **0.002 ± 0.001**	n/a	0.17 0.001 ± 0.001	0.41 0.0003 ± 0.0004
Fat mass US 2SF (%)	n/a	n/a	**0.049** **0.029 ± 0.009**	n/a	0.11 0.013 ± 0.007	0.60 0.003 ± 0.006

[a] *p*-values, [b] parameter estimates and standard errors of estimate for significant associations between feeding frequency at given time points and the changes in measured variables between different months after birth. [c] Results are presented only for variables with at least one significant raw *p*-value ($p < 0.05$, indicated by the bold text); after the false discovery rate adjustment, the predictor *p*-values were considered to be significant at <0.0004 for 24-h milk intake (none are significant). [d] BIS—bioimpedance spectroscopy; BMI—body mass index; US 2SF—ultrasound 2-skinfolds; US 4SF—ultrasound 4-skinfolds. [e] 24-h milk intake was measured at 24-h milk production between 2 and 5 months ($n = 17$) and within 2 weeks of 9 ($n = 8$) and 12 months ($n = 8$). [f] Results are not presented for impractical combinations, n/a—not applicable.

Table A4. Associations between feeding frequency at given time points and infant body composition changes between time points.

Changes in Infant Characteristic	Months after Birth					
	5 and 2	9 and 2	12 and 2	9 and 5	12 and 5	12 and 9
	Self-reported feeding frequency at 2 months [e]					
BMI [d] (kg/m^2)	0.83 [a] 0.14 ± 064 [b]	0.067 −1.95 ± 0.92	0.42 −0.99 ± 1.15	**0.013** [c] **−2.09 ± 0.66**	0.25 −1.13 ± 0.87	**0.027** **1.03 ± 0.37**
Fat mass US 4SF [d] (%)	0.55 1.34 ± 2.14	0.058 −7.19 ± 3.25	0.25 −4.67 ± 3.79	**0.027** **−9.11 ± 3.37**	0.13 −5.80 ± 3.40	0.28 3.20 ± 2.74
Fat mass US 4SF (kg)	0.37 0.14 ± 0.15	0.12 −0.59 ± 0.34	0.23 −0.44 ± 0.33	**0.028** **−0.76 ± 0.28**	0.076 −0.56 ± 0.28	0.42 0.17 ± 0.20
Fat mass index US 4SF (kg/m^2)	0.28 0.40 ± 0.35	**0.039** **−1.73 ± 0.70**	0.27 −0.97 ± 0.81	**0.009** **−2.13 ± 0.62**	0.094 −1.35 ± 0.70	0.14 0.83 ± 0.49

Table A4. *Cont.*

Changes in Infant Characteristic	Months after Birth					
	5 and 2	9 and 2	12 and 2	9 and 5	12 and 5	12 and 9
Self-reported feeding frequency at 9 months [e]						
Fat-free mass US 4SF (kg)	n/a [g]	0.055 0.21 ± 0.10	0.25 0.21 ± 0.17	**0.003** **0.25 ± 0.07**	0.13 0.18 ± 0.11	0.93 −0.01 ± 0.09
Fat-free mass index US 4SF (kg/m²)	n/a	0.10 0.29 ± 0.16	0.37 0.29 ± 0.31	**0.014** **0.36 ± 0.13**	**0.025** **0.48 ± 0.19**	0.49 0.13 ± 0.18
Self-reported feeding frequency at 12 months [e]						
BMI (kg/m²)	n/a [g]	n/a [g]	0.45 0.15 ± 0.18	n/a [g]	0.12 0.21 ± 0.12	**0.044** **0.14 ± 0.06**
Fat-free mass US 2SF [d] (kg)	n/a	n/a	**0.031** **0.13 ± 0.04**	n/a	**0.022** **0.12 ± 0.05**	0.43 0.03 ± 0.03
Fat-free mass US 4SF (kg)	n/a	n/a	**0.047** **0.15 ± 0.06**	n/a	**0.001** **0.15 ± 0.03**	0.21 0.04 ± 0.03
Fat-free mass index US 2SF (kg/m²)	n/a	n/a	**0.024** **0.24 ± 0.07**	n/a	**0.020** **0.24 ± 0.09**	0.052 0.12 ± 0.06
Fat-free mass index US 4SF (kg/m²)	n/a	n/a	**0.043** **0.31 ± 0.10**	n/a	**0.003** **0.27 ± 0.07**	0.073 0.15 ± 0.08
Fat-free mass index BIS [d] (kg/m²)	n/a	n/a	0.051 0.25 ± 0.09	n/a	**0.030** **0.16 ± 0.06**	0.37 0.07 ± 0.07
Fat mass US 4SF (%)	n/a	n/a	**0.043** **−1.05 ± 0.39**	n/a	0.11 −0.67 ± 0.38	0.44 −0.26 ± 0.32
24-h MP feeding frequency between 2 and 5 months [f]						
Fat-free mass index US 2SF (kg/m²)	**0.028** **0.45 ± 0.17**	0.16 −0.27 ± 0.17	0.52 −0.17 ± 0.25	0.13 −0.28 ± 0.17	0.29 −0.21 ± 0.19	0.64 0.06 ± 0.12
Fat-free mass index US 4SF (kg/m²)	**0.012** **0.45 ± 0.13**	0.51 −0.16 ± 0.23	0.80 −0.09 ± 0.36	0.065 −0.25 ± 0.12	0.63 −0.09 ± 0.18	0.46 0.11 ± 0.15
Fat mass US 2SF (%)	0.39 −1.60 ± 1.75	0.24 1.20 ± 0.94	0.48 1.34 ± 1.81	**0.012** **2.23 ± 0.78**	0.068 1.70 ± 0.86	0.21 −0.51 ± 0.38
Fat mass US 4SF (%)	0.23 −0.96 ± 0.73	0.53 0.93 ± 1.38	0.62 0.90 ± 1.73	**0.010** **2.09 ± 0.69**	0.12 1.26 ± 0.77	0.086 −0.76 ± 0.41
Fat mass US 2SF (kg)	0.62 −0.08 ± 0.15	0.23 0.14 ±0.10	0.48 0.13 ± 0.17	**0.007** **0.21 ± 0.07**	**0.033** **0.17 ± 0.07**	0.34 −0.04 ± 0.04
Fat mass US 4SF (kg)	0.81 −0.01 ± 0.05	0.24 0.14 ± 0.11	0.38 0.12 ± 0.13	**0.006** **0.21 ± 0.06**	0.054 0.14 ± 0.07	0.17 −0.05 ± 0.04
Fat mass index US 2SF (kg/m²)	0.64 −0.16 ± 0.32	0.40 0.20 ± 0.23	0.40 0.30 ± 0.34	**0.016** **0.44 ± 0.16**	0.11 0.33 ± 0.19	0.22 −0.11 ± 0.08
Fat mass index US 4SF (kg/m²)	0.81 −0.03 ± 0.13	0.53 0.19 ± 0.28	0.60 0.20 ± 0.36	**0.023** **0.42 ± 0.16**	0.17 0.26 ± 0.18	0.053 −0.16 ± 0.08

Table A4. *Cont.*

Changes in Infant Characteristic	Months after Birth					
	5 and 2	9 and 2	12 and 2	9 and 5	12 and 5	12 and 9
24-h MP feeding frequency at 9 months [f]						
Fat-free mass US 2SF (kg)	n/a [g]	**0.030** **−0.28 ± 0.05**	0.33 −0.32 ± 0.28	**0.013** **−0.33 ± 0.09**	0.16 −0.33 ± 0.20	0.85 −0.03 ± 0.15
Fat-free mass index US 4SF (kg/m^2)	n/a	0.33 −0.45 ± 0.35	0.43 −0.55 ± 0.57	0.14 −0.35 ± 0.19	**0.044** **−0.68 ± 0.23**	0.15 −0.35 ± 0.20
24-h MP feeding frequency at 12 months [f]						
Fat-free mass US 2SF (kg)	n/a [g]	n/a [g]	**0.029** **−0.23 ± 0.06**	n/a [g]	0.097 −0.20 ± 0.11	0.55 −0.05 ± 0.07
Fat-free mass index US 2SF (kg/m^2)	n/a	n/a	0.070 −0.41 ± 0.12	n/a	**0.037** **−0.48 ± 0.18**	0.45 −0.13 ± 0.15
Fat mass US 2SF (%)	n/a	n/a	0.13 2.00 ± 0.97	n/a	**0.004** **2.12 ± 0.52**	0.96 0.03 ± 0.61
Fat mass US 2SF (kg)	n/a	n/a	0.090 0.15 ± 0.06	n/a	**0.009** **0.19 ± 0.05**	0.90 0.01 ± 0.04
Fat mass index US 2SF (kg/m^2)	n/a	n/a	0.30 0.24 ± 0.17	n/a	**0.015** **0.41 ± 0.12**	0.75 −0.04 ± 0.11

[a] *p*-values, [b] parameter estimates and standard errors of estimate for significant associations between feeding frequency at given time points and the changes in measured variables between different months after birth. [c] Results are presented only for variables with at least one significant raw *p*-value ($p < 0.05$, indicated by the bold text); after the false discovery rate adjustment, the predictor *p*-values were considered to be significant at <0.001 for self-reported feeding frequency, and <0.004 for 24-h milk production feeding frequency (none are significant). [d] BIS—bioimpedance spectroscopy; BMI—body mass index; MP—milk production; US 2SF—ultrasound 2-skinfolds; US 4SF—ultrasound 4-skinfolds. [e] Feeding frequency was self-reported by mothers at the time of the visit as a typical time between feeds (e.g., each 2 h) (n = 11, n = 19, n = 17, n = 13 at 2, 5, 9 and 12 months respectively). [f] Feeding frequency as meals per 24-h was measured at 24-h milk production between 2 and 5 months (presented at 5 months here, n = 17) and within 2 weeks of 9 (n = 8) and 12 months (n = 9). [g] Results are not presented for impractical combinations, n/a—not applicable.

Table A5. Associations between breastfeeding parameters at given time points and maternal body composition changes between time points.

Changes in Maternal Characteristic	Months after Birth					
	5 and 2	9 and 2	12 and 2	9 and 5	12 and 5	12 and 9
24-h milk intake at 9 months [e]						
Fat mass BIS [d] (%)	n/a [g]	0.075 [a] 0.04 ± 0.01 [b]	0.33 0.01 ± 0.01	**0.042** [c] **−0.01 ± 0.004**	**0.013** **−0.02 ± 0.005**	0.16 −0.007 ± 0.004
Fat mass BIS (kg)	n/a	**0.026** **0.04 ± 0.01**	0.28 0.01 ± 0.01	0.10 −0.006 ± 0.003	**0.011** **−0.01 ± 0.003**	0.16 −0.005 ± 0.003
Fat mass index BIS (kg/m^2)	n/a	**0.020** **0.02 ± 0.002**	0.26 0.003 ± 0.002	0.11 −0.002 ± 0.001	**0.009** **−0.004 ± 0.001**	0.15 −0.002 ± 0.001

Table A5. *Cont.*

Changes in Maternal Characteristic	Months after Birth					
	5 and 2	9 and 2	12 and 2	9 and 5	12 and 5	12 and 9
			Self-reported feeding frequency at 12 months [f]			
BMI [d] (kg/m^2)	n/a [g]	n/a [g]	**0.025** **0.15 ± 0.05**	n/a [g]	0.96 −0.003 ± 0.05	0.74 0.02 ± 0.05
Fat mass BIS (%)	n/a	n/a	**0.048** **0.38 ± 0.15**	n/a	0.83 0.07 ± 0.32	0.63 0.10 ± 0.20
Fat mass BIS (kg)	n/a	n/a	**0.020** **0.38 ± 0.11**	n/a	0.71 0.08 ± 0.20	0.59 0.08 ± 0.15
Fat mass index BIS (kg/m^2)	n/a	n/a	**0.014** **0.12 ± 0.03**	n/a	0.78 0.02 ± 0.07	0.58 0.03 ± 0.05

[a] *p*-values, [b] parameter estimates and standard errors of estimate for significant associations between breastfeeding parameters at given time points and the changes in measured variables between different months after birth. [c] Results are presented only for variables with at least one significant raw *p*-value ($p < 0.05$; indicated by the bold text; none were significant for 24-h milk production feeding frequency); after the false discovery rate adjustment, the predictor *p*-values were considered to be significant at <0.009 for 24-h milk intake and <0.014 for self-reported feeding frequency (none are significant). [d] BIS—bioimpedance spectroscopy; BMI—body mass index. [e] 24-h milk intake was measured at 24-h milk production between 2 and 5 months ($n = 17$) and within 2 weeks of 9 ($n = 8$) and 12 months ($n = 8$). [f] Feeding frequency was self-reported by mothers at the time of the visit as a typical time between feeds (e.g., each 2 h) ($n = 11$, $n = 19$, $n = 17$, $n = 13$ at 2, 5, 9 and 12 months respectively). [g] Results are not presented for impractical combinations, n/a—not applicable.

References

1. Geddes, D.; Prescott, S. Developmental origins of health and disease: The role of human milk in preventing disease in the 21(st) century. *J. Hum. Lact.* **2013**, *29*, 123–127. [CrossRef] [PubMed]
2. Prescott, S.L. Early nutrition as a major determinant of 'immune health': Implications for allergy, obesity and other noncommunicable diseases. In *Preventive Aspects of Early Nutrition*; Fewtrell, M.S., Haschke, F., Prescott, S.L., Eds.; Vevey/S. Kager AG: Basel, Switzerland, 2016; Volume 85, pp. 1–17.
3. Socha, P.; Hellmuth, C.; Gruszfeld, D.; Demmelmair, H.; Rzehak, P.; Grote, V.; Weber, M.; Escribano, J.; Closa-Monasterolo, R.; Dain, E.; et al. Endocrine and metabolic biomarkers predicting early childhood obesity risk. In *Preventive Aspects of Early Nutrition*; Fewtrell, M.S., Haschke, F., Prescott, S.L., Eds.; Vevey/S. Kager AG: Basel, Switzerland, 2016; Volume 85, pp. 81–88.
4. Kelishadi, R.; Farajian, S. The protective effects of breastfeeding on chronic non-communicable diseases in adulthood: A review of evidence. *Adv. Biomed. Res.* **2014**, *3*, 3:1–3:5. [CrossRef] [PubMed]
5. Godfrey, K.M.; Costello, P.M.; Lillycrop, K.A. Development, epigenetics and metabolic programming. In *Preventive Aspects of Early Nutrition*; Fewtrell, M.S., Haschke, F., Prescott, S.L., Eds.; Vevey/S. Kager AG: Basel, Switzerland, 2016; Volume 85, pp. 71–80.
6. Wells, J.C.; Chomoto, S.; Fewtrell, M.S. Programming of body composition by early growth and nutrition. *Proc. Nutr. Soc.* **2007**, *66*, 423–434. [CrossRef] [PubMed]
7. Sievers, E.; Oldigs, H.D.; Santer, R.; Schaub, J. Feeding patterns in breast-fed and formula-fed infants. *Ann. Nutr. Metab.* **2002**, *46*, 243–248. [CrossRef] [PubMed]
8. Savino, F.; Liguori, S.A.; Fissore, M.F.; Oggero, R. Breast milk hormones and their protective effect on obesity. *Int. J. Pediatr. Endocrinol.* **2009**, *2009*, 327505:1–327505:8. [CrossRef]
9. Bartok, C. Babies fed breastmilk by breast versus by bottle: A pilot study evaluating early growth patterns. *Breastfeed. Med.* **2011**, *6*, 117–124. [CrossRef] [PubMed]
10. Luque, V.; Closa-Monasterolo, R.; Escribano, J.; Ferre, N. Early programming by protein intake: The effect of protein on adiposity development and the growth and functionality of vital organs. *Nutr. Metab. Insights* **2015**, *8*, 49–56. [CrossRef] [PubMed]
11. Butte, N.; Wong, W.; Hopkinson, J.; Smith, E.; Ellis, K. Infant feeding mode affects early growth and body composition. *Pediatrics* **2000**, *16*, 1355–1366. [CrossRef]
12. Kent, J.; Mitoulas, L.; Cox, D.B.; Owens, R.; Hartmann, P. Breast volume and milk production during extended lactation in women. *Exp. Physiol.* **1999**, *84*, 435–447. [CrossRef] [PubMed]

13. Mitoulas, L.R.; Kent, J.C.; Cox, D.B.; Owens, R.A.; Sherriff, J.L.; Hartmann, P.E. Variation in fat, lactose and protein in human milk over 24 h and throughout the first year of lactation. *Br. J. Nutr.* **2002**, *88*, 29–37. [CrossRef] [PubMed]
14. Leddy, M.A.; Power, M.L.; Schulkin, J. The impact of maternal obesity on maternal and fetal health. *Rev. Obstet. Gynecol.* **2008**, *1*, 170–178. [PubMed]
15. Nahar, S.; Mascie-Taylor, C.G.; Begum, H.A. Maternal anthropometry as a predictor of birth weight. *Public Health Nutr.* **2007**, *10*, 965–970. [CrossRef] [PubMed]
16. Yu, Z.; Han, S.; Zhu, J.; Sun, X.; Ji, C.; Guo, X. Pre-pregnancy body mass index in relation to infant birth weight and offspring overweight/obesity: A systematic review and meta-analysis. *PLoS ONE* **2013**, *8*, e61627. [CrossRef] [PubMed]
17. Rossner, S.; Ohlin, A. Maternal body weight and relation to birth weight. *Acta Obstet. Gynaecol Scand.* **1990**, *69*, 475–478. [CrossRef]
18. Moussa, H.N.; Alrais, M.A.; Leon, M.G.; Abbas, E.L.; Sibai, B.M. Obesity epidemic: Impact from preconception to postpartum. *Future Sci. OA* **2016**, *2*, FSO137:1–FSO137:12. [CrossRef] [PubMed]
19. Sewell, M.F.; Huston-Presley, L.; Super, D.M.; Catalano, P. Increased neonatal fat mass, not lean body mass, is associated with maternal obesity. *Am. J. Obstet. Gynecol.* **2006**, *195*, 1100–1103. [CrossRef] [PubMed]
20. Castillo-Laura, H.; Santos, I.S.; Quadros, L.C.M.; Matijasevich, A. Maternal obesity and offspring body composition by indirect methods: A systematic review and meta-analysis. *Cad. Saude Publica* **2015**, *31*, 2073–2092. [CrossRef] [PubMed]
21. Kugananthan, S.; Gridneva, Z.; Lai, C.T.; Hepworth, A.R.; Mark, P.J.; Kakulas, F.; Geddes, D.T. Associations between maternal body composition and appetite hormones and macronutrients in human milk. *Nutrients* **2017**, *9*, 252. [CrossRef] [PubMed]
22. Fields, D.A.; Schneider, C.R.; Pavela, G. A narrative review of the associations between six bioactive components in breast milk and infant adiposity. *Obesity* **2016**, *24*, 1213–1221. [CrossRef] [PubMed]
23. Kent, E.; O'Dwyer, V.; Fattah, C.; Farah, N.; O'Connor, C.; Turner, M.J. Correlation between birth weight and maternal body composition. *Obstet. Gynecol.* **2013**, *121*, 46–50. [CrossRef] [PubMed]
24. O'Connor, C.; O'Higgins, A.; Segurado, R.; Turner, M.J.; Stuart, B.; Kennelly, M.M. Maternal body composition and birth weight. *Prenat. Diagn.* **2014**, *34*, 605–607. [PubMed]
25. Larciprete, G.; Valensise, H.; Vasapollo, B.; Di Pierro, G.; Menghini, S.; Magnani, F.; De Lorenzo, A.; Arduini, D. Maternal body composition at term gestation and birth weight: Is there a link? *Acta Diabetol.* **2003**, *40*, 222–224. [CrossRef] [PubMed]
26. Sanin Aguirre, L.H.; Reza-Lopez, S.; Levario-Carrillo, M. Relation between maternal body composition and birth weight. *Biol. Neonate* **2004**, *86*, 55–62. [CrossRef] [PubMed]
27. Ejlerskov, K.T.; Christensen, L.B.; Ritz, C.; Jensen, S.M.; Molgaard, C.; Michaelsen, K.F. The impact of early growth patterns and infant feeding on body composition at 3 years of age. *Br. J. Nutr.* **2015**, *114*, 316–327. [CrossRef] [PubMed]
28. Holliday, M.A. Metabolic rate and organ size during growth from infancy to maturity and during late gestation and early infancy. *Pediatrics* **1971**, *47*, 169–179.
29. Elia, M. Organ and tissue contribution to metabolic rate. In *Energy Metabolism. Tissue Determinants and Cellular Corollaries*; Kinney, J.M., Tucker, H.N., Eds.; Raven: New York, NY, USA, 1992; pp. 61–79.
30. Dewey, K.; Heinig, M.; Nommsen, L.; Lonnerdal, B. Maternal versus infant factors related to breast milk intake and residual milk volume: The DARLING study. *Pediatrics* **1991**, *87*, 829–837. [PubMed]
31. Kent, J.C.; Mitoulas, L.R.; Cregan, M.D.; Ramsay, D.T.; Doherty, D.A.; Hartmann, P.E. Volume and frequency of breastfeedings and fat content of breast milk throughout the day. *Pediatrics* **2006**, *117*, e387–e395. [CrossRef] [PubMed]
32. Gridneva, Z.; Kugananthan, S.; Hepworth, A.R.; Tie, W.J.; Lai, C.T.; Ward, L.C.; Hartmann, P.E.; Geddes, D.T. Effect of human milk appetite hormones, macronutrients, and infant characteristics on gastric emptying and breastfeeding patterns of term fully breastfed infants. *Nutrients* **2017**, *9*, 15. [CrossRef] [PubMed]
33. Binns, C.W.; Fraser, M.L.; Lee, A.H.; Scott, J. Defining exclusive breastfeeding in Australia. *J. Paediatr. Child Health* **2009**, *45*, 174–180. [CrossRef] [PubMed]
34. Gridneva, Z.; Hepworth, A.; Ward, L.; Lai, C.T.; Hartmann, P.; Geddes, D.T. Bioimpedance spectroscopy in the infant: Effect of milk intake and extracellular fluid reservoirs on resistance measurements in term breastfed infants. *Eur. J. Clin. Nutr.* **2016**, *70*, 843–851. [CrossRef] [PubMed]

35. Gridneva, Z.; Hepworth, A.R.; Ward, L.C.; Lai, C.T.; Hartmann, P.E.; Geddes, D.T. Determinants of body composition in breastfed infants using bioimpedance spectroscopy and ultrasound skinfolds—Methods comparison. *Pediatr. Res.* **2016**, *81*, 423–433. [CrossRef] [PubMed]
36. Lingwood, B.E.; van Leeuwen, A.M.S.; Carberry, A.E.; Fitzgerald, E.C.; Callaway, L.K.; Colditz, P.B.; Ward, L.C. Prediction of fat-free mass and percentage of body fat in neonates using biolelectrical impedance analysis and anthropometric measures: Validation against Pea Pod. *Br. J. Nutr.* **2012**, *107*, 1545–1552. [CrossRef] [PubMed]
37. Bocage, C. Impedance Measurements of Body Composition in Children. Master's Thesis, University of West Indies, Kingston, Jamaica, 1988.
38. Butte, N.; Hopkinson, J.; Wong, W.; Smith, E.; Ellis, K. Body composition during the first 2 years of life: An updated reference. *Pediatr. Res.* **2000**, *47*, 578–585. [CrossRef] [PubMed]
39. McLeod, G.; Geddes, D.; Nathan, E.; Sherriff, J.; Simmer, K.; Hartmann, P. Feasibility of using ultrasound to measure preterm body composition and to assess macronutrient influences on tissue accretion rates. *Early Hum. Dev.* **2013**, *89*, 577–582. [CrossRef] [PubMed]
40. Ulbricht, L.; Neves, E.; Ripka, W.; Romaneli, E. Comparison between Body Fat Measurements Obtained by Portable Ultrasound and Caliper in Young Adults. In Proceedings of the 2012 Annual International Conference of the IEEE Engineering in Medicine and Biology Society (EMBS), San Diego, CA, USA, 28 August–1 September 2012; pp. 1952–1955.
41. Slaughter, M.; Lohman, T.; Boileau, R.; Horswill, C.; Stillman, R.; Van Loan, M.; Bemben, D. Skinfold equations for estimation of body fatness in children and youth. *Hum. Biol.* **1988**, *60*, 709–723. [PubMed]
42. Brook, C. Determination of body composition of children from skinfold measurements. *Arch. Dis. Child.* **1971**, *46*, 182–184. [CrossRef] [PubMed]
43. Lohman, T. Body composition in children and youth. In *Advances in Pediatric Sport Sciences*; Boileau, R.A., Ed.; Human Kinetics Publishers: Champaign, IL, USA, 1984; pp. 29–57.
44. Van Itallie, T.B.; Yang, M.U.; Heymsfield, S.B.; Funk, R.C.; Boileau, R.A. Height-normalized indices of the body's fat-free mass and fat mass: Potentially useful indicators of nutritional status. *Am. J. Clin. Nutr.* **1990**, *52*, 953–959.
45. Arthur, P.; Hartmann, P.; Smith, M. Measurement of the milk intake of breast-fed infants. *J. Pediatr. Gastroenterol. Nutr.* **1987**, *6*, 758–763. [CrossRef] [PubMed]
46. R Core Team. *R: A Language and Environment for Statistical Computing*; R Foundation for Statistical Computing: Vienna, Austria, 2017.
47. Pinheiro, J.B.; Bates, D.; DebRoy, S.; Sarkar, D.; R Development Core Team. *nlme: Linear and Nonlinear Mixed Effects Models*; R Package Version 3.1–131; R Foundation for Statistical Computing: Vienna, Austria, 2017.
48. Bates, D.; Maechler, M.; Bolker, B.; Walker, S. *Lme4: Linear Mixed-Efects Models Using Eigen and S4*; R Package Version 1.1–7; R Foundation for Statistical Computing: Vienna, Austria, 2014.
49. Fox, J.; Weisberg, S. *An R Companion to Applied Regression*; Sage: Thousand Oaks, CA, USA, 2011.
50. Gamer, M.; Lemon, J.; Fellows, I.; Singh, P. *Various Coefficients of Interrater Reliability and Agreement*; R Package Version 0.84; R Foundation for Statistical Computing: Vienna, Austria, 2012.
51. Hothorn, T.; Bretz, F.; Westfall, P. Simultaneous inference in general parametric models. *Biom. J.* **2008**, *50*, 346–363. [CrossRef] [PubMed]
52. Wickham, H. *ggplot2: Elegant Graphics for Data Analysis*; Springer: New York, NY, USA, 2009.
53. Faul, F.; Erdfelder, E.; Buchner, A.; Lang, A.-G. Statistical power analyses using G*Power 3.1: Tests for correlation and regression analyses. *Behav. Res. Methods* **2009**, *41*, 1149–1160. [CrossRef] [PubMed]
54. Diggle, P.J.; Heagerty, P.J.; Liang, K.-Y.; Zeger, S.L. *Analysis of Longitudinal Data*; Oxford University Press Inc.: New York, NY, USA, 2002.
55. Institute of Medicine; Subcommittee on Nutrition During Lactation. *Nutrition During Lactation*; National Academy Press: Washington, DC, USA, 1991.
56. Nommsen, L.A.; Lovelady, C.A.; Heinig, M.; Lonnerdal, B.; Dewey, K.G. Determinants of energy, protein, lipid, and lactose concentrations in human milk during the first 12 mo of lactation: The DARLING study. *Am. J. Clin. Nutr.* **1991**, *53*, 457–465. [PubMed]
57. Curran-Everett, D. Multiple comparisons: Philosophies and illustrations. *Am. J. Physiol. Regul. Integr. Comp. Physiol.* **2000**, *279*, R1–R8. [CrossRef] [PubMed]

58. Gallagher, D.; Heymsfield, S.B.; Heo, M.; Jebb, S.A.; Murgatroyd, P.R.; Sakamoto, Y. Healthy percentage body fat ranges: An approach for developing guidelines based on body mass index. *Am. J. Clin. Nutr.* **2000**, *72*, 694–701. [PubMed]
59. Rzehak, P.; Oddy, W.H.; Mearin, M.L.; Grote, V.; Mori, T.A.; Szajewska, H.; Shamir, R.; Koletzko, S.; Weber, M.; Beilin, L.J.; et al. Infant feeding and growth trajectory patterns in childhood and body composition in young adulthood. *Am. J. Clin. Nutr.* **2017**, *106*, 568–580. [CrossRef] [PubMed]
60. Nazlee, N.; Bilal, R.; Latif, Z.; Bluck, L. Maternal body composition and its relationship to infant breast milk intake in rural Pakistan. *Food Nutr. Sci.* **2011**, *2*, 932–937. [CrossRef] [PubMed]
61. Galpin, L.; Thakwalakwa, C.; Phuka, J.; Ashorn, P.; Maleta, K.; Wong, W.W.; Manary, M.J. Breast milk intake is not reduced more by the introduction of energy dense complementary food than by typical infant porridge. *J. Nutr.* **2007**, *137*, 1828–1833. [PubMed]
62. Butte, N.F.; Wills, C.; Jean, C.A.; Smith, E.O.; Garza, C. Feeding patterns of exclusively breast-fed infants during the first four months of life. *Early Hum. Dev.* **1985**, *12*, 291–300. [CrossRef]
63. Rattigan, S.; Ghisalberti, A.V.; Hartmann, P.E. Breast-milk production in Australian women. *Br. J. Nutr.* **1981**, *45*, 243–249. [CrossRef] [PubMed]
64. Kent, J.; Hepworth, A.; Sherriff, J.; Cox, D.; Mitoulas, L.; Hartmann, P. Longitudinal changes in breastfeeding patterns from 1 to 6 months of lactation. *Breastfeed. Med.* **2013**, *8*, 401–407. [CrossRef] [PubMed]
65. Ay, L.; Van Houten, V.A.; Steegers, E.A.; Hofman, A.; Witteman, J.C.; Jaddoe, V.W.; Hokken-Koelega, A.C. Fetal and postnatal growth and body composition at 6 months of age. *J. Clin. Endocrinol. Metab.* **2009**, *94*, 2023–2030. [CrossRef] [PubMed]
66. Forsum, E.; Lof, M.; Olausson, H.; Olhager, E. Maternal body composition in relation to infant birth weight and subcutaneous adipose tissue. *Br. J. Nutr.* **2006**, *96*, 408–414. [CrossRef] [PubMed]
67. Hull, H.R.; Dinger, M.K.; Knehans, A.W.; Thompson, D.M.; Fields, D.A. Impact of maternal body mass index on neonate birthweight and body composition. *Am. J. Obstet. Gynecol.* **2008**, *198*, 416.e411–416.e416. [CrossRef] [PubMed]
68. Dulloo, A.G.; Jacquet, J.; Miles-Chan, J.L.; Schutz, Y. Passive and active roles of fat-free mass in the control of energy intake and body composition regulation. *Eur. J. Clin. Nutr.* **2017**, *71*, 353–357. [CrossRef] [PubMed]
69. Haroun, D.; Wells, J.C.K.; Williams, J.E.; Fuller, N.J.; Fewtrell, M.S.; Lawson, M.S. Composition of the fat-free mass in obese and nonobese children: Matched case-control analyses. *Int. J. Obes.* **2005**, *29*, 29–36. [CrossRef] [PubMed]
70. Catalano, P.M.; Tyzbir, E.D.; Allen, S.R.; McBean, J.H.; McAuliffe, T.L. Evaluation of fetal growth by estimation of neonatal body composition. *Obstet. Gynecol.* **1992**, *79*, 46–50. [PubMed]
71. Singh, K.A.; Huston-Presley, L.P.; Mencin, P.; Thomas, A.; Amini, S.B.; Catalano, P.M. Birth weight and body composition of neonates born to Caucasian compared with African-American mothers. *Obstet. Gynecol.* **2010**, *115*, 998–1002. [CrossRef] [PubMed]
72. Andersen, G.S.; Girma, T.; Wells, J.C.K.; Kastel, P.; Michaelsen, K.F.; Friis, H. Fat and fat-free mass at birth: Air displacement plethysmography measurements on 350 Ethiopian newborns. *Pediatr. Res.* **2011**, *70*, 501–506. [CrossRef] [PubMed]
73. Chomtho, S.; Wells, J.C.K.; Davies, P.S.; Lucas, A.; Fewtrell, M.S. Early growth and body composition in infancy. In *Early Nutrition Programming and Health Outcomes in Later Life. Advances in Experimental Medicine and Biology*; Koletzko, B., Decsi, T., Molnar, D., de la Hunty, A., Eds.; Springer: Dordrecht, The Netherlands, 2009; Volume 646, pp. 165–168.
74. Andres, A.; Hull, H.R.; Shankar, K.; Casey, P.H.; Cleves, M.A.; Badger, T.M. Longitudinal body composition of children born to mothers with normal weight, overweight, and obesity. *Obesity* **2015**, *23*, 1252–1258. [CrossRef] [PubMed]
75. Silliman, K.; Kretchmer, N. Maternal obesity and body composition of the neonate. *Biol. Neonate* **1995**, *68*, 384–393. [CrossRef] [PubMed]
76. Breij, L.M.; Abrahamse-Berkeveld, M.; Acton, D.; De Lucia Rolfe, E.; Ong, K.K.; Hokken-Koelega, A.C.S. Impact of early infant growth, duration of breastfeeding and maternal factors on total body fat mass and visceral fat at 3 and 6 months of age. *Ann. Nutr. Metab.* **2017**, *71*, 203–210. [CrossRef] [PubMed]
77. Badon, S.E.; Dyer, A.R.; Josefson, J.L.; HAPO Study Coopwrative Research Group. Gestational weight gain and neonatal adiposity in the hyperglycemia and adverse pregnancy outcome study—North American region. *Obesity* **2014**, *22*, 1731–1738. [CrossRef] [PubMed]

78. Anne, D.; O'Higgins, A.; O'Connor, C.; Mullaney, L.; Bennet, A.M.; Sheridan-Pereira, M.; Turner, M.J. PS-275 The relationship between infant birth weight and neonatal body composition. *Arch. Dis. Child.* **2014**, *99*, A211. [CrossRef]
79. Fomon, S.; Nelson, S. Body composition of the male and female reference infants. *Ann. Rev. Nutr.* **2002**, *22*, 1–17. [CrossRef] [PubMed]
80. Jensen, S.M.; Ritz, C.; Ejlerskov, K.; Molgaard, C.; Michaelsen, K.F. Infant BMI peak, breastfeeding, and body composition at age 3 years. *Am. J. Clin. Nutr.* **2015**, *101*, 319–325. [CrossRef] [PubMed]
81. Roy, S.M.; Spivack, J.G.; Faith, M.S.; Chesi, A.; Mitchell, J.A.; Kelly, A.; Grant, S.F.; McCormack, S.E.; Zemel, B.S. Infant BMI or weight-for-length and obesity risk in early childhood. *Pediatrics* **2016**, *137*, e20153492:1–e20153492:9. [CrossRef] [PubMed]
82. Gale, C.; Logan, K.; Santhakumaran, S.; Parkinson, J.; Hyde, M.; Modi, N. Effect of breastfeeding compared with formula feeding on infant body composition: A systematic review and meta-analysis. *Am. J. Clin. Nutr.* **2012**, *95*, 656–669. [CrossRef] [PubMed]
83. Lee, H.; Park, H.; Ha, E.; Hong, Y.-C.; Ha, M.; Park, H.; Kim, B.-N.; Lee, B.; Lee, S.-J.; Lee, K.Y.; et al. Effect of breastfeeding duration on cognitive development in infants: 3-year follow-up study. *J. Korean Med. Sci.* **2016**, *31*, 579–584. [CrossRef] [PubMed]
84. Booth, A.; Magnuson, A.; Foster, M. Detrimental and protective fat: Body fat distribution and its relation to metabolic disease. *Horm. Mol. Biol. Clin. Investig.* **2014**, *17*, 13–27. [CrossRef] [PubMed]
85. Roggero, P.; Gianni, M.; Orsi, A.; Piemontese, P.; Amato, O.; Liotto, N.; Morlacchi, L.; Taroni, F.; Fields, D.; Catalano, P.; et al. Quality of growth in exclusively breast-fed infants in the first six months of life: An Italian study. *Pediatr. Res.* **2010**, *68*, 542–544. [CrossRef] [PubMed]
86. Gilchrist, J. Body Composition Reference Data for Exclusively Breast-Fed Infants. In Proceedings of the Pediatric Academic Society Annual Meeting, Toronto, ON, Canada, 5–7 May 2007.
87. Carberry, A.; Golditz, P.; Lingwood, B. Body composition from birth to 4.5 months in infants born to non-obese women. *Pediatr. Res.* **2010**, *68*, 84–88. [CrossRef] [PubMed]
88. Gilchrist, J.; Andres, A.; Badger, T. Body composition of infants fed breast-milk, milk-based formula or soy-based formula during the first 6 months of life. *Obesity* **2008**, *16*, 434.
89. Twigger, A.J.; Hepworth, A.R.; Lai, C.T.; Chetwynd, E.; Stuebe, A.M.; Blancafort, P.; Hartmann, P.E.; Geddes, D.T.; Kakulas, F. Gene expression in breastmilk cells is associated with maternal and infant characteristics. *Sci. Rep.* **2015**, *5*, 12933:1–12933:14. [CrossRef] [PubMed]
90. Lepe, M.; Bacardi Gascon, M.; Castaneda-Gonzalez, L.M.; Perez Morales, M.E.; Jimenez Cruz, A. Effect of maternal obesity on lactation: Systematic review. *Nutr. Hosp.* **2011**, *26*, 1266–1269. [PubMed]
91. Villalpando, S.F.; Butte, N.F.; Wong, W.W.; Flores-Huerta, S.; Hernandez-Beltran, M.J.; Smith, E.O.; Garza, C. Lactation performance of rural Mesoamerindians. *Eur. J. Clin. Nutr.* **1992**, *46*, 337–348. [PubMed]
92. World Health Organization. Child Growth Standards: Weight-for-Age Pecentiles. Available online: http://www.who.int/childgrowth/standards/weight_for_age/en/ (accessed on 21 December 2017).
93. Hatsu, I.E.; McDougald, D.M.; Anderson, A.K. Effect of infant feeding on maternal body composition. *Int. Breastfeed. J.* **2008**, *3*, 18:1–18:8. [CrossRef] [PubMed]
94. Quandt, S.A. Changes in maternal postpartum adiposity and infant feeding patterns. *Am. J. Phys. Anthropol.* **1983**, *60*, 455–461. [CrossRef] [PubMed]
95. Stuebe, A.M.; Rich-Edwards, J.W. The reset hypothesis: Lactation and maternal metabolism. *Am. J. Perinatol.* **2009**, *26*, 81–88. [CrossRef] [PubMed]
96. National Health and Medical Research Council. *Infant Feeding Guidelines Information for Health Workers*; National Health and Medical Research Council: Canberra, Australia, 2012.
97. World Health Organization. *Planning Guide for National Implementation of the Global Strategy for Infant and Young Child Feeding*; World Health Organization: Geneva, Switzerland, 2007.
98. Han, S.-Y.; Brewis, A.A. Influence of weight concerns on breastfeeding: Evidence from the Norwegian mother and child cohort study. *Am. J. Hum. Biol.* **2017**, e23086:1–e23086:4. [CrossRef] [PubMed]

3

Longitudinal Analysis of Macronutrient Composition in Preterm and Term Human Milk

Céline J. Fischer Fumeaux [1], Clara L. Garcia-Rodenas [2], Carlos A. De Castro [3], Marie-Claude Courtet-Compondu [4], Sagar K. Thakkar [5], Lydie Beauport [1], Jean-François Tolsa [1] and Michael Affolter [4,*]

[1] Clinic of Neonatology, Department Woman Mother Child, University Hospital of Lausanne, 1011 Lausanne, Switzerland
[2] Nestlé Institute of Health Sciences, Nestlé Research, 1000 Lausanne, Switzerland
[3] Clinical Development Unit, Nestlé Research Asia, Singapore 138567, Singapore
[4] Nestlé Institute of Food Safety & Analytical Science, Nestlé Research, 1000 Lausanne, Switzerland
[5] Nestlé Research Asia, Singapore 138567, Singapore
* Correspondence: Michael.Affolter@rdls.nestle.com

Abstract: Background: Mother's own milk is the optimal source of nutrients and provides numerous health advantages for mothers and infants. As they have supplementary nutritional needs, very preterm infants may require fortification of human milk (HM). Addressing HM composition and variations is essential to optimize HM fortification strategies for these vulnerable infants. Aims: To analyze and compare macronutrient composition in HM of mothers lactating very preterm (PT) (28 0/7 to 32 6/7 weeks of gestational age, GA) and term (T) infants (37 0/7 to 41 6/7 weeks of GA) over time, both at similar postnatal and postmenstrual ages, and to investigate other potential factors of variations. Methods: Milk samples from 27 mothers of the PT infants and 34 mothers of the T infants were collected longitudinally at 12 points in time during four months for the PT HM and eight points in time during two months for the T HM. Macronutrient composition (proteins, fat, and lactose) and energy were measured using a mid-infrared milk analyzer, corrected by bicinchoninic acid (BCA) assay for total protein content. Results: Analysis of 500 HM samples revealed large inter- and intra-subject variations in both groups. Proteins decreased from birth to four months in the PT and the T HM without significant differences at any postnatal time point, while it was lower around term equivalent age in PT HM. Lactose content remained stable and comparable over time. The PT HM contained significantly more fat and tended to be more caloric in the first two weeks of lactation, while the T HM revealed higher fat and higher energy content later during lactation (three to eight weeks). In both groups, male gender was associated with more fat and energy content. The gender association was stronger in the PT group, and it remained significant after adjustments. Conclusion: Longitudinal measurements of macronutrients compositions of the PT and the T HM showed only small differences at similar postnatal stages in our population. However, numerous differences exist at similar postmenstrual ages. Male gender seems to be associated with a higher content in fat, especially in the PT HM. This study provides original information on macronutrient composition and variations of HM, which is important to consider for the optimization of nutrition and growth of PT infants.

Keywords: human milk; preterm; term; neonate; infant; macronutrients; protein; fat; lactose; nutrition

1. Introduction

Human milk (HM) is a highly complex, dynamic and species-specific system that incorporates numerous nutritional and bioactive elements. Despite progress in analytical technologies enabling the growth of data over the past decade, HM composition remains only partially elucidated [1–4]. Recent studies revealed countless inter- and intra-individual factors influencing HM composition, such as maternal, circadian, pregnancy, delivery, infantile, chronological and environmental variables [5–9]. Among these factors, temporal changes of HM composition before and after term equivalent time are of particular interest considering the critical challenges of preterm (PT) infants' nutrition and the critical importance of HM for this vulnerable population [10,11].

As for healthy term (T) babies, breastfeeding provides numerous health advantages for PT infants and their mothers, and is thus strongly recommended [12–16]. In addition, for very PT at risk neonates, mother's own milk appears particularly protective against several severe complications, such as necrotizing enterocolitis, sepsis, bronchopulmonary dysplasia, retinopathy of prematurity, and reduces duration of hospital stay or incidence of rehospitalizations [17–20]. Furthermore, it may improve brain growth and the development of these fragile infants [21–24].

Despite these crucial protective effects, HM may not fully meet some specific additional nutritional requirements of very PT infants to avoid growth flattening, nutritional deficits, and related complications [25–27]. Therefore, human milk fortification is often recommended in very PT neonates, however controversies exist and optimal, feasible fortification strategies remain to be identified [11,16]. Nevertheless, even with the development of HM fortification practices, growth failure remains frequent in neonatal intensive care units (NICUs), affecting up to half of very low birthweight neonates [28].

In this context, we need to have better knowledge and understanding of HM composition and its variations, and especially temporal changes, in order to enhance nutritional enteral strategies, mainly human milk fortification and/or formula complements according to the situation [11]. Currently, studies on HM composition after very PT delivery remain scarce and are mostly based on cross-sectional studies. Only a few studies have longitudinally measured the trajectory of HM composition and its time variations in both T and PT infants, and the data remain controversial [10].

In this prospective cohort study, we aimed: (i) to quantify macronutrient composition in very PT and T HM over time; (ii) to compare macronutrient composition between PT and T milk, at similar lactation stages (postnatal ages) and gestational stages (postmenstrual ages); and (iii) to investigate other factors potentially associated with macronutrient variations in HM.

2. Materials and Methods

2.1. Study Design, Subjects, and Setting

This study was a part of a prospective, monocentric, cohort study aiming to analyze various components of HM over time and to compare their contents in the PT HM versus the T HM. We previously published the study design and the description of the population in detail [29].

The study was conducted between October 2013 and July 2014 at the University Hospital of Lausanne, Switzerland. Eligible mothers were those older than 18 years of age, intending to breastfeed their offspring, and who delivered either (i) very prematurely (PT group), from 28 0/7 to 32 6/7 weeks of gestational age (GA) or (ii) at term (T group), between 37 0/7 to 41 6/7 weeks of GA.

Exclusion criteria included any counter-indication to breastfeeding, maternal diabetes (type I or II) before pregnancy, alcohol or drug consumption, and insufficient French language skills.

The mothers who were included in the study were followed until postnatal week 16 for the PT group, and week 8 for the T group, or until lactation discontinuation (whichever came first).

2.2. Data Collection

The main clinical and sociodemographic maternal and neonatal characteristics were prospectively collected. All data were recorded in electronic case report forms in a dedicated database.

2.3. Milk Sampling and Processing

Sequential, iterative samples of milk were collected according to the following schedule, illustrated in Figure 1:

(i) Preterm group: 1–10 mL of milk was collected at the end of the 1st week, then weekly for the first 8 weeks, then every 2 weeks for an additional 8 weeks; this corresponded thus to a maximum of 12 samples during the 16 weeks.

(ii) Term group: 10 mL of milk were collected weekly for 8 weeks, starting at the end of week 1.

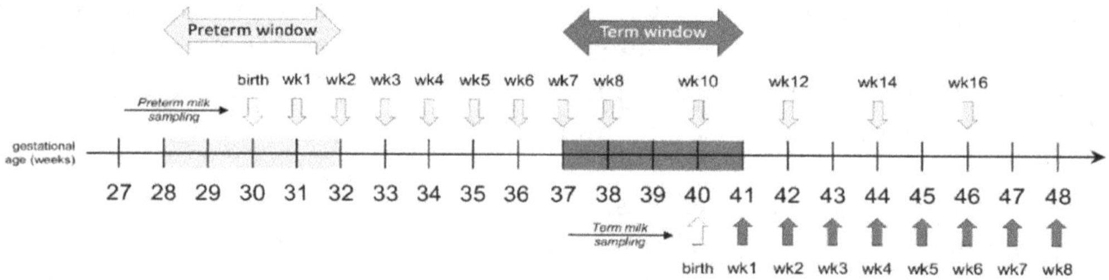

Figure 1. Milk sampling schedule (reprinted from Garcia-Rodenas et al. 2018, with permission from Elsevier).

Standardized milk sampling relied on a single sampling of a single breast in the morning (first morning expression). Milk samples were expressed between 6–12 a.m., using an electric breast pump (Symphony®, Medela, Baar, Switzerland). After the breast was entirely emptied, the milk was homogenized and an aliquot of maximum 10 mL of milk (1–10 mL for the first two time points in the PT group) was collected. Each sample aliquot was immediately transferred to dedicated freezing tubes (15 mL polypropylene tubes, Falcon™, Fisher Scientific, Reinach, Switzerland), and stored at −18 °C in the home freezer for a maximum of 1 week until frozen transfer to the hospital. At the hospital, samples were temporarily kept at −80 °C and then transferred to the Nestlé Research Centre (NRC, Lausanne, Switzerland). The frozen milk samples were thawed for splitting into 15 aliquots and stored at −80 °C until analysis of macronutrient and other HM components (reported in independent publications).

2.4. Measurement of HM Macronutrient Composition

The macronutrient content (total protein, fat, and carbohydrate, i.e., lactose) and energy density were measured using a human milk analyzer (MIRIS AB, Uppsala, Sweden) based on mid-infrared transmission spectroscopy (www.mirissolutions.com). One mL of each milk sample was thawed and warmed to 40 °C in a water bath. Prior to the measurement, each sample was homogenized using the MIRIS sonicator to avoid protein aggregation and lipid phase separation. A daily calibration check (MIRIS check solution) was performed according to the manufacturer's recommendations. Macronutrient quantities were measured in a single run and the energy content was calculated automatically by the MIRIS instrument (protein 4.4 kcal/g, carbohydrate 4 kcal/g, fat 9 kcal/g) [30].

We used a MIRIS measure validation process that had been previously published [31]. As in other literature reports, this validation showed that the MIRIS was not accurate enough for the measurement of total protein in human milk as compared with the Kjeldahl reference method (AOAC International, method number 991.22), while no differences were observed for fat and carbohydrate content as compared with the corresponding reference methods. To address this issue, we used colorimetric bicinchoninic acid (BCA, ThermoFisher Scientific) assay, which produced accurate human milk protein values as compared with those obtained with the reference Kjeldahl method. In order to include this more accurate protein information in the energy density value of the human milk samples, energy density was recalculated for each milk sample using the same formula as the MIRIS instrument: Energy (kcal/L) = protein (g/L) × 4.4 + fat (g/L) × 9.25 + carbohydrate (g/L) × 4.

2.5. Statistics

The paucity of quantitative data on the macronutrient content in the PT HM precluded a proper power calculation in this exploratory study. The study size was initially set at $n = 20$ subjects per group (preterm and term infant mothers) according to the estimated recruitment feasibility at the study center within a one-year period.

The temporal changes of macronutrient contents were compared in the PT and T HM at equivalent infant (1) postpartum ages and (2) postmenstrual ages. For both comparisons, mixed linear models were used to estimate the differences between preterm and term infants. The models used age (either postpartum or postmenstrual), term/preterm status, and interaction between age and term/preterm status. Within subject variability was accounted for by declaring the subject ID as a random effect. Contrast estimates of the model were calculated by comparing the PT and T HM groups at each time point. No imputation method was applied for missing data (both in between visits and loss to follow up) as the method used does not require a complete dataset. A conventional two-sided 5% error rate was used without adjusting for multiplicity as this exploratory trial is for hypothesis generation purposes.

Similar methods were used to analyze the effects of gender and delivery mode and their interaction with age (both postpartum and postmenstrual and also both in the PT and the T populations together and separately). Statistical analyses were done using SAS 9.3 (SAS Institute, Cary, North Carolina, USA) and R 3.2.1 (R Foundation for Statistical Computing, Vienna, Austria; https://www.R-project.org).

2.6. Ethics

The study was approved by the local Ethical Board (Commission cantonal d'éthique de la recherche sur l'être humain du Canton de Vaud) (Protocol 69/13, clinical study 11.39.NRC; April 9, 2013). Maternal written consent was obtained. The study was registered at ClinicalTrials.gov with the identifier NCT02052245.

3. Results

3.1. Study Population

The detailed study flow chart and study population description has been published elsewhere [29]. They are presented in the supplementary material (see Figure S1 and Table S1).

Sixty-one mothers were included in the study: 27 mothers of 33 PT neonates, and 34 mothers of 34 T neonates. In the PT group, 25/27 mothers (93%) completed the study (one neonatal death, one withdrawal). In the T group, 28/34 mothers (82.4%) completed the study (one maternal illness, two withdrawals, three early breastfeeding disruption). In all, we collected 500 HM samples (280 PT and 220 T samples).

Mothers of the two groups were comparable in age (mean ± SD: 32.4 ± 5.6 years in the PT group, versus 31.2 ± 4.2 years in the T group, $p = 0.3173$) and body mass index before pregnancy and at delivery. The mean ± SD gestational age and birthweight of the PT and T neonates differed as expected (30.8 ± 1.4 weeks versus 39.5 ± 1.0 weeks, $p < 0.0001$, and 1421 ± 373 g versus 3278 ± 354 g, $p < 0.0001$), and more PT neonates were born by caesarean section (63% versus 23%, $p = 0.0019$). The sex ratio was similar in the two groups (54% versus 53% of males, $p = 0.8952$).

3.2. HM Macronutrient Composition

Overall, we noticed a substantial intra- and inter-individual variability in data for all macronutrients, indicating a large heterogeneity between macronutrient content for milk samples. Maximal/minimal ratios reached up to 16 for fat, 5.4 for protein, 4.1 for energy, and 3.4 for lactose content.

Detailed numerical values of each macronutrient according to postnatal age (A) and postmenstrual age (B) are reported in the corresponding supplemental Tables.

3.2.1. Total Protein

The values of total protein content in the PT and T HM according to postnatal age are depicted in Figure 2A. The total protein content gradually decreases from birth to four months, from (mean ± SD) 2.2 ± 0.3 g/100 mL to 1.5 ± 0.5 g/100 mL in preterm and from 2.5 ± 0.8 g/100 mL to 1.7 ± 0.3 g/100 mL in T HM, without significant differences between the PT and T groups at any point in time.

Figure 2B shows the total protein content in the PT and T HM according to postmenstrual age. There were significant differences ($p < 0.005$) at gestational ages of 38–40 and 42 weeks, with T HM containing higher amounts of protein. These differences peaked at 39 weeks with T values up to 1.7 times higher than PT values. Later postmenstrual ages (>43 weeks) did not show any significant differences in protein content.

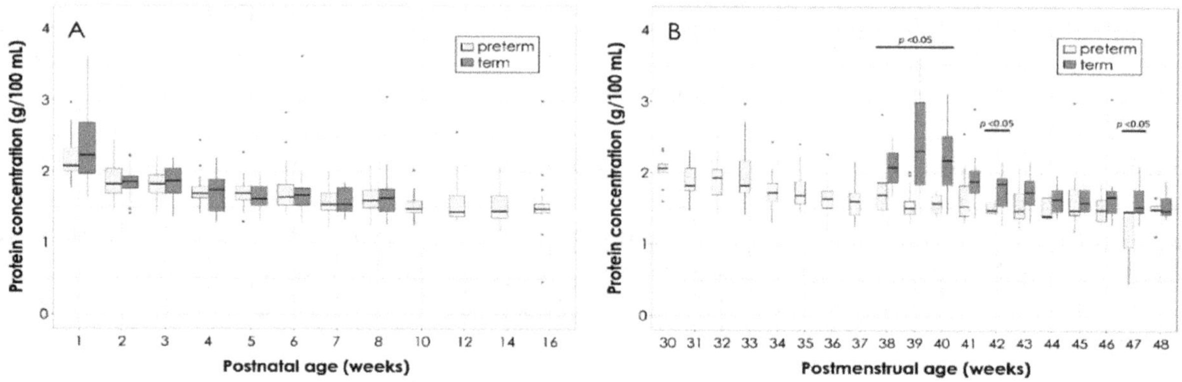

Figure 2. Total protein content in the preterm (PT) and the term (T) human milk (HM) according to postnatal age (**A**) and postmenstrual age (**B**). Box plots represent medians with 25th and 75th percentile, minimal-maximal range, and outliers (values >4.5 are excluded from the graph). Statistically significant p-values are indicated in the graph.

3.2.2. Total Fat

The mean values for total fat content in the PT and T HM slightly increase in early lactation and then remain constant over time (Figure 3A). As compared to the T HM, the PT HM contained significantly more fat (mean ± SD, 2.8 ± 1.1 g/100 mL in PT HM versus 2.1 ± 1.0 g/100 mL in T HM; $p = 0.04$) in the first week of lactation, but less in the later stages of lactation (week three to eight).

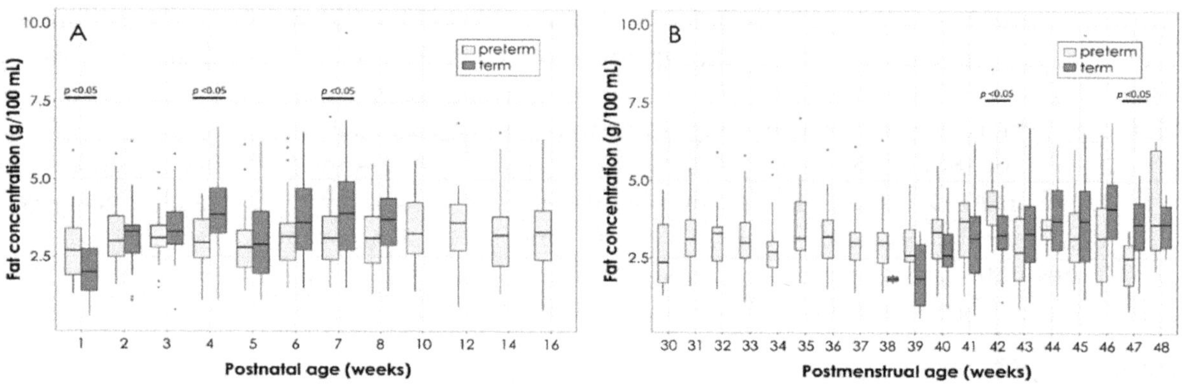

Figure 3. Total fat content in PT and T HM according to postnatal age (**A**) and postmenstrual age (**B**). Box plots represent medians with 25th and 75th percentile, minimal-maximal range, and outliers. Statistically significant p-values are indicated in the graph.

When comparing the fat content according to postmenstrual age (Figure 3B), two significant differences were observed for gestational age of 42 and 47 weeks, respectively, with higher fat content at week 42 and lower fat content at week 47 in the PT HM as compared to the T HM.

3.2.3. Total Lactose

The mean values for lactose content remained stable over postnatal time in both groups with a consistent, but not significant, higher content in the PT versus the T HM (mean ± SD over all lactation stages: 5.9 ± 0.2 g/100 mL versus 5.8 ± 0.1 g/100 mL) (Figure 4A). A significant difference was observed at week 7 with the PT HM containing higher amounts of lactose (6.1 ± 0.5 g/100 mL versus 5.6 ± 0.9 g/100 mL, $p = 0.0233$).

When comparing lactose contents according to gestational age (Figure 4B), significant variations were found for week 45 and 47, where lactose content was lower in the PT HM than in the T HM.

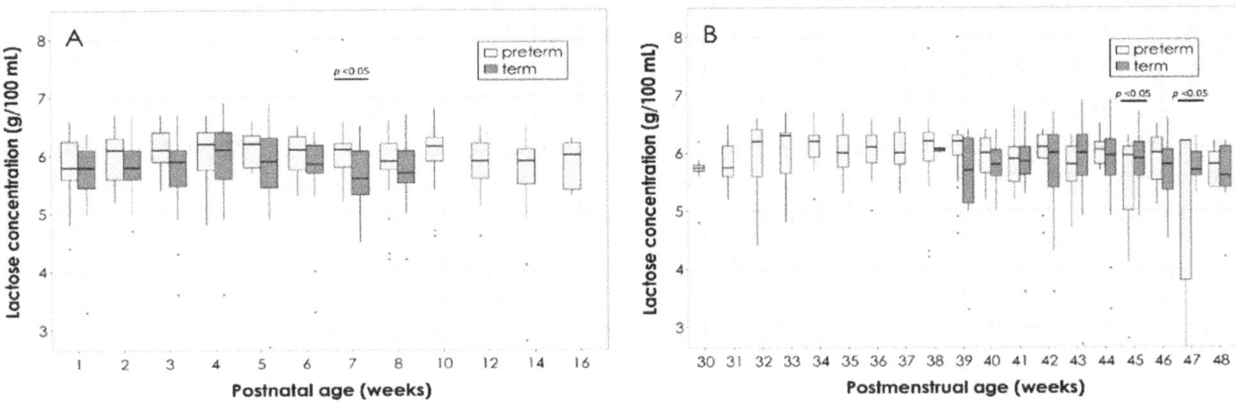

Figure 4. Total lactose content in the PT and T HM according to postpartum age (**A**) and postmenstrual age (**B**). Box plots represent medians with 25th and 75th percentile, minimal-maximal range, and outliers. Statistically significant p-values are indicated in the graph.

3.2.4. Energy Density

The mean ± SD values for energy density tended to be higher in the PT HM (58.7 ± 10.2 kcal/100 mL versus 53.1 ± 8.8 kcal/100 mL; $p = 0.08$) in the first week of lactation, whereas in weeks three to eight postpartum, energy density in the T HM was higher (Figure 5A).

When comparing the energy density according to postmenstrual age (Figure 5B), there were punctual variations between the PT and T HM, but trajectory over lactation remained relatively constant.

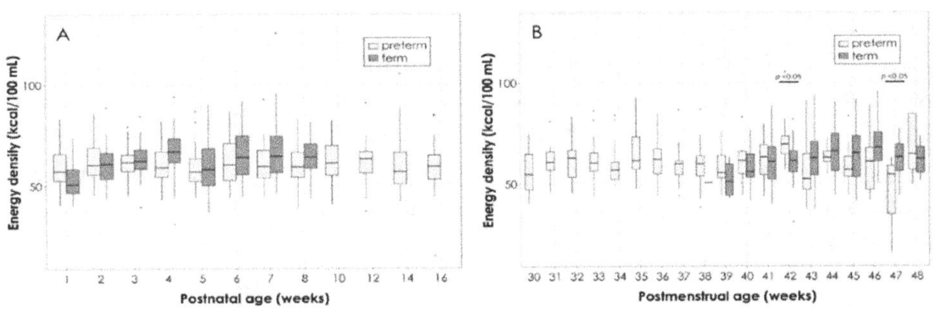

Figure 5. Calculated energy density in the PT and T HM according to postpartum age (**A**) and postmenstrual age (**B**). Box plots represent medians with 25th and 75th percentile, minimal-maximal range, and outliers. Statistically significant p-values are indicated in the graph.

3.2.5. Other Factors Influencing HM Macronutrient Composition

The composition of macronutrients was also compared over time in the population and in each T and PT subgroup separately, according to infant gender or mode of delivery (see Figures in supplementary material).

Milk of mothers with male infants was consistently higher in fat and energy as compared to milk of mothers with female infants, reaching statistical significance at postnatal weeks five and seven (estimated differences of 0.89 g/100 mL and 1.07 g/100 mL of fat, respectively). The difference at five weeks was more pronounced in the PT group (estimated difference of 1.04 g/100 mL) and the difference at seven weeks was more pronounced for the T group (1.58 g/100 mL). There was also a trend of increased content of total protein in milk for male as compared to female infants in both the T and the PT groups, but the differences were not significant. We did not observe a gender difference for lactose content. Regarding the mode of delivery, it was not associated with consistent nor significant changes in HM macronutrients contents in our population.

A mixed linear model, taking into account the variables T or PT, postpartum age, interaction between T/PT and postpartum age, gender, and mode of delivery, was assessed in order to have an indication of which variables affect macronutrient concentration. It was observed that in general, the postpartum age has a significant effect on the macronutrient concentration of milk. Carbohydrate content was significantly higher for premature infants globally (all time points combined) while differences in proteins, energy, and fat depended on the postpartum age. Energy and fat concentration were significantly affected by the gender of the infant.

4. Discussion

This study provides substantial longitudinal data on the macronutrient compositions of 500 HM samples from 61 mothers delivering either very prematurely (n = 27) or at term (n = 34), during a time period of up to 16 and eight weeks for a PT and a T group, respectively. The original milk sampling design enabled the comparison of the PT and T HM composition not only at similar postnatal ages, corresponding to similar maternal lactation stages, but also at similar postmenstrual ages, corresponding to a similar infant developmental stage.

In this cohort, HM iterative macronutrients analysis showed notably: (i) large inter- and intra-subject variations, most marked for fat content; (ii) little differences between the PT and T HM at similar postnatal ages/lactation stages, while there were more significant differences between the PT and T HM at similar postmenstrual ages/developmental stages; (iii) an overall decrease in total protein content over time, whereas lactose, fat, and energy density remained stable; and (iv) some gender differences in HM composition, as HM dedicated to male infants tended to be richer in fat and energy.

First, we have emphasis on the magnitude of the variations observed in our cohort. Differences between minimal and maximal measurements reached up to more than 10 times for fat. These variations are more important, on the whole, than those reported in other studies [10,11,32]. Extreme values were verified and confirmed. An effect of milk preservation or homogenization is unlikely, as the procedure was standardized [33]. An impact of the method of collection (first morning one single breast, rather than 24 h two breasts collections) is possible [5]. Nevertheless, these results confirm and underline how much a unique "standard" HM composition basis of calculation cannot fit all individual situations, and that more accurate alternatives for estimations of nutritional intake are required, notably for fortification issues [34].

Among factors of variations, temporal changes in HM macronutrient composition have been previously reported [10,35–37]. The study plan allowed us to investigate the HM composition changes according to both postnatal and gestational ages, related to adaptive and developmental stages, respectively. Interestingly, in our study, macronutrient composition changes were overall more pronounced according to postnatal time than to gestational age, which is in line with other recent observations [38]. Consequently, there were fewer differences between the PT and the T HM at similar postnatal ages, than at similar gestational ages. Its final implication, however, remains to be further explored. This finding should also be considered regarding the definition of nutritional needs of the PT infants and establishment of fortification targets.

Concerning the protein composition, the observed trajectory in our cohort follows a progressive decrease, which is consistent with previous observations [10,35,39]. Our protein values align well with published results for the first four weeks of lactation, and then seem to remain slightly higher than reported values (week 6 to 12) [10,37]. Unlike most existing data, we did not find a higher protein content in the PT HM than in the T HM, and there were no significant differences in the PT and T HM protein contents at any point. By contrast, the longitudinal trajectory of the protein content according to postmenstrual age revealed some significant differences between PT and T HM, which culminate between weeks 38 and 42. This implies that a preterm breastfed infant arriving at term equivalent age receives lower amounts of protein as compared with a breastfed term infant.

Concerning the fat composition, the changes of the PT and T HM contents follow a very similar trajectory as described previously, with an initial slight increase in fat content from week one to week two, followed by a constant level over the remaining lactation period. Initially at week one, the PT HM contained a higher fat content, and then, until the end of the sampling period, the T HM contained slightly higher fat levels, which also effectively matches published data [10].

Concerning the lactose content, we observed stable concentrations over time with a trend of higher content in the PT versus T HM. Our results are in line with most of the previous reported data, although some studies described an increase in lactose concentration during the first month of lactation [10,35,39]. As lactose constitutes the major energy source among total carbohydrates, it is an acceptable proxy for digestible carbohydrates [35].

Finally, the energy density was not directly measured in our study, but it was calculated and corrected for adjusted protein content for each milk sample, using the formula published by Polberg and Lönnerdal [30]. Overall, values of our cohort tended to be generally slightly lower than those reported in the literature [10,35,39]. The single morning HM sampling procedure could have contributed to this observation, as fat content has been reported to be higher in the evening [5].

Besides these temporal factors of variations, we also investigated the influence of other factors, such as gender and mode of delivery. We noticed that HM for male infants was more concentrated in fat and energy as compared with female infants. This was observed both in the T and PT group, but it was more marked in the PT group. A multivariate analysis confirmed that the infant's male gender was significantly and independently associated with higher concentrations of fat and energy in HM. So far, this phenomenon of "sex bias" milk synthesis, possibly already partly conditioned in utero, has mainly been studied and discussed in other mammals, such as cows, horses, monkeys, and hamsters [40,41]. In humans, by contrast, only a small number of studies have reported a possible gender specificity of the HM composition. In 2010, Powe et al. observed an increase in energy value of 25% for male infants of well-fed American women [42]. In a study conducted in Singapore, Thakkar et al. found similar differences in term newborns (energy + 24% and fat + 39% for boys), with a lipid profile that also varied by gender [43]. More recently, in a term delivering population of mothers living in Seoul, Hahn also observed an increased energy density in HM for male infants, related to a higher carbohydrates content. By contrast, Quinn et al. did not observe any gender difference in the milk of 103 Filipino women [7,44]. Interaction with environmental and/or nutritional conditions is possible, as suggested by Fujita et al. [45]. According to an evolutionary perspective, these authors hypothesize that economically disadvantaged mothers produce richer milk for girls, while well-nourished women produce richer milk for boys [45]. According to BMI indicators, our population was rather well nourished [29]. The reasons for these observed differences remain unclear. One can hypothesize that, due to their different growth trajectories and hormonal environment, male and female infants may have different energy requirements. The implications of such differences, if confirmed, could be important. On the other hand, the effect of delivery mode reported by Dizdar et al. was not verified in our population [8]. However, due to the relatively limited number of subjects and the important variability of data, these results should be interpreted cautiously.

This work has some limitations to consider: (i) as mentioned above, the method of sampling (first milk of the morning rather than pooled over 24 h) could have increased the measured variations, especially for lipids; (ii) variations in milk volumes, that may have also contributed to the important variability observed, were not recorded and thus could not be taken into account; (iii) the method of measuring macronutrients (MIRIS ©) is a method whose reliability is open to criticism [46]. We attempted to enhance its accuracy through validation methods and protein correction strategy [31]; (iv) finally, the small number of patients in each group limited the power of the study, and allowed only a limited number of associated factors to be analyzed. However, the influence of other factors, such as intrauterine growth restriction, twinning, antenatal steroids, smoking, and maternal comorbidities, for example, also deserves to be further investigated.

Despite this, our results emphasize that, although pragmatic, a unique definition of a "standard" nutritional composition of HM, as traditionally applied, can be insufficient and inaccurate for the nutritionally vulnerable infants, such as preterm infants [47]. These infants may require more individualized nutritional approaches, such as "targeted" fortification based on regular measurements of HM composition, or "adjusted" fortification according to serum urea values [11,30,48]. However, so far, targeted approaches remain challenging and expensive in daily care practices, without enthusiastic durable results on growth or development. Thus, future research should aim to develop optimized, efficient and feasible fortification strategies. Recent progresses in bioengineering should help in these issues [49]. Importantly, studies should also investigate other maternal and infant factors interacting with HM composition, including offspring gender.

Meanwhile, it would be good to consider changing the way nutritional intakes are calculated for clinical or research purposes. Currently, when direct measurements of HM composition are not available, a unique HM composition is generally assumed. However, it would be preferable to use a model that adjusts the assumed composition according to the T/PT status and/or postnatal age as recently proposed by an expert group [34].

5. Conclusions

Macronutrient composition and energy density in human milk change over time, with important inter- and intra- individual variations. The original design of this longitudinal study allowed us to compare term and preterm mother milk composition both at similar postnatal stages, corresponding to similar adaptive stages after birth, and at similar gestational ages, corresponding to similar developmental stages after conception. This original approach revealed that differences between the PT and T HM were more preponderant at equivalent gestational ages, especially around term, than at equivalent postpartum lactation stages. Moreover, our results suggest a possible gender adaptation of HM, with a more caloric milk for male infants. This is also a rather novel and compelling issue that deserves additional research.

Accordingly, there is definitely not one, but a multitude of human milk compositions and breastfeeding appears to be a powerful preventive and personalized medicine. Whereas HM use is strongly encouraged in preterm as well as in term infants, there is a need to further explore HM composition and variations to assess whether more individualized nutritional approaches may help in optimizing growth and development of more vulnerable infants.

Author Contributions: C.J.F.F. and M.A. contributed to the study design and to the development of the overall research plan, conducted the research, contributed to the interpretation of the results, and drafted the manuscript; C.L.G.-R. and S.K.T. contributed to the interpretation of the results, reviewed the manuscript, and approved the final version; C.A.D.C. performed the statistical analysis, participated in manuscript writing, and approved the final version; M.-C.C.-C. conducted the research, reviewed the manuscript, and approved the final version; L.B. and J.-F.T. contributed to the study design and to the development of the overall research plan, conducted the research, reviewed the manuscript, and approved the final version.

Acknowledgments: Sincere thanks to all mothers who enthusiastically participated in this study, to Nassima Grari, the study lactation nurse who admirably cared about all mothers during the full study duration, and to Céline Romagny and Emilie Darcillon who managed the organizational and operational part of the clinical study and the data management in perfection. We are grateful to Sean Austin for English language corrections and proof-reading of the manuscript.

References

1. Andreas, N.J.; Kampmann, B.; Mehring Le-Doare, K. Human breast milk: A review on its composition and bioactivity. *Early Hum. Dev.* **2015**, *91*, 629–635. [CrossRef] [PubMed]
2. Jakaitis, B.M.; Denning, P.W. Human breast milk and the gastrointestinal innate immune system. *Clin. Perinatol.* **2014**, *41*, 423–435. [CrossRef] [PubMed]
3. Ballard, O.; Morrow, A.L. Human milk composition: Nutrients and bioactive factors. *Pediatr. Clin. N. Am.* **2013**, *60*, 49–74. [CrossRef] [PubMed]
4. Picciano, M.F. Nutrient composition of human milk. *Pediatr. Clin. N. Am.* **2001**, *48*, 53–67. [CrossRef]
5. Moran-Lev, H.; Mimouni, F.B.; Ovental, A.; Mangel, L.; Mandel, D.; Lubetzky, R. Circadian Macronutrients Variations over the First 7 Weeks of Human Milk Feeding of Preterm Infants. *Breastfeed. Med.* **2015**, *10*, 366–370. [CrossRef] [PubMed]
6. Çetinkaya, A.K.; Dizdar, E.A.; Yarcı, E.; Sari, F.N.; Oguz, S.S.; Uras, N.; Canpolat, F.E. Does Circadian Variation of Mothers Affect Macronutrients of Breast Milk? *Am. J. Perinatol.* **2017**, *34*, 693–696. [PubMed]
7. Quinn, E.A. No evidence for sex biases in milk macronutrients, energy, or breastfeeding frequency in a sample of Filipino mothers. *Am. J. Phys. Anthropol.* **2013**, *152*, 209–216. [CrossRef] [PubMed]
8. Dizdar, E.A.; Sari, F.N.; Degirmencioglu, H.; Canpolat, F.E.; Oguz, S.S.; Uras, N.; Dilmen, U. Effect of mode of delivery on macronutrient content of breast milk. *J. Matern. Fetal Neonatal Med.* **2014**, *27*, 1099–1102. [CrossRef]
9. Affolter, M.; Garcia-Rodenas, C.L.; Vinyes-Pares, G.; Jenni, R.; Roggero, I.; Avanti-Nigro, O.; de Castro, C.A.; Zhao, A.; Zhang, Y.; Wang, P.; et al. Temporal Changes of Protein Composition in Breast Milk of Chinese Urban Mothers and Impact of Caesarean Section Delivery. *Nutrients* **2016**, *17*, 8. [CrossRef]
10. Gidrewicz, D.A.; Fenton, T.R. A systematic review and meta-analysis of the nutrient content of preterm and term breast milk. *BMC Pediatr.* **2014**, *14*, 216. [CrossRef]
11. Rochow, N.; Landau-Crangle, E.; Fusch, C. Challenges in breast milk fortification for preterm infants. *Curr. Opin. Clin. Nutr. Metab. Care* **2015**, *18*, 276–284. [CrossRef] [PubMed]
12. Gibertoni, D.; Corvaglia, L.; Vandini, S.; Rucci, P.; Savini, S.; Alessandroni, R.; Sansavini, A.; Fantini, M.P.; Faldella, G. Positive effect of human milk feeding during NICU hospitalization on 24 month neurodevelopment of very low birth weight infants: An Italian cohort study. *PLoS ONE* **2015**, *10*, e0116552. [CrossRef] [PubMed]
13. Section on Breastfeeding. Breastfeeding and the use of human milk. *Pediatrics* **2012**, *129*, e827–e841. [CrossRef] [PubMed]
14. WHO. Evidence on the Long-Term Effects of Breastfeeding. Systematic Reviews and Meta-Analyses. 2007. Available online: http://www.who.int/maternal_child_adolescent/documents/9241595230/en/ (accessed on 20 February 2019).
15. WHO; Edmond, K.; Bahl, R. Optimal Feeding of Low-Birth-Weight Infants. Technical Review. ISBN 9241595094. Available online: http://www.who.int/maternal_child_adolescent/documents/9241595094/en/ (accessed on 20 February 2019).

16. Moro, G.E.; Arslanoglu, S.; Bertino, E.; Corvaglia, L.; Montirosso, R.; Picaud, J.C.; Polberger, S.; Schanler, R.J.; Steel, C.; van Goudoever, J.; et al. XII. Human Milk in Feeding Premature Infants: Consensus Statement. *J. Pediatr. Gastroenterol. Nutr.* **2015**, *61*, S16–S19. [CrossRef] [PubMed]
17. Miller, J.; Tonkin, E.; Damarell, R.A.; McPhee, A.J.; Suganuma, M.; Suganuma, H.; Middleton, P.F.; Makrides, M.; Collins, C.T. A Systematic Review and Meta-Analysis of Human Milk Feeding and Morbidity in Very Low Birth Weight Infants. *Nutrients* **2018**, *31*, 10. [CrossRef] [PubMed]
18. Boquien, C.Y. Human Milk: An Ideal Food for Nutrition of Preterm Newborn. *Front. Pediatr.* **2018**, *6*, 295. [CrossRef] [PubMed]
19. Underwood, M.A. Human milk for the premature infant. *Pediatr. Clin. N. Am.* **2013**, *60*, 189–207. [CrossRef]
20. Menon, G.; Williams, T.C. Human milk for preterm infants: Why, what, when and how? *Arch. Dis. Child. Fetal Neonatal Ed.* **2013**, *98*, F559–F562. [CrossRef]
21. Vohr, B.R.; Poindexter, B.B.; Dusick, A.M.; McKinley, L.T.; Higgins, R.D.; Langer, J.C.; Poole, W.K.; National Institute of Child Health and Human Development National Research Network. Persistent beneficial effects of breast milk ingested in the neonatal intensive care unit on outcomes of extremely low birth weight infants at 30 months of age. *Pediatrics* **2007**, *120*, e953–e959. [CrossRef]
22. Belfort, M.B.; Anderson, P.J.; Nowak, V.A.; Lee, K.J.; Molesworth, C.; Thompson, D.K.; Doyle, L.Y.; Inder, T.F. Breast Milk Feeding, Brain Development, and Neurocognitive Outcomes: A 7-Year Longitudinal Study in Infants Born at Less Than 30 Weeks' Gestation. *J. Pediatr.* **2016**, *177*, 133–139. [CrossRef]
23. Belfort, M.B.; Ehrenkranz, R.A. Neurodevelopmental outcomes and nutritional strategies in very low birth weight infants. *Semin. Fetal Neonatal Med.* **2017**, *22*, 42–48. [CrossRef] [PubMed]
24. Blesa, M.; Sullivan, G.; Anblagan, D.; Telford, E.J.; Quigley, A.J.; Sparrow, S.A.; Serag, A.; Semple, S.I.; Bastin, M.E.; Boardman, J.P. Early breast milk exposure modifies brain connectivity in preterm infants. *NeuroImage* **2018**, *18*, 431–439. [CrossRef] [PubMed]
25. Henderson, G.; Anthony, M.Y.; McGuire, W. Formula milk versus maternal breast milk for feeding preterm or low birth weight infants. *Cochrane Database Syst. Rev.* **2007**, *4*. [CrossRef] [PubMed]
26. Kuschel, C.A.; Harding, J.E. Multicomponent fortified human milk for promoting growth in preterm infants. *Cochrane Database Syst. Rev.* **2004**, *1*. [CrossRef]
27. Tudehope, D.I. Human milk and the nutritional needs of preterm infants. *J. Pediatr.* **2013**, *162*, S17–S25. [CrossRef] [PubMed]
28. Horbar, J.D.; Ehrenkranz, R.A.; Badger, G.J.; Edwards, E.M.; Morrow, K.A.; Soll, R.F.; Buzas, J.S.; Bertino, E.; Gagliardi, L.; Bellù, R. Weight Growth Velocity and Postnatal Growth Failure in Infants 501 to 1500 Grams: 2000–2013. *Pediatrics* **2015**, *136*, e84–e92. [CrossRef] [PubMed]
29. Garcia-Rodenas, C.L.; De Castro, C.A.; Jenni, R.; Thakkar, S.K.; Beauport, L.; Tolsa, J.F.; Fischer-Fumeaux, C.J.; Affolter, M. Temporal changes of major protein concentrations in preterm and term human milk. A prospective cohort study. *Clin. Nutr. Edinb. Scotl.* **2018**, *38*, 1844–1852. [CrossRef]
30. Polberger, S.; Lönnerdal, B. Simple and rapid macronutrient analysis of human milk for individualized fortification: Basis for improved nutritional management of very-low-birth-weight infants? *J. Pediatr. Gastroenterol. Nutr.* **1993**, *17*, 283–290. [CrossRef]
31. Giuffrida, F.; Austin, S.; Cuany, D.; Sanchez-Bridge, B.; Longet, K.; Bertschy, E.; Sauser, J.; Thakkar, S.K.; Lee, L.Y.; Affolter, M. Comparison of macronutrient content in human milk measured by mid-infrared human milk analyzer and reference methods. *J. Perinatol.* **2018**, *14*, 497–503. [CrossRef]
32. Cooper, A.R.; Barnett, D.; Gentles, E.; Cairns, L.; Simpson, J.H. Macronutrient content of donor human breast milk. *Arch. Dis. Child. Fetal Neonatal. Ed.* **2013**, *98*, F539–F541. [CrossRef]
33. García-Lara, N.R.; Escuder-Vieco, D.; García-Algar, O.; De la Cruz, J.; Lora, D.; Pallás-Alonso, C. Effect of freezing time on macronutrients and energy content of breastmilk. *Breastfeed. Med.* **2012**, *7*, 295–301. [CrossRef] [PubMed]
34. Cormack, B.E.; Embleton, N.D.; van Goudoever, J.B.; Hay, W.W.; Bloomfield, F.H. Comparing apples with apples: It is time for standardized reporting of neonatal nutrition and growth studies. *Pediatr. Res.* **2016**, *79*, 810–820. [CrossRef] [PubMed]
35. Boyce, C.; Watson, M.; Lazidis, G.; Reeve, S.; Dods, K.; Simmer, K.; McLeod, G. Preterm human milk composition: A systematic literature review. *Br. J. Nutr.* **2016**, *116*, 1033–1045. [CrossRef] [PubMed]
36. Hsu, Y.C.; Chen, C.H.; Lin, M.C.; Tsai, C.R.; Liang, J.T.; Wang, T.M. Changes in preterm breast milk nutrient content in the first month. *Pediatr. Neonatol.* **2014**, *55*, 449–454. [CrossRef] [PubMed]

37. Bauer, J.; Gerss, J. Longitudinal analysis of macronutrients and minerals in human milk produced by mothers of preterm infants. *Clin. Nutr. Edinb. Scotl.* **2011**, *30*, 215–220. [CrossRef] [PubMed]
38. Maly, J.; Burianova, I.; Vitkova, V.; Ticha, E.; Navratilova, M.; Cermakova, E.; Premature Milk Study Group. Preterm human milk macronutrient concentration is independent of gestational age at birth. *Arch. Dis. Child. Fetal Neonatal Ed.* **2019**, *104*, F50–F56. [CrossRef] [PubMed]
39. Tsang, R.; Uauy, R.; Koletzko, B.; Zlotkin, S. Nutrition of the preterm infant. *Early Hum. Dev.* **2005**, *88*, S5–S7.
40. Hinde, K. Richer milk for sons but more milk for daughters: Sex-biased investment during lactation varies with maternal life history in rhesus macaques. *Am. J. Hum. Biol.* **2009**, *21*, 512–519. [CrossRef] [PubMed]
41. Hinde, K.; Carpenter, A.J.; Clay, J.S.; Bradford, B.J. Holsteins favor heifers, not bulls: Biased milk production programmed during pregnancy as a function of fetal sex. *PLoS ONE* **2014**, *9*, e86169. [CrossRef] [PubMed]
42. Powe, C.E.; Knott, C.D.; Conklin-Brittain, N. Infant sex predicts breast milk energy content. *Am. J. Hum. Biol.* **2010**, *22*, 50–54. [CrossRef] [PubMed]
43. Thakkar, S.K.; Giuffrida, F.; Cristina, C.H.; De Castro, C.A.; Mukherjee, R.; Tran, L.A.; Steenhout, P.; Lee, L.Y.; Destaillats, F. Dynamics of human milk nutrient composition of women from Singapore with a special focus on lipids. *Am. J. Hum. Biol.* **2013**, *25*, 770–779. [CrossRef] [PubMed]
44. Hahn, W.H.; Song, J.H.; Song, S.; Kang, N.M. Do gender and birth height of infant affect calorie of human milk? An association study between human milk macronutrient and various birth factors. *J. Matern. Fetal Neonatal Med.* **2017**, *30*, 1608–1612. [CrossRef] [PubMed]
45. Fujita, M.; Roth, E.; Lo, Y.J.; Hurst, C.; Vollner, J.; Kendell, A. In poor families, mothers' milk is richer for daughters than sons: A test of Trivers-Willard hypothesis in agropastoral settlements in Northern Kenya. *Am. J. Phys. Anthropol.* **2012**, *149*, 52–59. [CrossRef] [PubMed]
46. Fusch, G.; Rochow, N.; Choi, A.; Fusch, S.; Poeschl, S.; Ubah, A.O.; Lee, S.Y.; Raja, P.; Fusch, C. Rapid measurement of macronutrients in breast milk: How reliable are infrared milk analyzers? *Clin. Nutr. Edinb. Scotl.* **2015**, *34*, 465–476. [CrossRef] [PubMed]
47. American Academy of Pediatrics. Committee on Nutrition. Nutritional Needs of Preterm Infants. In *Pediatric Nutrition Handbook*; Kleinman, R.E., Ed.; American Academy of Pediatrics: Elk Grove Village, IL, USA, 2004.
48. Arslanoglu, S. IV. Individualized Fortification of Human Milk: Adjustable Fortification. *J. Pediatr. Gastroenterol. Nutr.* **2015**, *61*, S4–S5. [CrossRef] [PubMed]
49. Van Goudoever, J. VI. Bioengineering Human Milk: Why? *J. Pediatr. Gastroenterol. Nutr.* **2015**, *61*, S7–S9. [CrossRef] [PubMed]

4

Hourly Breast Expression to Estimate the Rate of Synthesis of Milk and Fat

Jacqueline C. Kent [1,*], Hazel Gardner [1], Ching-Tat Lai [1], Peter E. Hartmann [1], Kevin Murray [2], Alethea Rea [3] and Donna T. Geddes [1]

1 School of Molecular Sciences, The University of Western Australia, 35 Stirling Hwy, Crawley, WA 6009, Australia; Hazel.Gardner@uwa.edu.au (H.G.); Ching-Tat.Lai@uwa.edu.au (C.-T.L.); Peter.Hartmann@uwa.edu.au (P.E.H.); Donna.Geddes@uwa.edu.au (D.T.G.)
2 School of Population and Global Health, The University of Western Australia, 35 Stirling Hwy, Crawley, WA 6009, Australia; Kevin.Murray@uwa.edu.au
3 Centre of Applied Statistics, The University of Western Australia, 35 Stirling Hwy, Crawley, WA 6009, Australia; Alethea.Rea@uwa.edu.au
* Correspondence: Jacqueline.Kent@uwa.edu.au

Abstract: Objective measurement of the rate of synthesis of breast milk and fat in breastfeeding mothers requires test-weighing of each breastfeed and the measurement of each expression from each breast over 24 h, with the collection of milk samples before and after each breastfeed and expression. We sought an abbreviated technique for measuring these rates of synthesis. Participants completed a 24-h breastfeeding milk profile, and expressed their breasts on arrival at the research room and each hour thereafter for 3 h (4 expressions). The hourly rate of milk synthesis, as measured by the yield of milk from the fourth expression, was closely related to the hourly rate of milk synthesis calculated from the 24-h milk profile. The hourly rate of fat synthesis, calculated from the fat content of small samples of the first and last milk expressed during the fourth expression, was different from the rate of fat synthesis calculated from the fat content and volumes of all the breastfeeds and expressions during the 24-h milk profile. The study confirms the use of an abbreviated technique to measure the rate of breast milk synthesis, but is not reliable as a measure of the rate of fat synthesis for an individual.

Keywords: human lactation; expressing; milk synthesis; fat synthesis

1. Introduction

Many mothers are not achieving the recommendations of the World Health Organization, the National Health and Medical Research Council, and the American Academy of Pediatrics of exclusive breastfeeding for 6 months [1–5]. Over 90% of mothers in Perth, Western Australia commence breastfeeding, but fewer than 1% are exclusively breastfeeding at 6 months [3]. In the United States 81% of mothers ever breastfed, and 22% are exclusively breastfeeding at 6 months [5]. A common reason given for early weaning is a perception of insufficient milk [6] that in turn is associated with a lack of confidence in breastfeeding [7]. Clinical indications of infants receiving enough breast milk include sufficient bowel movements and urine output [8] and satisfactory weight gains [9]. These are believed to be sufficient to provide reassurance for both parents and health professionals. However, the high frequency mothers who have a perception of insufficient milk indicates that further objective measures of milk production are required.

Objective measurement of milk supply can be made by carrying out a 24-h milk profile that involves weighing the fully-clothed infant before and after every breastfeed at home and recording volumes of milk expressed (if applicable) for 24–26 h [10]. This allows calculation of both the total daily milk intake of the infant over 24 h, and the total daily milk production of each breast [10]. The average hourly rate of milk synthesis can then be calculated from the total milk production in 24 h divided by 24. If a mother is reluctant to measure her milk profile over a full 24 h, a small study has demonstrated that when the breasts are expressed using an electric breast pump each hour, the hourly rate of milk production from the 2nd to the 7th hour (the 3rd to the 8th expression) represents the longer-term physiological rate of milk synthesis [11]. The authors suggested that further studies are required to confirm this finding.

In addition to the volume of milk ingested by the infant, total caloric intake is important for energy expenditure and growth. Fat provides 49% of the energy in breast milk [12], and therefore the contribution of fat to the energy intake of the infant is significant. The daily fat intake of breastfed infants has been underestimated when unsuitable sampling regimes have been used. For example, calculations based on daily milk intake by test-weighing and fat content of milk samples collected before and after the first breastfeed of the morning [13] will underestimate the daily fat intake of the breastfed infant, because the fat content of milk in the morning is less than during the day and afternoon [14]. Another approach was to feed the infant from one breast only at each breastfeeding session and pump the other breast, alternating the breasts, for a 24-h period and measure the fat content of the pooled pumped milk [12]. The yield of milk from the pumping sessions averaged 49% of the 24-h milk production determined by test-weighing, but some were <40% and others >60% [12], indicating that this technique may be sufficiently accurate for a population study, but not useful to predict the daily fat intake for an individual infant.

When mothers collect small samples (<1 mL) of breast milk before and after each breastfeed during the 24-h milk profile, the total fat intake can be calculated from the fat content of the samples and the volume of each breastfeed. If the mother is also expressing breast milk, the measurement of the fat content of small samples (<1 mL) of breast milk collected before and after each expression and the volume of each expression, in addition to the data from the 24-h breastfeeds, allows calculation of the mother's total daily fat production. The hourly rate of fat synthesis can then be calculated by dividing the total fat production in 24 h by 24.

We aimed to provide further data to investigate if the technique of hourly pumping can be used to estimate the rate of milk synthesis, and ascertain if the same technique could be used to estimate the rate of milk fat synthesis if mothers prefer this technique to 24-h test-weighing with milk samples.

2. Materials and Methods

We recruited lactating mothers between 5 and 11 months from birth of term singleton infants who agreed to measure their 24-h milk profile with milk samples, and come to the research room at The University of Western Australia for a three-and-a-half-hour study session. Participants were only included in the study if their infants had previously accepted breast milk from a bottle. The study was approved by the Human Research Ethics Committee of The University of Western Australia (RA/4/1/4492) and all participants provided written informed consent.

Demographics were recorded and the participants were loaned accurate digital scales (BabyWeigh™, Medela Inc., McHenry, IL, USA, resolution 2 g, accuracy ± 0.034%) to measure their 24-h milk profile. All measurements of breastfeed volumes and milk production were made in grams but expressed in mL because the density of milk is 1.03 g/mL [15]. Data were recorded either on paper or entered on a secure password-protected website accessed by invitation only. The corrected 24-h milk production, for participants who were either exclusively breastfeeding or breastfeeding and expressing, was calculated by the method of Arthur et al. [10]. However, no correction for infant insensible water loss was made, and therefore milk production may be underestimated by an average of 10% (range 3–55%) [10]. The mean rate of milk production for each breast was calculated by dividing the corrected 24-h milk production for each breast by 24.

During this 24-h period, the mothers hand-expressed small milk samples (<1 mL) into 5-mL polypropylene plastic vials (Disposable Products, Adelaide, SA, Australia), immediately before and after each breastfeed or expression from each breast. Samples were frozen as soon as possible and kept at -15°C until analyzed. The cream content was measured using the creamatocrit method [16]. The cream content of the milk of each feed or expression during the measurement of milk profile was calculated as ([0.53 × pre-feed creamatocrit + 0.47 × post-feed creamatocrit]/2) [17]. The creamatocrit was converted to fat using the following formula: fat (g/L) = 3.968 + (5.917 × creamatocrit) [16]. The amount of fat in each breastfeed or expression was calculated from the fat content of the milk and the volume of the feed or expression. The total amount of fat synthesized by each breast in the 24-h period was calculated by summing amount of fat in all the breastfeeds and expressions from that breast, and the mean rate of fat synthesis was calculated by dividing the total amount of fat synthesized for each breast by 24.

For the hourly-pumping study the participants pumped either both breasts simultaneously or one breast only according to the preference of the participant. On arrival at the research room at The University of Western Australia, the mothers expressed their breast(s) using a Medela Symphony breast pump at their own maximum comfortable vacuum for 10 min after milk ejection was detected by an increase in milk flow. For each breast, milk was conveyed via a connecting tube from the breast shield to one of three bottles placed on the weigh platform of a continuous weigh balance (ShowMilk, Carag AG, Baar, Switzerland). The first 1 mL (first milk) was collected into the first bottle, the bulk of the expressed milk was collected into the second bottle (pooled milk), and the last milk expressed (~1 mL) was collected into the third bottle (last milk). The ShowMilk device measures the cumulative weight of milk at 50 Hz with a resolution of 0.1 g and accuracy 0.02% to a maximum of 2 kg [18]. The expression was repeated 1, 2 and 3 h after the commencement of the first expression. The total volume of each expression (mL) from each breast was recorded.

The creamatocrit of the first, pooled, and last milk of each expression was measured as above and converted to fat content (g/L) [16]. This, with the total volume of milk expressed, was used to calculate the total amount of fat in the expressed milk for each hour.

From the 24-h milk profile, the fat content of all the milk samples and the volumes of all the breastfeeds were used to estimate the breastfeeding storage capacity of the breasts [19]. If the participants expressed their breast milk on one or more occasions during the 24 h, the data from the expressions were included with the breastfeeding data to calculate the potential storage capacity of the breasts [20]. The fat content of the first milk samples was used to calculate the degree of fullness of the breast before the expression [21].

Statistics

Data are presented as mean ± SD or median (IQR). A paired *t*-test was used to compare fat content of first milk and last milk for each expression, and unpaired *t*-test was used to compare total milk production of participants who were exclusively breastfeeding with those who were breastfeeding and expressing. Linear mixed models were used to analyse the responses volume of fourth expression, rate of synthesis, amount of fat fourth expression, and rate of fat synthesis using a fixed effect of method (hourly pumping vs. 24-h profile) and random effects of participant and breast within participant. The volume of each expression, and the fat content of the first and last milk at time points 0, 1, 2, and 3 h of the hourly pumping study were included in the fixed effect of method. Key comparisons were considered using general linear hypothesis tests (with a Tukeys adjustment). Significance was set at the 5% level, and data were analysed using the R environment for statistical computing [22].

3. Results

Data were collected from 15 participants, of whom 10 were feeding male infants and 5 female infants. A 24-h milk profile was measured by 11 participants on a day during which they were exclusively breastfeeding and 4 participants on a day during which they were breastfeeding and expressing (1 participant on two occasions). The demographics of the participants are presented in Table 1. A single study session occurred within 11 weeks of the measurement of 24-h milk profile for 14 of the participants. One participant measured her 24-h milk profile when her infant was 5 weeks old and participated in a study session 6 weeks later. She measured her 24-h milk profile again when her infant was 17 weeks old and participated in a second study session 4 weeks later. During the study sessions 3 participants expressed from one breast, 11 expressed from both breasts, and 1 expressed from both breasts for 2 study sessions, providing data for 29 breasts. Milk samples before and after each breastfeeding or expression during the 24-h milk profile were collected by 11 of the participants, and 4 participants did not collect milk samples. The breastfeeding storage capacity [20] (calculated from the fat content of samples collected before and after breastfeeds only) was 165 ± 42 mL. When the fat content of all samples from all breastfeeds and expressions, including those from the study sessions, was included the potential storage capacity [20] was 182 ± 58 mL. On average, the breastfeeding infants took 67 ± 11% of the milk that was available in the breast when the 24-h milk profile was measured.

Table 1. Demographics of participants (n = 15).

	Median (IQR)
Infant	
Age (weeks)	22 (12)
Birth weight (g)	3650 (726)
Fat intake (g/24h) (n = 11)	34 (13)
Mother	
Age (years)	35 (37)
Exclusive breastfeeding during 24-h milk profile measurement (n = 11)	
24-h milk production (mL)	860 (237)
Breastfeeding and expressing during 24-h milk profile measurement (n = 5 *)	
Milk transfer breastfeeding (breast to infant) (mL)	565 (311)
Milk transfer (breast to bottle) (mL)	180 (124)
Total 24-h milk production (mL)	810 (224)

* 1 participant measured her 24-h milk profile on 2 occasions.

There was no significant difference in 24-h milk production between participants who were exclusively breastfeeding and those who were breastfeeding and expressing (difference = 68.6 mL, 95% CI: 101.9–239.1, p = 0.400)

The yield of milk from each expression during the study session and the hourly rate of milk synthesis calculated from the 24-h milk profile data are presented in Figure 1.

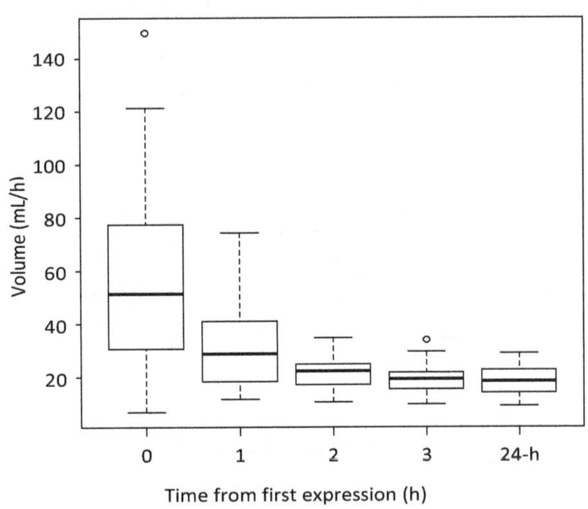

Figure 1. The yield of milk from hourly expressions, and the hourly rate of milk synthesis calculated from the 24-h milk profile data (24-h). n = 29 breasts.

On average the yield of milk from each of the second, third and fourth expressions (1, 2 and 3 h after the first expression) was lower than for the expression the hour before (mean expression 59.0 mL at time 0, 32.0 mL at time 1, 22.0 mL at time 2 and 18.9 mL at time 3).

The yield of milk from the fourth expression (3 h after the first expression) (18.9 ± 5.8 mL) was not significantly different from the hourly rate of milk synthesis (18.2 ± 5.4 mL/h) calculated from the 24-h milk profile data (mean difference = 0.966, SE = 0.995, $p = 0.997$). There was also a statistically significant relationship between the volume of the fourth expression and rate of synthesis ($p = 0.002$) (Figure 2).

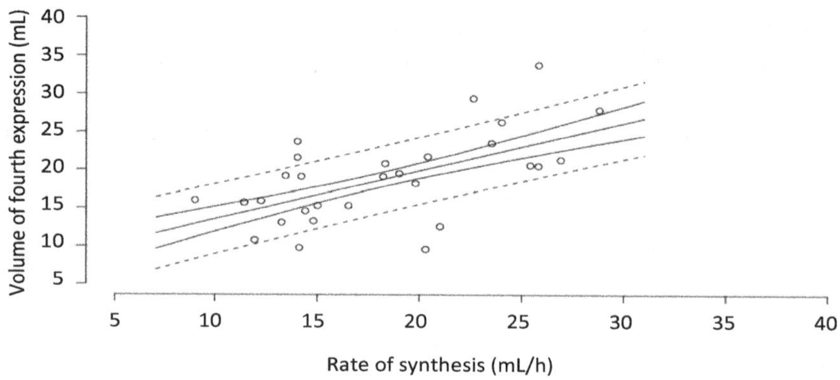

Figure 2. Relationship between the volume of milk from the fourth expression (3 h after the first expression) and the hourly rate of milk synthesis calculated from the 24-h milk profile data. Fitted model (solid line), with the confidence (solid line) and prediction intervals (dashed lines). $n = 29$ breasts.

The fat content of the first and last milk collected at each expression and the average fat content of milk samples collected during the 24-h milk profile are presented in Figure 3. The fat content of the last milk was higher than the first milk for each expression but not statistically different at time 3 (time 0: mean difference = 34.9 g/L, SE = 8.1, $p = 0.001$; time 1: mean difference = 22.0 g/L, SE = 8.1, $p < 0.001$; time 2: mean difference = 17.8 g/L, SE = 8.1, $p = 0.021$; time 3: mean difference = 15.7 g/L, SE = 8.1, $p = 0.092$). There was no significant difference in the fat content of milk collected at the end of each of the first, second, third or fourth expressions (63.7 ± 27.6 g/L, 69.1 ± 28.2 g/L, 69.1 ± 29.4 g/L, 58.4 ± 27.0 g/L respectively). There was no significant difference between the fat content of pooled milk from the fourth expression (52.5 ± 23.5 g/L) and the average fat content of milk collected over the 24-h period (46.6 ± 8.1 g/L) (mean difference = 10.5 g/L, 95% CI: 7.2–20.1, $p = 0.18$).

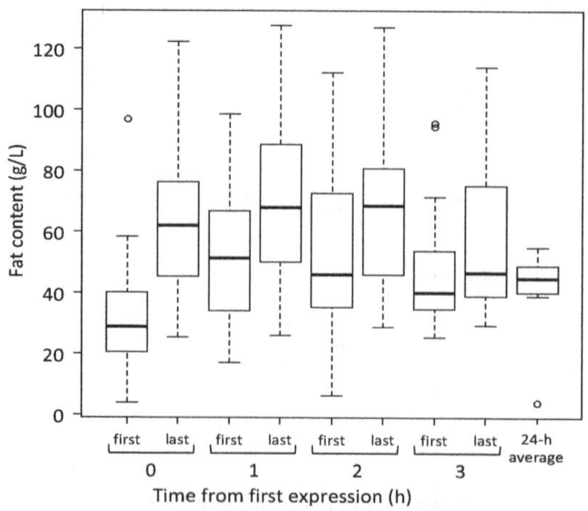

Figure 3. The fat content of first and last milk collected at each expression and the average fat content of milk samples collected during the 24-h milk profile data (24-h average). $n = 29$ breasts.

The amount of fat in the milk from the fourth expression was 1.02 ± 0.50 g. This was different from the hourly rate of fat synthesis (0.79 ± 0.23 g/h) calculated from the 24-h milk profile (mean difference = 0.23 g/h, SE = 0.10, $p = 0.034$). There was no significant relationship between the two measurements ($p = 0.054$) (Figure 4).

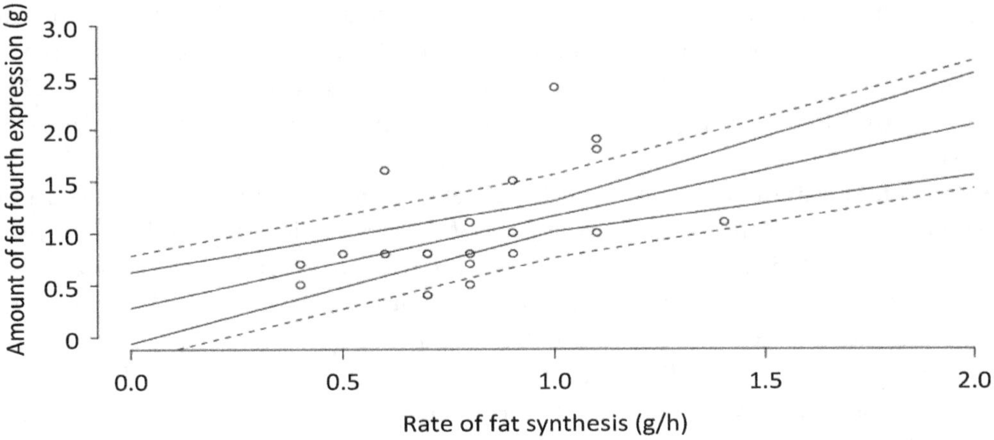

Figure 4. Relationship between the amount of fat from the fourth expression and the hourly rate of milk fat synthesis calculated from the 24-h milk profile data ($p = 0.054$). Fitted model (solid line), with the confidence (solid line) and prediction interval (dashed line). $n = 29$ breasts.

The degree of fullness of the breast before the first expression (time 0), calculated from the fat content of the first milk and the potential storage capacity of the breast, was 0.6 ± 0.2. The first expression removed 53 ± 26% of the available milk, with 6 sessions classified as low outcome (<40% of the available milk removed), and 5 sessions classified as high outcome (>70% of the available milk removed).

4. Discussion

The data suggest that all the milk from the fourth expression had been synthesized since the end of the third expression, and the yield of milk from that hour (50 minutes after the last expression plus 10 minutes expressing) was closely related to the hourly rate of milk synthesis calculated from the 24-h milk profile data. Therefore, this study has confirmed the findings of Lai et al. [11] that for mothers who are fully breastfeeding the technique of hourly pumping for 4 expressions can be used as a measure of the hourly rate of milk synthesis. It was established by Lai et al. that hourly pumping for a further 3 h yielded the same volume as the fourth expression, indicating that the steady state of milk synthesis and removal had been reached, and more than three hourly expressions after the first expression are not required. It has been established that an accurate measure of 24-h breast milk production cannot be calculated by test-weighing an infant for a 12-h period (6 a.m. to 6 p.m.) and doubling the total [14,23], nor by taking the mean milk intake for two consecutive feedings and multiplying it by the number of feedings in the 24-h period [23]. If mothers are reluctant to weigh their infants before and after every breastfeed for a full 24 h, or if they urgently need to know their rate of breast milk synthesis and are prepared to express their breasts every hour for 3 h after the first expression, this technique can provide reliable information. If milk production is less than optimal, early intervention is beneficial [24]. An objective measurement of the rate of milk synthesis can guide advice from a clinician on increasing milk production if required. It must be borne in mind that the infant will probably need to be given milk by another means unless there is usually an interval between breastfeeds of more than 3 h.

The proportion of mothers in Australia who combine breastfeeding and expressing is increasing [25], either to leave expressed breast milk with a carer, or to increase milk supply [26].

Mothers with concerns about their infants' transfer of milk from the breast need to undertake a full 24-h period of test-weighing to determine the efficacy of their breastfeeding. Using the hourly pumping technique will provide information about their current total rate of milk production, and can be used to monitor the effects of alterations in their expression regime to increase milk production.

The finding that the milk removed during the fourth expression represents the hourly rate of milk secretion suggests that the yield of fat should represent the hourly rate of fat secretion. Although there was a trend towards a relationship between the amount of fat in the last expression and the hourly rate of fat synthesis calculated from the 24-h profile data, the mean difference was 0.23 (a reduction of 23%), indicating that this technique is not reliable for predicting the rate of fat synthesis for an individual mother.

The changes in fat content before and after each expression are interesting, and an explanation is worthwhile. The breast reaches its maximum degree of fullness following the longest interval after the previous removal of milk. This long interval allows time for the fat globules in the alveoli to partition, as they tend to adhere to the surface of the lactocytes, resulting in the first milk expressed being low in fat content [27]. The wide range in fat content before the first expression is a result of both the variable time since the previous removal of milk from the breast and inter-individual differences in fat content of milk [28]. The fat content increases as milk is removed from the breast, reaching a maximum when the breast is fully drained [27,29]. The wide range in fat content after the first expression is a result of the variability between mothers and the effectiveness of milk removal by a breast pump [18]. In the 50 min between the end of the first expression and the start of the second expression, the fat content of the milk within the alveoli (69.1 g/L) was diluted by the newly-secreted milk with an average fat content of (41.1 g/L) [14] to reach 51.3 g/L (Figure 3). Compared with the previous interval, there was less time for the fat globules to partition between the lumen of the alveoli and the luminal wall of the lactocytes, resulting in a smaller difference between the first and last milk of the second expression (Figure 3). The higher fat content of the last milk of the second expression occurred because the first expression did not drain the breast completely (53% of the available milk removed), leaving milk with a high fat content in the alveoli. The wide variability is the result of the 6 sessions that were low outcome (<40% of the available milk removed). The yield of milk from the third expression was significantly higher than from the fourth expression, indicating that the third expression did not quite drain the breast, and only the fourth expression comprised only milk secreted in the previous hour. This is consistent with the fat content of the last milk from the third expression remaining elevated (Figure 3). There was a small difference in the fat content between the first and last milk from the fourth expression, which was consistent with some partitioning of the fat globules during the 50 min after the end of the third expression.

It is puzzling that, although the volume of the last expression was closely related to the hourly rate of milk synthesis calculated from the 24-h milk profile data, the amount of fat in the last expression was not an accurate reflection of the rate of fat synthesis for an individual. We suggest that it is the result of the steep rise in fat content as the breast is drained [29,30] such that the final small volume of milk expressed makes a disproportionately large contribution to the fat content of the final milk sample.

The higher fat content of the second expression could make it suitable for feeding low-birth-weight infants when the mother has an abundant supply, with the milk from the first expression being stored for later use. This may be an alternative to fractionating an expression [31].

5. Conclusions

These data confirm that the fourth hourly expression can be used to estimate the average rate of breast milk synthesis for individuals and may be useful when low milk production is suspected. However, while there is a tendency to an overall relationship between hourly pumping and 24-h milk profile for estimating the rate of synthesis of milk fat, this technique is less accurate for individuals.

Author Contributions: Conceptualization, P.E.H., C.-T.L. and J.C.K.; Methodology, P.E.H., C.-T.L. and J.C.K.; Formal Analysis, A.R. and K.M.; Investigation, J.C.K., C.-T.L., H.G.; Resources, P.E.H. and D.T.G. Data Curation,

J.C.K.; Writing-Original Draft Preparation, J.C.K.; Writing-Review & Editing, D.T.G., C.-T.L., H.G., P.E.H. and A.R.; Supervision, P.E.H. and D.G.; Project Administration, P.E.H. and D.G.; Funding Acquisition, P.E.H. and D.T.G.

Acknowledgments: We thank the participants, and the Australian Breastfeeding Association (WA Branch) for their support (Approval 2016-4).

References

1. Gartner, L.M.; Morton, J.; Lawrence, R.A.; Naylor, A.J.; O'Hare, D.; Schanler, R.J.; Eidelman, A.I. American Academy of Pediatrics. Breastfeeding and the use of human milk. *Pediatrics* **2005**, *115*, 496–506. [PubMed]
2. National Health and Medical Research Council. *Dietary Guidelines for Children and Adolescents in Australia*; Australian Government Publishing Service: Canberra, Australia, 2003.
3. Scott, J.A.; Binns, C.W.; Oddy, W.H.; Graham, K.I. Predictors of breastfeeding duration: Evidence from a cohort study. *Pediatrics* **2006**, *117*, e646–e655. [CrossRef] [PubMed]
4. World Health Organization. *Global Strategy for Infant and Young Child Feeding*; World Health Organization: Geneva, Switzerland, 2003; p. 30.
5. Centers for Disease Control and Prevention CDC Breastfeeding Report Card 2016. Available online: www.cdc.gov/breastfeeding/pdf/2016breastfeedingreportcard.pdf (accessed on 10 July 2018).
6. Gatti, L. Maternal perceptions of insufficient milk supply in breastfeeding. *J. Nurs. Scholarsh.* **2008**, *40*, 355–363. [CrossRef] [PubMed]
7. Dennis, C.L. The breastfeeding self-efficacy scale: Psychometric assessment of the short form. *J. Obstet. Gynecol. Neonatal Nurs.* **2003**, *32*, 734–744. [CrossRef] [PubMed]
8. Neifert, M.R. Prevention of breastfeeding tragedies. *Pediatr. Clin. N. Am.* **2001**, *48*, 273–297. [CrossRef]
9. WHO Multicentre Growth Reference Study Group. *WHO Child Growth Standards: Growth Velocity Based on Weight, Length and Head Circumference. Methods and Development*; World Health Oragnization: Geneva, Switzerland, 2009.
10. Arthur, P.G.; Hartmann, P.E.; Smith, M. Measurement of the milk intake of breast-fed infants. *J. Pediatr. Gastroenterol. Nutr.* **1987**, *6*, 758–763. [CrossRef] [PubMed]
11. Lai, C.T.; Hale, T.W.; Simmer, K.; Hartmann, P.E. Measuring milk synthesis in breastfeeding mothers. *Breastfeed. Med.* **2010**, *5*, 103–107. [CrossRef] [PubMed]
12. Butte, N.F.; Garza, C.; Smith, E.O.; Nichols, B.L. Human milk intake and growth in exclusively breast-fed infants. *J. Pediatr.* **1984**, *104*, 187–195. [CrossRef]
13. Grote, V.; Verduci, E.; Scaglioni, S.; Vecchi, F.; Contarini, G.; Giovannini, M.; Koletzko, B.; Agostoni, C. Breast milk composition and infant nutrient intakes during the first 12 months of life. *Eur. J. Clin. Nutr.* **2016**, *70*, 250–256. [CrossRef] [PubMed]
14. Kent, J.C.; Mitoulas, L.R.; Cregan, M.D.; Ramsay, D.T.; Doherty, D.A.; Hartmann, P.E. Volume and frequency of breastfeedings and fat content of breast milk throughout the day. *Pediatrics* **2006**, *117*, e387–e395. [CrossRef] [PubMed]
15. Moya, J.; Phillips, L.; Schuda, L.; Wood, P.; Diaz, A.; Lee, R.; Clickner, R.; Birch, R.J.; Adjei, N.; Blood, P. Human Milk Intake. In *Exposure Factors Handbook*; US Environmental Protection Agency: Washington, WA, USA, 2011.
16. Meier, P.P.; Engstrom, J.L.; Zuleger, J.L.; Motykowski, J.E.; Vasan, U.; Meier, W.A.; Hartmann, P.E.; Williams, T.M. Accuracy of a user-friendly centrifuge for measuring creamatocrits on mothers' milk in the clinical setting. *Breastfeed. Med.* **2006**, *1*, 79–87. [CrossRef] [PubMed]
17. Mitoulas, L.R. Short- and Long-term Variation in the Production, Content and Composition of Human Milk Fat. Ph.D. Thesis, The University of Western Australia, Perth, WA, Austalia, 2000.
18. Prime, D.K.; Garbin, C.P.; Hartmann, P.E.; Kent, J.C. Simultaneous breast expression in breastfeeding women is more efficacious than sequential breast expression. *Breastfeed. Med.* **2012**, *7*, 442–447. [CrossRef] [PubMed]
19. Cox, D.B.; Kent, J.C.; Casey, T.M.; Owens, R.A.; Hartmann, P.E. Breast growth and the urinary excretion of lactose during human pregnancy and early lactation: Endocrine relationships. *Exp. Physiol.* **1999**, *84*, 421–434. [CrossRef] [PubMed]

20. Kent, J.C.; Mitoulas, L.R.; Cregan, M.D.; Geddes, D.T.; Larsson, M.; Doherty, D.A.; Hartmann, P.E. Importance of vacuum for breastmilk expression. *Breastfeed. Med.* **2008**, *3*, 11–19. [CrossRef] [PubMed]
21. Cox, D.B.; Owens, R.A.; Hartmann, P.E. Blood and milk prolactin and the rate of milk synthesis in women. *Exp. Physiol.* **1996**, *81*, 1007–1020. [CrossRef] [PubMed]
22. R: A Language and Environment for Statistical Computing. Available online: https://www.gbif.org/tool/81287/r-a-language-and-environment-for-statistical-computing (accessed on 10 July 2018).
23. Matheny, R.J.; Picciano, M.F. Assessment of abbreviated techniques for determination of milk volume intake in the human milk-fed infant. *J. Pediatr. Gastroenterol. Nutr.* **1985**, *4*, 808–812. [CrossRef] [PubMed]
24. Hill, P.D.; Aldag, J.C.; Chatterton, R.T.; Zinaman, M. Comparison of milk output between mothers of preterm and term infants: The first 6 weeks after birth. *J. Hum. Lact.* **2005**, *21*, 22–30. [CrossRef] [PubMed]
25. Johns, H.M.; Forster, D.A.; Amir, L.H.; McLachlan, H.L. Prevalence and outcomes of breast milk expressing in women with healthy term infants: A systematic review. *BMC Pregnancy Childbirth* **2013**, *13*, 212. [CrossRef] [PubMed]
26. Johns, H.M.; Amir, L.H.; McLachlan, H.L.; Forster, D.A. Breast pump use amongst mothers of healthy term infants in Melbourne, Australia: A prospective cohort study. *Midwifery* **2016**, *33*, 82–89. [CrossRef] [PubMed]
27. Atwood, C.S.; Hartmann, P.E. Collection of fore and hind milk from the sow and the changes in milk composition during suckling. *J. Dairy Res.* **1992**, *59*, 287–298. [CrossRef] [PubMed]
28. Neville, M.C.; Keller, R.P.; Seacat, J.; Casey, C.E.; Allen, J.C.; Archer, P. Studies on human lactation. I. Within-feed and between-breast variation in selected components of human milk. *Am. J. Clin. Nutr.* **1984**, *40*, 635–646. [CrossRef] [PubMed]
29. Hytten, F.E. Clinical and chemical studies in human lactation. I. Collection of milk samples. *Br. Med. J.* **1954**, *23*, 175–182. [CrossRef]
30. Daly, S.E.; Di Rosso, A.; Owens, R.A.; Hartmann, P.E. Degree of breast emptying explains changes in the fat content, but not fatty acid composition, of human milk. *Exp. Physiol.* **1993**, *78*, 741–755. [CrossRef] [PubMed]
31. Valentine, C.J.; Hurst, N.M.; Schanler, R.J. Hindmilk improves weight gain in low-birth-weight infants fed human milk. *J. Pediatr. Gastroenterol. Nutr.* **1994**, *18*, 474–477. [CrossRef] [PubMed]

5

DNA Methylation Signatures of Breastfeeding in Buccal Cells Collected in Mid-Childhood

Veronika V. Odintsova [1,2,3,*], Fiona A. Hagenbeek [1,2], Matthew Suderman [4], Doretta Caramaschi [4], Catharina E. M. van Beijsterveldt [1], Noah A. Kallsen [5], Erik A. Ehli [5], Gareth E. Davies [5], Gennady T. Sukhikh [3], Vassilios Fanos [6], Caroline Relton [4], Meike Bartels [1,2], Dorret I. Boomsma [1,2] and Jenny van Dongen [1,2,*]

1 Department of Biological Psychology, Vrije Universiteit Amsterdam, 1081 BT Amsterdam, The Netherlands; f.a.hagenbeek@vu.nl (F.A.H.); t.van.beijsterveldt@vu.nl (C.E.M.v.B.); m.bartels@vu.nl (M.B.); di.boomsma@vu.nl (D.I.B.)

2 Amsterdam Public Health Research Institute, 1081 BT Amsterdam, The Netherlands

3 Kulakov National Medical Research Center for Obstetrics, Gynecology and Perinatology, Moscow 101000, Russia; inter_otdel@mail.ru

4 MRC Integrative Epidemiology Unit, Bristol Medical School, Population Health Science, University of Bristol, Bristol BS8 1TH, UK; matthew.suderman@bristol.ac.uk (M.S.); d.Caramaschi@bristol.ac.uk (D.C.); caroline.relton@bristol.ac.uk (C.R.)

5 Avera Institute for Human Genetics, Sioux Falls, SD 57101, USA; Noah.Kallsen@avera.org (N.A.K.); Erik.Ehli@avera.org (E.A.E.); Gareth.Davies@avera.org (G.E.D.)

6 Neonatal Intensive Care Unit, Department of Surgical Sciences, AOU and University of Cagliari, 09121 Cagliari, Italy; vafanos@tin.it

* Correspondence: v.v.odintsova@vu.nl (V.V.O.); j.van.dongen@vu.nl (J.v.D.)

Abstract: Breastfeeding has long-term benefits for children that may be mediated via the epigenome. This pathway has been hypothesized, but the number of empirical studies in humans is small and mostly done by using peripheral blood as the DNA source. We performed an epigenome-wide association study (EWAS) in buccal cells collected around age nine (mean = 9.5) from 1006 twins recruited by the Netherlands Twin Register (NTR). An age-stratified analysis examined if effects attenuate with age (median split at 10 years; $n_{<10} = 517$, mean age = 7.9; $n_{>10} = 489$, mean age = 11.2). We performed replication analyses in two independent cohorts from the NTR (buccal cells) and the Avon Longitudinal Study of Parents and Children (ALSPAC) (peripheral blood), and we tested loci previously associated with breastfeeding in epigenetic studies. Genome-wide DNA methylation was assessed with the Illumina Infinium MethylationEPIC BeadChip (Illumina, San Diego, CA, USA) in the NTR and with the HumanMethylation450 Bead Chip in the ALSPAC. The duration of breastfeeding was dichotomized ('never' vs. 'ever'). In the total sample, no robustly associated epigenome-wide significant CpGs were identified ($\alpha = 6.34 \times 10^{-8}$). In the sub-group of children younger than 10 years, four significant CpGs were associated with breastfeeding after adjusting for child and maternal characteristics. In children older than 10 years, methylation differences at these CpGs were smaller and non-significant. The findings did not replicate in the NTR sample ($n = 98$; mean age = 7.5 years), and no nearby sites were associated with breastfeeding in the ALSPAC study ($n = 938$; mean age = 7.4). Of the CpG sites previously reported in the literature, three were associated with breastfeeding in children younger than 10 years, thus showing that these CpGs are associated with breastfeeding in buccal and blood cells. Our study is the first to show that breastfeeding is associated with epigenetic variation in buccal cells in children. Further studies are needed to investigate if methylation differences at these loci are caused by breastfeeding or by other unmeasured confounders, as well as what mechanism drives changes in associations with age.

Keywords: breastfeeding; EWAS; DNA methylation; twins; EPIC; NTR; ALSPAC

1. Introduction

Early life environmental influences are associated with development and disease. One mechanism that has been hypothesized to account for the association is through the "epigenetic programming" of genes, some of which may act to confer plasticity to developmental processes [1,2]. Nutrition in early life may play a crucial role in modulating gene expression [3,4]. It has been hypothesized that nutrition-induced epigenetic variation may result in different development trajectories and may be associated with metabolic and immune development during critical periods of early life [5–8]. Epigenetic mechanisms are a key element in understanding the developmental origins of later life disease risk [9–11]. One of the best studied epigenetic mechanisms is DNA methylation—the modification of a cytosine base, usually at CpG dinucleotides, with a methyl group, which regulates gene expression and seems to already be sensitive to nutrition during the prenatal period [12–17].

In humans, prenatal maternal famine has been associated with long-term DNA methylation changes that are still observable in middle-aged individuals [18,19]. The early postnatal period is also believed to be a critical period at which permanent long-term changes may be induced by environmental exposures that affect the child's susceptibility to chronic disease [20]; however, whether similar long-term changes in the human epigenome may be induced in this period is unexplored. The first nutrition period, including breastfeeding, has long-term effects on children [3]. Human breast milk has a unique composition that differs from other lactating animals and that is quite impossible to reproduce in artificial production; in fact, breast milk contains a unique mixture of microorganisms (the microbiome) [21], metabolites [22], multipotent stem cells [23], growth factors [24] and other components that render it unique and individualized for each newborn [25]. Moreover, breast milk varies its composition according to the lactation period and circadian rhythm, and it even varies from the start till the end of one feeding [26]. The benefits of breastfeeding on the health of children are widely described [27–29] and may involve the transmission of nutrients, hormones, and antibodies from mother to child [24,30,31]. These benefits also include the process of interaction and attachment of a child to their mother, although the effect of bonding may also be achieved through formula feeding [32,33].

Balanced newborn feeding is the basis for the adequate growth and development in childhood and beyond [25,28,34]. Breast milk is important for sensory, neurological and cognitive development [35–37], especially in preterm infants [38], but its effects on cognition are confounded by maternal education [39]. The association between breastfeeding duration and a lower risk of infectious diseases, obesity, cancer, coronary heart disease, some allergies, autoimmune disease, diabetes mellitus, inflammatory bowel diseases, and metabolic syndrome at later age has been widely studied [27,40–49]. Even though a protective effect of breastfeeding in hypertension, diabetes, obesity, and metabolic syndrome has not been evident in some large studies [30,50], the benefits of breastfeeding are well recognized, and the understanding of the biological mechanisms of its influence is of interest. Previous studies on the association between breastfeeding and child outcomes have used a variety of definitions of breastfeeding, including: never vs. ever breastfeeding, breastfeeding duration which has been assessed as a continuous measure in months or weeks, or as a categorical variable (e.g., long vs. short). Some studies have examined the percentage of breastfed meals, exclusive breastfeeding duration (when a child is exclusively breastfed until formula feed and/or solid foods are introduced). In a meta-analysis by Victora et al. [27], breastfeeding never vs. ever was associated with a reduction in sudden infant deaths, a reduction of acute otitis during the first few years of life, a protection against allergic rhinitis in children <5 years, a higher child Intelligence Quotient (IQ) of about three IQ points. More versus less breastfeeding has been associated with major protection against diarrhea morbidity, a reduction in severe respiratory infection, and effects on deciduous teeth. Exclusive breastfeeding has been associated with a strong protective result against infectious disease and allergic rhinitis in children <5 years. A dose–response association with duration of breastfeeding was found for a higher IQ and a decreased risk for overweight and obesity.

Epigenome-wide association studies (EWASs) can offer new insights into DNA–environment interactions in determining child development and health [51]. To our knowledge, seven association studies (two candidate gene studies, two EWASs with breastfeeding as covariate and three EWASs of breastfeeding) have been performed on breastfeeding and DNA methylation in humans to date (see Table S1). A candidate gene study of Obermann-Borst et al. found a negative association between the duration of breastfeeding (in categories) and methylation level in blood cells from 120 children (mean age 1.4 years) at seven CpG sites in the promoter of the *LEP* gene; a hormone that regulates energy homeostasis [52]. A suggestive positive association of the methylation level of 2201 CpGs and a negative association of the methylation level of 2075 CpGs with the duration of breastfeeding (continuous measure in weeks) were reported in blood samples from 37 infants (mean age 25.7 months) [53]. These CpGs were annotated to genes predominantly involved in the control of cell signaling systems, the development of anatomical structures and cells, and the development and function of the immune and central nervous systems [53]. The impact of breastfeeding duration (continuous measure in months) on DNA methylation patterns in 200 children (mean age 11.6 years) was suggested in a study of asthma [54]. An EWAS of Sherwood et al. on exclusive breastfeeding supported the findings of Obermann-Borst et al. at a later stage in childhood (10 years, n = 297) but not in young adulthood (18 years, n = 305) [55]. This suggests that methylation changes induced by breastfeeding may change with time and may be more evident at an early age. Similarly, it has been observed that associations between DNA methylation and maternal smoking and birthweight attenuate during childhood [56,57]. Nevertheless, a long-lasting modulating effect of breastfeeding (continuous measure in weeks) on the effects of methylation quantitative trait loci (mQTLs) for CpG sites at the 17q21 locus, where the *IL4R* (interleukin-4) gene is located, has been suggested at age 18 (n = 245) [58]. Not having been breastfed has been associated with an increase in methylation of the promoter of the tumor suppressor gene *CDKN2A* (cyclin dependent kinase inhibitor 2A) in premenopausal breast tumors of 639 women (mean age of 57.6 years) [59]. In a more recent EWAS study, breastfeeding (dichotomized as never vs. ever) was associated with changes in the *TTC34* gene at age 7 (n = 640), which were still evident in adolescence (n = 709) [60]. These previous epigenetic studies of breastfeeding were often conducted with relatively small samples (average sample size = 307, range = 37–640). In all studies, DNA was extracted from peripheral blood [52–55,58], or from tumor tissues in adults [59].

We aimed to carry out an EWAS of breastfeeding in 1006 children around nine years of age recruited by the Netherlands Twin Register (NTR) based on buccal cell DNA and a replication analysis of loci previously associated with breastfeeding in aforementioned epigenetic studies. Buccal samples typically consist of a large proportion of epithelial cells, which might serve as a surrogate tissue for other ectodermal tissues, including the brain [61,62]. Buccal samples also consist of a smaller proportion of leukocytes [63]. To date, few EWASs have been performed on buccal DNA. As some studies have suggested that the effects of early life exposures, including breastfeeding [55–58], may fade away during childhood, we also performed an EWAS on younger children (age <10 years; where 10 corresponds to the median age of the sample) and compared effect sizes in this group with effect sizes in children older than 10 years. We applied a median split of the sample by age to achieve equal sample sizes in both groups. We hypothesized that if effects of breastfeeding attenuate with age, associations would be strongest in the younger age group. We performed replication in an independent buccal-cells DNA methylation dataset from the NTR (n = 98) and in a blood-DNA-methylation dataset from the Avon Longitudinal Study of Parents and Children (ALSPAC) (n = 938). We also examined the correlation between methylation levels of twins for the significant CpGs associated with breastfeeding. We hypothesized that the equal exposure to breastfeeding of co-twins should cause resemblance in their methylation profiles.

2. Materials and Methods

2.1. Overview

We carried out an EWAS in the NTR in 1006 children from 496 complete pairs and 14 twins from incomplete pairs with DNA methylation in buccal cells, testing 787,711 methylation sites (α = 0.05/787771 = 6.34×10^{-8}). The EWAS analyses in different age groups were performed following the median-split of the sample by age (age <10 years: n = 517, age range = 5–9; age ≥ 10 years: n = 489, age range = 10–12). Two models were applied with different covariates (Model 1 = "basic model" and Model 2 = "adjusted model") (see Table S2). Epigenome-wide significant results were taken forward, after checking effects of outliers, for a replication analysis in an independent sample, consisting of 98 NTR children with DNA methylation in buccal cells and in 938 ALSPAC children with DNA methylation in peripheral blood cells. Lastly, we performed a follow-up analysis of the results of previous studies (3859 CpGs) in the discovery cohort (NTR) in the total sample (n = 1006) and the younger age group (n = 517). A flowchart of the analyses is provided in Figure 1.

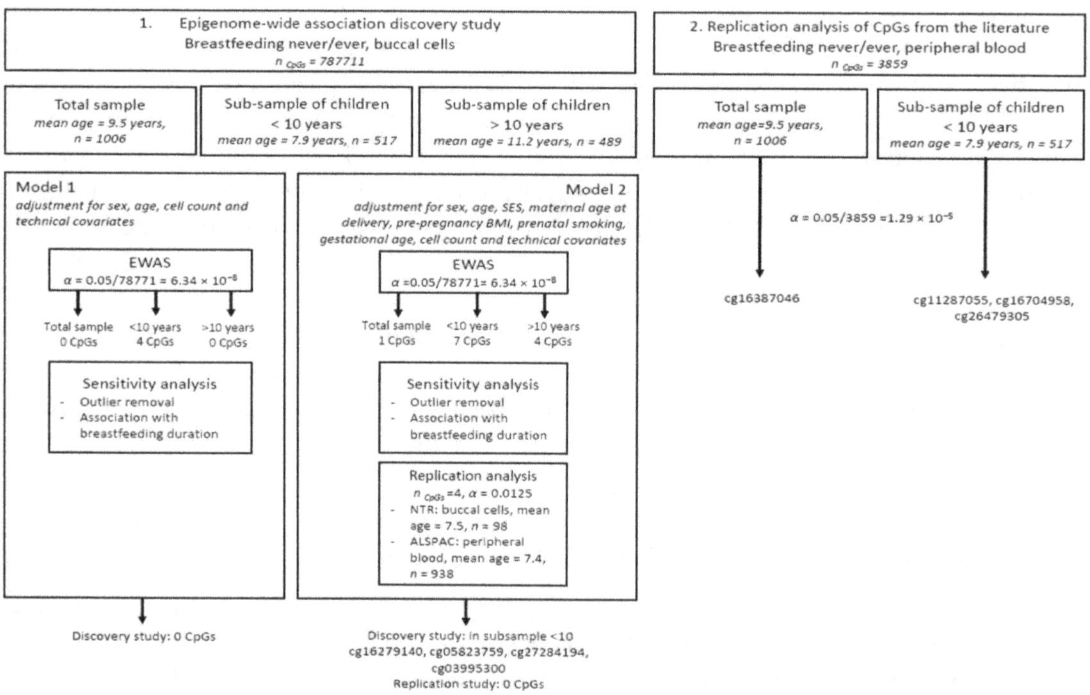

Figure 1. Flowchart of analyses.

2.2. Subjects and Samples

2.2.1. Discovery Study

The subjects were enrolled in the NTR [64] a few weeks to months after birth. Informed consent was obtained from parents. Data on breastfeeding collected around the age of 2 years of the children and good quality DNA methylation data around 9 years of age (mean = 9.5, standard deviation (SD) = 1.89, range = 5–12) were available for 1006 children. The dataset included 51.6% girls and 86% monozygotic twins. This study is embedded in a larger project on childhood aggression: Aggression in Children: Unraveling gene-environment interplay to inform Treatment and InterventiON strategies (ACTION) [65,66]. From the population-based NTR, the ACTION study identified twins who at least once scored higher or lower on a sum score for aggression [67,68].

2.2.2. NTR Replication Study

An independent group of children from the NTR for whom EPIC array methylation data were previously described [63] were included as replication study. This cohort was also embedded in the ACTION project and were comprised of 98 monozygotic twins with available data on breastfeeding duration and DNA methylation from buccal swabs (mean age = 7.5 years, SD = 2.4, age range = 1–10). The NTR studies were approved by the Central Ethics Committee on Research Involving Human Subjects of the VU University Medical Centre, Amsterdam, an Institutional Review Board certified by the U.S. Office of Human Research Protections (IRB number IRB00002991 under federal-wide Assurance-FWA00017598; IRB/institute codes, NTR 03–180).

2.2.3. ALSPAC Replication Study

Data came from the ALSPAC [69,70], a population-based birth cohort. All pregnant women living in the geographical area of Avon (UK) with expected delivery date between 1 April 1991 and 31 December 1992 were invited to participate. Approximately 85% of the eligible population was enrolled, totaling 14,541 pregnant women who gave informed and written consent. The study website contains details of all the data that are available through a fully searchable data dictionary and variable search tool (http://www.bris.ac.uk/alspac/researchers/data-access/data-dictionary/). Ethical approval for the study was obtained from the ALSPAC Ethics and Law Committee and the Local Research Ethics Committees. Of these, 938 children had information on breastfeeding duration and DNA methylation from peripheral blood cells measured on the Infinium HumanMethylation450 BeadChip (mean age = 7.4, SD = 0.13, age range = 7.1–8.8) within the Accessible Resource for Integrated Epigenomics Studies (ARIES) project [71].

2.3. *Phenotype Data*

In the NTR, breastfeeding was assessed in a questionnaire sent to mothers 2 years after the twins were born. Mothers were separately asked about breastfeeding for the first and second born twin. There were six answer categories: 'no', 'less than 2 weeks', '2–6 weeks', '6 weeks to 3 months', '3–6 months', and 'more than 6 months', For the main analyses, breastfeeding as exposure was recoded into 2 categories: 'ever' and 'never', No information on exclusive and mixed breastfeeding was available. The duration of breastfeeding was used in a secondary analysis based on the 6 categories from the original questionnaire coded from 0 (no) to 5 (more than 6 months). Socio-economic status (SES) was determined in two ways (depending on the version of the survey): (1) SES was obtained from a full description of the occupation of the parents and was subsequently coded according to the Standard Classification of Occupations [72]; (2) SES was obtained by the Erikson-Goldthorpe-Portocarero (EPG)-classification scheme [73], combined with information on parental education. The self-reported maternal pre-pregnancy weight just before pregnancy (in kilograms) divided by the square of height (in meters) was used to obtain the maternal pre-pregnancy body mass index (BMI) (weight/height^2). Maternal smoking during pregnancy was reported by mothers for three trimesters of pregnancy and was coded as non-smoking if the mother did not smoke during the entire pregnancy and smoking if the mother smoked at least during one trimester [74]. The mode of conception was classified in three groups: naturally conceived, conceived through stimulation, and conceived via in vitro fertilization (IVF) or intracytoplasmic sperm injection (ICSI) [75]. The mode of delivery was assessed as vaginal delivery, caesarean section (planned and urgent), and vaginal delivery with urgent intervention with forceps or vacuum extraction. Apgar scores at the 1st and 5th minute were presented in 3 conventional categories 0–6 (low), 7–9 (intermediate), and 10 (high) [76]. Gestational age, birthweight, parental age at birth were categorized in groups for descriptive statistics and treated as continuous z-scores in the analyses.

ALSPAC Replication Study

Breastfeeding was assessed via a questionnaire sent to mothers when the study children were approximately 6 months old. Breastfeeding was coded as 'ever' or 'never'. Information on sample characteristics and covariates was obtained by questionnaires completed by the mother during pregnancy and from medical birth records. Socio-economic status was determined by the highest level of maternal education (grouped as follows: certificate of secondary education or not, vocational, O-level, A-level, or university degree). Maternal characteristics included age at birth, pre-pregnancy height and weight, and smoking during pregnancy (any or none). Gestational characteristics included caesarean delivery, gestational age and birthweight.

2.4. DNA Sample Collection

2.4.1. NTR (Discovery and Replication Study)

DNA samples were collected from buccal swabs, as described previously [77]. In short, 16 cotton mouth swabs were individually rubbed against the inside of the cheek on 2 days (morning and evening) and placed in four separate 15 mL conical tubes containing 0.5 mL of a Sodium Chloride-Tris-Ethylenediaminetetraacetic acid (STE) buffer (100 mM sodium chloride, 10 mM Tris hydrochloride (pH 8.0), and 10 mM ethylenediaminetetraacetic acid) with proteinase K (0.1 mg/mL) and sodium dodecyl sulfate (SDS) (0.5%) per swab. Individuals were asked to refrain from eating or drinking 1 h prior to sampling. High molecular weight genomic DNA was extracted by standard DNA extraction techniques. The DNA samples were quantified using the Quant-iT PicoGreen dsDNA Assay Kit (ThermoFisher Scientific, Waltham, MA, USA).

2.4.2. ALSPAC Replication Study

The ALSPAC blood-based DNA methylation profiles were generated at age 7 as part of the ARIES [71], a subsample of approximately 1000 mother-child pairs from the ALSPAC study.

2.5. DNA-Methylation Measurements

2.5.1. NTR Discovery Study

The genome-wide DNA methylation in buccal cells [68] was assessed with the Infinium MethylationEPIC BeadChip (Illumina, San Diego, CA, USA) [78] by the Human Genotyping facility (HugeF) of ErasmusMC, the Netherlands (http://www.glimdna.org/). Five hundred nanograms of genomic DNA from buccal swabs were bisulfite treated using the ZymoResearch EZ DNA Methylation kit (Zymo Research Corp, Irvine, CA, USA). The quality control of the methylation data are described in detail elsewhere [68]. In brief, the quality control (QC) and normalization of the methylation data were performed using a pipeline developed by the Biobank-based Integrative Omics Study (BIOS) consortium [79], which includes sample quality control using the R package MethylAid [80] and probe filtering and functional normalization as implemented in the R package DNAmArray. We previously and successfully applied this pipeline in a pilot study of EPIC array data from buccal samples [63], which was used as replication sample in the current paper. MethylAid was applied with the default EPIC array-specific quality filter thresholds for EPIC arrays. The R package omicsPrint [81] was used to call genotypes based on methylation probes and to verify sample relationships based on those single nucleotide polymorphisms (SNPs) (e.g., the zygosity of twins and samples from the same individual). We checked for sample mismatches between methylation data and genotype data by computing the correlation between SNP genotypes called by omicsPrint based on methylation probes and genotypes based on genome-wide SNP arrays. DNAmArray and meffil [82] were used to identify sex mismatches (both packages identified the same mismatches).

Functional normalization was performed based on five control probe principal components (PCs). The following probe filters were applied: Probes were set to missing (NA) in a sample if they had an intensity value of exactly zero, detection p-value > 0.01, or bead count <3. Probes were excluded from all samples if they mapped to multiple locations in the genome, if they overlapped with an SNP or insertion/deletion (INDEL), or if they had a success rate <0.95 across samples. Annotations of ambiguous mapping probes (based on an overlap of at least 47 bases per probe) and probes where genetic variants (SNPs or INDELS) with a minor allele frequency >0.01 in Europeans overlap with the targeted CpG or single base extension site (SBE) were obtained from Pidsley et al. [83]. After probe filtering, the success rate of probes for each sample was checked: All samples had a success rate above 0.95 after removal of low-performing samples detected by MethylAid. Only the autosomal methylation sites were analyzed, leaving 787,711 out of 865,859 sites for analysis.

2.5.2. NTR Replication Study

Genome-wide DNA methylation in buccal cells was assessed with the Infinium MethylationEPIC BeadChip (Illumina, San Diego, CA, USA) [78] by the Avera Institute for Human Genetics. The quality control, processing and normalization of the data were performed with the same pipeline as for the NTR discovery cohort, a pipeline which has previously been described in detail [63].

2.5.3. ALSPAC Replication Study

DNA methylation wet laboratory procedures, preprocessing analyses, and quality control were performed at the University of Bristol, as previously described [71]. DNA methylation outliers were identified as those three times the inter-quartile range from the nearest of the first and third quartiles. Outliers were replaced with missing values.

2.6. Cellular Proportions

2.6.1. NTR Discovery and Replication Study

Cellular proportions were predicted with hierarchical epigenetic dissection of intra-sample-heterogeneity (HepiDISH) with the RPC method (reduced partial correlation), as described by Zheng et al. [84] and implemented in the R package HepiDISH. HepiDISH is a cell-type deconvolution algorithm that was specifically developed for estimating cellular proportions in epithelial tissues based on genome-wide methylation profiles and that makes use of reference DNA methylation data from epithelial cells, fibroblast and seven leukocyte subtypes. This was applied to the data after data QC and normalization.

2.6.2. ALSPAC Replication Study

Cell count estimates were estimated from DNA methylation profiles using a deconvolution algorithm [85] and included in statistical models to adjust for cell count heterogeneity.

2.7. Data Analyses

2.7.1. Associations between Breastfeeding and Pre- and Perinatal Factors

The association between covariates and breastfeeding was tested in the discovery cohort using a generalized estimating equations (GEE) model that accounted for the correlation structure within families. Six breastfeeding duration categories were included as the continuous outcome variable. The predictors consisted of variables previously described as covariates in EWASs of maternal smoking and birth weight [56,57], i.e., parental SES, maternal smoking during pregnancy (yes/no), gestational age (z-scores), maternal age at birth (z-score), maternal pre-pregnancy BMI (z-scores), cell counts of epithelial cells and natural killer (NK) cells, child's sex, and child's age at DNA-methylation (see Table S3). This analysis was performed in SPSS version 25.

2.7.2. EWAS

Discovery Study

The association between DNA methylation level and breastfeeding was tested using a generalized estimating equations (GEE) model that accounted for the correlation structure within families with DNA methylation β-value as the outcome variable (see Table S2). All analyses in the NTR were performed with GEE models, which were fitted with the R package 'gee.' The following settings were used: Gaussian link function (for continuous outcome variables), 100 iterations, and the 'exchangeable' option to account for the correlation structure within families. To examine and adjust (where applicable) for the inflation of test statistics, the R package bacon was used [86]. We first fitted a basic model with the following predictors: breastfeeding, sex, age at sample collection, the percentages of epithelial and natural killer cells, EPIC array row and bisulfite sample plate (using dummy coding). For the primary EWAS, the breastfeeding outcome was dichotomized (yes/no). Secondly, we fitted a model in which we adjusted for additional covariates (SES, maternal smoking, mother's age at birth, mother's BMI at pregnancy, and gestational age). These covariates were selected on the base of adjustments done in recent meta-analyses of maternal smoking and birthweight [56,57]. We also considered the effects of the duration of breastfeeding by evaluating the same model with the original six categories (not-breastfed; <2 weeks; 2–6 weeks; 6 weeks to 3 months; >6 months). Thirdly, we repeated the EWAS in children younger than 10 years and older than 10 years. To this end, we split up the sample into two groups (median age split) to have two equally-sized groups: children younger than 10 years and children older than 10 years. Epigenome-wide significance was assessed following Bonferroni correction for the number of methylation sites tested ($\alpha = 0.05/787{,}711 = 6.34 \times 10^{-8}$).

We carefully checked if epigenome-wide significant associations were influenced by outliers. As a sensitivity analysis, we repeated the association analysis in the discovery sample for significant CpGs without outliers defined using the Tukey method [87], in which an outlier is any value greater than the upper quartile plus three-times the interquartile range or any value lower than the lower quartile minus three-times the interquartile ranges.

Twin Correlations

The correlation between DNA methylation levels of monozygotic (MZ) and dizygotic (DZ) twins was computed for CpGs that were significant in the discovery study and which were robust to outliers. The methylation beta-values were adjusted for the set of covariates as included in the basic EWAS model with a linear model, and residuals were saved. Next, the MZ and DZ twin correlations were computed on the residuals.

Replication

CpGs that were significant in the discovery study and which were robust to outliers were selected for replication. The basic and adjusted models were applied as in the discovery sample: in the NTR, the GEE model had the same covariates; in the ALSPAC, cell count estimates for peripheral blood were included instead of the epithelium cells count; the sex, age of the child at blood collection around age 7 and the same covariates from the adjusted Model 2 were included; no siblings were included. In the ALSPAC, DNA methylation variation due to technical artefacts or unknown confounders were handled by including 20 surrogate variables generated from the DNA methylation data using the 'sva' R package [88], and associations were tested with linear models implemented by the limma package [89].

2.8. Methylation Data Annotation

To examine previously reported associations for epigenome-wide significant CpGs associated with breastfeeding, we looked them up in the EWAS atlas (https://bigd.big.ac.cn/ewas/tools; accessed on 3 October 2019 [90]) and the EWAS catalog (http://www.ewascatalog.org; accessed on 3 October 2019).

To analyze the possible function of CpGs, we searched for overlaps with mQTLs in a study that analyzed EPIC array data from 102 buccal samples [63] to identify the associated SNPs, and we looked up these SNPs and genes in the genome-wide association study (GWAS) catalog (https://www.ebi.ac.uk/gwas/; accessed on 4 October 2019).

2.9. Overlap with Previous Findings

The follow-up analyses were done for CpGs that were previously associated with breastfeeding in EWASs or candidate gene studies. These included all CpGs on the EPIC array that were annotated to the genes *LEP* ($n_{\text{CpGs}} = 23$) [52–55,58], *IL4R* ($n_{\text{CpGs}} = 37$) [58], *CDKN2A* ($n_{\text{CpGs}} = 32$) [59], 1 CpG from the study of Hartwig et al. [60], and 4297 suggestive CpGs from the study of Naumova et al. [53]. In total, this resulted in a list of 4370 CpGs, of which 3859 CpGs were present (after QC) in our data. For these CpGs, we performed a look-up analysis in the total sample ($n = 1006$) and in the subsample younger than 10 years ($n = 517$) of the discovery NTR cohort. Significance was assessed after Bonferroni correction for the number of CpGs tested ($\alpha = 0.05/3858 = 1.29 \times 10^{-5}$).

3. Results

3.1. Descriptive Statistics

Descriptive statistics are presented in Table 1. The total discovery sample consisted of 1006 children (mean age 9.5, SD = 1.89); 73.7% of the children were breastfed with different duration, and 26.3% never received breastfeeding. Most of the children were breastfed at least one month: 189 (25.5%) were breastfed for 2 weeks to 1.5 months, 181 (24.4%) were breastfed for 1.5–3 months, 148 (20%) were breastfed for 2–6 months, and 148 (20%) were breastfed more than 6 months. The subsample of children younger than 10 years old included 517 twins (mean age 7.9, SD = 1.1) (see Table S4), and the group older than 10 years included 489 twins (mean age = 11.16, SD = 0.72) (see Table S5). The majority of twin pairs was concordant for breastfeeding (99.4%). Among the discordant twin pairs were three pairs, of which one twin was not breastfed while their co-twin received breastfeeding and three pairs of which the co-twins experienced different durations of breastfeeding.

Table 1. Early life characteristics and breastfeeding in the Netherlands Twin Register (NTR) discovery sample ($n = 1006$).

	Breastfeeding Never (n = 265)		Breastfeeding Ever (n = 741)		Total	
	n	%	n	%	n	%
Sex						
male	138	52.1%	349	47.1%	487	48.4%
female	127	47.9%	392	52.9%	519	51.6%
Zygosity						
Monozygotic (MZ)	226	85.3%	613	82.7%	839	83.4%
Dizygotic (DZ)	39	14.7%	128	17.3%	167	16.6%
Chorionicity						
MCMA	4	3.5%	21	7.3%	25	6.2%
MCDA	61	53.0%	144	50.3%	205	51.1%
DCDA	50	43.5%	121	42.3%	171	42.6%
Gestational Age (Weeks)						
Mean (SD)	36.2	(22.2)	35.8	(25.9)	35.9	(25.1)
≤ 32	12	4.8%	61	8.4%	73	7.5%
33–36	128	51.4%	359	49.4%	487	49.9%
≥ 37	109	43.8%	306	42.1%	415	42.6%
Mother's Age at Birth (Years)						
Mean (SD)	31.9	(4.5)	31.2	(4.2)	31.4	(4.3)
19–29	76	29.0%	288	39.0%	364	36.4%
30–39	175	66.8%	435	58.9%	610	61.0%
>40	11	4.2%	15	2.0%	26	2.6%
Mother's BMI Before Pregnancy						
Mean (SD)	24.3	(4.0)	24.2	(4.11)	24.2	(4.1)
<25	149	61.3%	470	66.1%	619	64.9%
25–29	70	28.8%	169	23.8%	239	25.1%
30–39	24	9.9%	65	9.1%	89	9.3%
>40	0	0.0%	7	1.0%	7	0.7%

Table 1. *Cont.*

	Breastfeeding Never (n = 265)		Breastfeeding Ever (n = 741)		Total	
	n	%	n	%	n	%
	Father's Age at Birth (Years)					
Mean (SD)	33.2	(4.4)	33.9	(5.4)	33.7	(5.2)
20–29	53	22.0%	146	20.3%	199	20.8%
30–39	163	67.6%	482	67.1%	645	67.3%
>40	25	10.4%	90	12.5%	115	12.0%
	Mode of Conception					
naturally	227	92.7%	623	86.5%	850	88.1%
stimulated	4	1.6%	26	3.6%	30	3.1%
IVF/ICSI	14	5.7%	71	9.9%	85	8.8%
	Maternal Smoking					
no smoking	205	86.1%	631	92.9%	836	91.2%
smoking	33	13.9%	48	7.1%	81	8.8%
	Parental SES					
low skill level	0	0.0%	8	1.2%	8	0.9%
lower secondary educational level	30	11.9%	41	6.1%	71	7.6%
upper secondary education level	99	39.3%	203	30.0%	302	32.5%
higher vocational level	89	35.3%	234	34.6%	323	34.8%
scientific level	34	13.5%	191	28.2%	225	24.2%
	Mode of Delivery					
vaginal	141	56.6%	416	57.1%	557	57.0%
caesarean planned	43	17.3%	97	13.3%	140	14.3%
urgent intervention (forceps, vacuum extraction)	20	8.0%	75	10.3%	95	9.7%
urgent caesarean section	45	18.1%	140	19.2%	185	18.9%
	Birth Weight					
Mean (SD)	2435.7	(444.8)	2394.6	(558)	2405	(531.7)
<1500	8	3.2%	52	7.1%	60	6.2%
1500–2500	123	49.8%	338	46.4%	461	47.3%
>2500	116	47.0%	338	46.4%	454	46.6%
	Apgar Score at 1st Minute					
0–6	17	12.3%	48	12.8%	65	12.7%
7–9	103	74.6%	290	77.5%	393	76.8%
10	18	13.0%	36	9.6%	54	10.5%
	Apgar Score at 5th Minute					
0–6	1	0.8%	14	3.9%	15	3.1%
7–9	41	31.1%	130	36.3%	171	34.9%
10	90	68.2%	214	59.8%	304	62.0%
	Breastfeeding Duration					
no	265	100.0%	0		265	26.3%
less than 2 weeks			75	10.1%	75	7.5%
2–6 weeks			189	25.5%	189	18.8%
6 weeks to 3 months			181	24.4%	181	18.0%
3–6 months			148	20.0%	148	14.7%
more than 6 months			148	20.0%	148	14.7%

Descriptive statistics of children included in the study. MCMA = monochorionic monoamniotic; MCDA = monochorionic diamniotic; DCDA = dichorionic diamniotic; SD = standard deviation; BMI = body mass index; IVF = in vitro fertilization; ICSI = intracytoplasmic sperm injection; and SES = socio-economic status.

Breastfeeding duration (six categories) was significantly positively associated with socio-economic status ($\beta = 0.353$, standard error (SE) = 0.09, and $p = 0.0004$) and inversely associated with maternal smoking ($\beta = -0.733$, SE = 0.32, and $p = 0.02$) and gestational age ($\beta = -0.194$, SE = 0.09, and $p = 0.03$) (see Table S3). Breastfeeding was not significantly correlated with maternal pre-pregnancy BMI ($\beta = -0.117$, SE = 0.75, and $p = 0.119$), maternal age at delivery ($\beta = -0.016$, SE = 0.09, and $p = 0.86$), and the cell composition of buccal swabs ($\beta = 1.27$, SE = 1.2, and $p = 0.25$ for count of epithelial cells; and $\beta = 14.78$, SE = 9.8, and $p = 0.13$ for count of natural killer cells).

3.2. *Association Analysis Findings*

First, genome-wide DNA-methylation analyses were performed to test the association between breastfeeding (never/ever) and DNA-methylation level while adjusting for sex, age at DNA sample collection, estimated proportion of epithelial cells, the estimated proportion of natural killer cells, the row of the sample on the chip, and the bisulfite plate (model 1). No epigenome-wide significant sites were identified (see Table S8). Genome-wide EWAS test statistics showed no inflation (see Figure S1). DNA methylation was also not associated with the duration of breastfeeding (see Table S9).

In the EWAS in children younger than 10 years with the same basic model, we identified four epigenome-wide significant CpGs (see Table S10): cg25178826 ($\beta = -0.026$, SE = 0.003, and $p = 8.04 \times 10^{-12}$) is located in the 5′ untranslated region (5′UTR) region of *PRLR* (prolactin receptor) gene, cg12087956 ($\beta = -0.03$, SE = 0.005, and $p = 1.8 \times 10^{-8}$) is in the gene body of *CDAN1* (codanin 1), cg24192772 ($\beta = -0.024$, SE = 0.004, and $p = 2.5 \times 10^{-8}$) is in the gene body of *FOXK2* (forkhead box K2), and cg10142656 ($\beta = -0.02$, SE = 0.004, and $p = 6.28 \times 10^{-8}$) is mapped to the transcription start site (TSS1500) of *TRMT10B* (tRNA methyltransferase 10B). These four CpGs were not strongly associated with breastfeeding duration (see Table S11). The plots of the methylation values for these four CpGs revealed several extreme methylation values in the data (see Figure S2 and Table S10), and the association with breastfeeding disappeared after outlier removal: cg25178826 $\beta = -0.00006$, SE = 0.001, and $p = 0.98$; cg12087956 $\beta = 0.00004$, SE = 0.0009, and $p = 0.5$; cg24192772 $\beta = 0.0009$, SE = 0.001, and $p = 0.15$; and cg10142656 $\beta = 0.0001$, SE = 0.0008, and $p = 0.13$ (see Table S10).

Next, we performed EWASs of breastfeeding never/ever with adjustments for SES, maternal age at delivery, maternal pre-pregnancy BMI, maternal prenatal smoking, and gestational age (Model 2). One CpG, cg22491379, was significant in the total sample ($\beta = -0.007$, SE = 0.001, and $p = 1.3 \times 10^{-9}$) (see Figure 2a, Figure S3, Table 2 and Table S12), and seven CpGs were significant in the children younger than 10 years (see Table 2 and Table S14). The Manhattan plot for the EWAS in children younger than 10 years showed a peak on chromosome 21, which contains a cluster of CpGs just below the epigenome-wide significance threshold (see Figure 2d). Results from the same analysis for breastfeeding duration are shown in Tables S13 and S15.

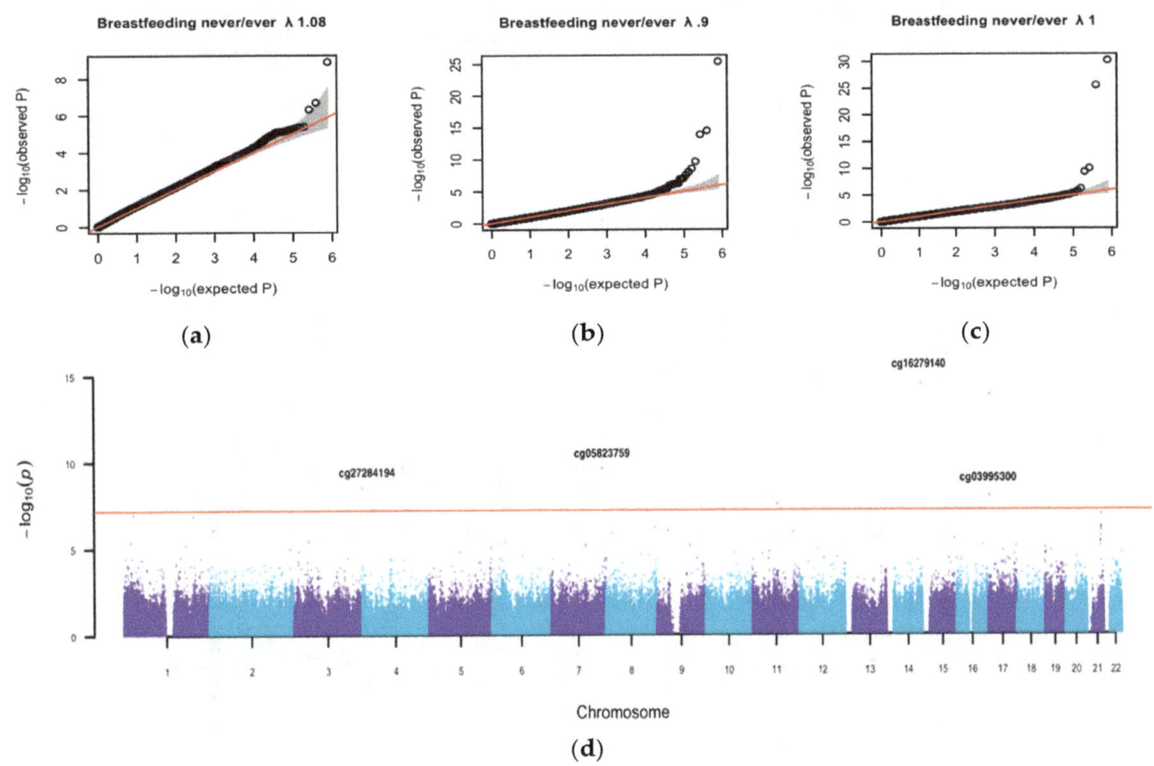

Figure 2. Quantile-Quantile (QQ) plots: (**a**) in the total sample; (**b**) in the subsample of children younger than 10 years old; and (**c**) in the subsample of children older than 10 years old. (**d**) Manhattan plot shows the epigenome-wide association study results of breastfeeding 'never'/'ever' in children younger than 10 years old. Covariates included sex, age, socio-economic status (SES), maternal age at delivery, maternal pre-pregnancy BMI, maternal prenatal smoking, gestational age, EPIC array row and bisulfite sample plate, and cell composition. In the Manhattan plot, the red line represents the Bonferroni threshold (6.34×10^{-8}). Given CpG names indicate significant loci after removal of outliers.

Table 2. Summary of epigenome-wide significant CpGs from the discovery epigenome-wide association study (EWAS) of DNA signatures of breastfeeding.

cgID	Chromosome	Position	Gene	Gene Region	Discovery Study			Discovery Study Without Outliers		
					Estimate	SE	p-Value	Estimate	SE	p-Value
Basic Model (1). Sub-Sample < 10 years (n = 517)										
cg25178826	chr5	35165447	*PRLR*	5′UTR	−0.026	0.004	8.04×10^{-12}	-6.04×10^{-5}	0.001	0.98
cg12087956	chr15	43022167	*CDAN1*	Body	−0.031	0.005	1.18×10^{-8}	4.92×10^{-5}	0.001	0.50
cg24192772	chr17	80536920	*FOXK2*	Body	−0.024	0.004	2.52×10^{-8}	9.17×10^{-4}	0.001	0.15
cg10142656	chr9	37753047	*TRMT10B*	TSS1500	−0.019	0.004	6.28×10^{-8}	9.98×10^{-5}	0.0007	0.14
Adjusted Model (2). Discovery Sample (n = 1006)										
cg22491379	chr2	120553625	*PTPN4*	5′UTR	−0.007	0.001	1.30×10^{-9}	−0.005	0.001	5.78×10^{-3}
Adjusted Model (2). Sub-Sample < 10 Years (n = 517)										
cg03463465	chr6	164143581			0.360	0.034	4.51×10^{-26}	−0.003	0.001	0.01
cg07670516	chr17	5019840	*ZNF232*	5′UTR	0.249	0.032	1.40×10^{-14}	0.006	0.014	0.65
cg20820810	chr11	71850130	*FOLR3*	Body	−0.300	0.054	2.82×10^{-8}	−0.001	0.001	0.21
cg16279140	chr14	103981749			−0.411	0.052	3.50×10^{-15}		no outliers	
cg05823759	chr7	149646627			0.205	0.032	2.35×10^{-10}		no outliers	
cg27284194	chr4	1044797			0.638	0.107	2.90×10^{-9}		no outliers	
cg03995300	chr17	5019989	*ZNF232*	5′UTR	0.229	0.040	1.02×10^{-8}		no outliers	

$\alpha = 0.05/787{,}711 = 6.34 \times 10^{-8}$. Basic Model 1 included breastfeeding coded as 'never' and 'ever' with adjustments for sex, age at DNA methylation, the count of epithelial cells, the count of natural killer cells, EPIC array row and bisulfite sample plate. Adjusted Model (2) included in additional to basic model covariates: SES, maternal smoking during pregnancy, maternal age at birth, maternal pre-pregnancy BMI, and gestational age. In bold: CpGs selected for replication.

Genome-wide EWAS test statistics from the analyses of Model 2 (in the total sample and in the children younger than 10 years) showed no inflation (see Figure 2a,b). For four out of the eight significant CpGs, the association disappeared after removal of outliers (see Figures S4 and S5). The four CpGs that were unaffected by outliers were selected for a replication analysis (see Figure S6): cg16279140 ($\beta = -0.4$, SE = 0.05, and $p = 3.5 \times 10^{-15}$), cg05823759 ($\beta = 0.2$, SE = 0.032, and $p = 2.35 \times 10^{-10}$), cg27284194($\beta = 0.64$, SE = 0.12, and $p = 2.9 \times 10^{-9}$), and cg03995300 ($\beta = 0.23$, SE = 0.04, and $p = 1.2 \times 10^{-8}$) (see Table S14). All four CpGs were significant in children younger than 10 years.

We next examined the association with breastfeeding in children older than 10 (Model 2). In this analysis, the genome-wide test statistics showed mild inflation (lambda = 1.11). After adjusting for inflation, four CpGs remained epigenome-wide significant, but none were significant after outlier removal. The four significant CpGs in the children younger than 10 years had smaller effects, and three CpGs showed inverse directions of effect in children older than 10: cg16279140 ($\beta = 0.04$, SE = 0.02, and $p = 0.04$), cg05823759 ($\beta = -0.002$, SE = 0.02, and $p = 0.92$), cg27284194 ($\beta = 0.18$, SE = 0.06, and $p = 0.002$), and cg03995300 ($\beta = -0.003$, SE = 0.02, and $p = 0.89$) (see Table S16). The quantile-quantile plots (see Figure 2b,c) suggested a stronger association signal for breastfeeding in children younger than 10 years than in the older group. We computed the correlations between the regression coefficients (i.e., the methylation difference associated with breastfeeding) for the top 100 CpGs from each age group. These correlations were weak ($r = 0.25$ and $p = 0.10$ for the top 100 CpG from the EWAS in children <10 years and from the EWAS in children >10 years). This suggests that methylation profiles associated with breastfeeding are different in children younger than 10 years and older than 10 years.

We computed the twin correlations in the MZ and DZ pairs for the significant CpGs, as we assumed that equal exposure to breastfeeding should cause similarity in methylation level of twins. The correlations of methylation levels of all four sites were very high in MZ twins and almost twice as high as in DZ twins: cg16279140 rMZ = 0.906, rDZ = 0.505; cg05823759 rMZ = 0.953, rDZ = 0.609; cg27284194 rMZ = 0.972, rDZ = 0.462; and cg03995300 rMZ = 0.902, rDZ = 0.453. This pattern suggests that there are heritable influences on DNA methylation at these CpGs, as previously shown by other studies of DNA methylation heritability.

3.3. Replication Analysis of Our Findings in Other Samples

Both replication datasets were comparable to the discovery subsample of children younger than 10 years old (see Tables S4, S6, and S7). As expected, the singleton children (ALSPAC) had a higher gestational age (~39 weeks vs. ~35.7), a higher birthweight (~3500 g vs. ~2400 g) and a lower proportion of caesarean deliveries (~9% vs. ~36.8%). We performed a replication analysis for significant CpGs unaffected by outliers from the adjusted Model 2 of the discovery analysis with the same set of covariates (see Table 3).

In the NTR replication cohort, for one CpG, the direction of effect changed (cg03995300, *ZNF232*, $\beta = -0.050$, SE = 0.033, and $p = 0.13$), and three other CpGs had the same direction of effect but were not significant: cg16279140 ($\beta = -0.03$, SE = 0.04, and $p = 0.43$), cg05823759 ($\beta = 0.03$, SE = 0.033, and $p = 0.32$), and cg27284194 ($\beta = 0.07$, SE = 0.054, and $p = 0.21$) (see Table 3, Figure S7).

In the ALSPAC, the most important difference to note were the different tissues used for DNA methylation profiling (peripheral blood) and the platform (the Illumina Infinium HumanMethylation450 Beadchip [Illumina, San Diego, CA, USA]). Because of the platform difference, roughly half of the CpG sites included in the discovery DNA methylation profiles were measured in the ALSPAC. In the adjusted Model 2, two of the four most strongly associated CpG sites were not included on the ALSPAC platform (cg16279140 and cg05823759), nor were any other sites within 1000 base pairs (bp) of these sites. The other two sites, cg27284194 and cg03995300, were included, but neither association was replicated ($p > 0.19$ and $p > 0.77$, respectively) in the adjusted model (see Table 3). An overall lack of replication was confirmed by low correlations between effect estimates in the discovery and the ALSPAC. In particular, we identified the 100 most strongly associated CpG sites in the discovery that were also present in the ALSPAC DNA methylation profiles. The correlation of effect estimates for these sites between studies was low (Pearson's $r = 0.13$ with $p = 0.2$ for the adjusted model).

Table 3. Summary of association between breastfeeding and significant in the discovery study CpGs in replication.

cgID	Direction of Effect in Discovery Study <10 Years	NTR Replication Study ($n = 98$)			ALSPAC Replication Study ($n = 938$)		
		Estimate	SE	*P*-Value [a]	Estimate	SE	*P*-Value
cg16279140	−	−0.0326	0.0412	0.43	NA	NA	NA
cg05823759	+	0.0329	0.0332	0.32	NA	NA	NA
cg27284194	+	0.0668	0.0542	0.21	0.0047	0.016	0.77
cg03995300	+	−0.0502	0.0334	0.13	0.0140	0.011	0.19

Adjusted Model 2 was used. [a] $\alpha = 0.05/4 = 0.01$. NA = not available on the 450k platform.

3.4. Replication Analysis of Findings from Previous EWAS

Of the 3858 CpGs from previous literature, four CpGs were associated with breastfeeding in our sample ($\alpha = 1.29 \times 10^{-5}$, see Table 4). One site was significant in the total sample (see Table S17): cg16387046 is located on chromosome 12 in the *MUCL1* (mucin like 1) gene ($\beta = 0.027$, SE = 0.005, and $p = 4.9 \times 10^{-7}$). Three sites were significant in the children younger than 10 years (see Table S18): cg16704958 ($\beta = 0.009$, SE = 0.002, and $p = 8.03 \times 10^{-6}$) and cg11287055 ($\beta = 0.056$, SE = 0.01, and $p = 4.9 \times 10^{-6}$), located on chromosome 21 in the *VPS26C* (endosomal protein sorting factor C; previous name *DSCR3*) gene, and cg26479305 ($\beta = 0.338$, SE = 0.07, and $p = 1.11 \times 10^{-5}$), located on chromosome 12 in the *ATG101* (autophagy related 101, previous name *C12orf44*) gene. All these CpGs were previously reported in the association study by Naumova et al. [53] that was carried out in infants around two years old (mean age 25.7 months) with DNA methylation profiling in peripheral blood with Illumina EPIC BeadChip (Illumina, San Diego, CA, USA). The direction of association was positive for all four CpGs in both studies. CpGs located in/nearby *LEP* [52,55], *IL4R* [58] and *CDKN2A* [59], previously discussed as candidate genes for association with breastfeeding, were not significant in our study.

Table 4. Replication of CpGs from previous literature.

cgID	Chromosome	Position	Gene	Gene Region	ESTIMATE	SE	*P*-Value
Total Sample ($n = 1006$)							
cg16387046	chr12	55248207	*MUCL1*	TSS200	0.027	0.005	4.93×10^{-7}
Sub-Sample <10 ($n = 517$)							
cg11287055	chr21	38630234	*VPS26C (DSCR3)*	Body	0.056	0.012	4.93×10^{-6}
cg16704958	chr21	38630728	*VPS26C (DSCR3)*	Body	0.009	0.002	8.03×10^{-6}
cg26479305	chr12	52470979	*ATG10 (C12orf44)*	3′UTR	0.338	0.077	1.11×10^{-5}

$\alpha = 0.05/3859 = 1.29 \times 10^{-5}$. The table shows all CpGs that were previously reported to be associated with breastfeeding and that were significantly replicated by our study.

3.5. Methylation Data Annotation

For the significant CpGs from discovery and follow-up studies, we looked up the associations with nearby genetic variants (mQTLs) in the results from a previously published mQTL study of buccal-derived DNA in monozygotic twins [63]. Four CpGs were associated with mQTLs (cg27284194, associated with SNPs on chromosome 4: 927973–1039876; cg16279140, associated with SNPs on chromosome 14: 103823243–104186876; cg16387046, associated with SNPs on chromosome 12: 54830518–54896008; and cg26479305, associated with SNPs on chromosome 12: 52492131). Additionally, no significant mQTLs were found for four CpGs (cg03995300, cg05823759, cg11287055, cg16704958).

Next, we compared our results against all previously associated traits in EWASs (the EWAS atlas and the EWAS catalog) and GWASs (the GWAS catalog). One CpG (cg03995300) is mapped to *ZNF232* and has been previously associated with prenatal maternal smoking, sex, and ancestry [56,91,92]. The *ZNF232* locus was associated with a family history of Alzheimer's disease in a GWA meta-analysis [93]. The intergenic CpG on chromosome 4 (cg27284194) has been previously associated with infertility [94,95]. In GWASs, the region 4: 927973–1039876 (harboring mQTLs for cg27284194) has been associated with a number of traits and diseases, including bone mineral density [96–100] and several metabolomic characteristics such as blood protein [101,102] and triglyceride [103] levels (See Table S19). The intergenic CpG on chromosome 14 (cg16279140) did not appear in previous EWASs. In GWASs, SNPs on chromosome 14: 103823243–104186876 have been linked to amino acids levels as biomarkers of metabolic disorders [104] and other blood metabolites [105], and some disease and addictions including multisite chronic pain [106], metabolite changes in chronic kidney disease [107], bipolar disorder [108], alcohol consumption [109] and risk-taking behavior [110] (See Table S19). The intergenic CpG on chromosome 7, cg05823759, has not been previously identified in an EWAS and is not associated with mQTLs.

Four CpGs that were replicated from previous studies on breastfeeding exposure have been reported in association with other traits and diseases. The *ATG10 (C12orf44)* gene, where cg26479305 is located, has been related to the autophagy pathway and cellular senescence in an EWAS [111]. It is related to regulators of inflammation (circulating cytokines and growth factors) [112], hematological traits in GWASs [113], and prenatal arsenic exposure [114].

CpGs (cg11287055, cg16704958) mapped to the *VPS26C (DSCR3)* have not been reported in other EWASs. *VPS26C* is a component of the retriever complex, which plays a role in cell surface processes such as cell migration, cell adhesion, nutrient supply and cell signaling [115].

4. Discussion

We aimed to study DNA methylation in buccal cells in mid-childhood in association with breastfeeding as an exposure. Associations were tested in the total sample and in groups stratified by age. The age distribution allowed us to analyze whether effects of breastfeeding can be attenuated with age, as this has been observed for other exposures in peripheral blood, including maternal smoking [56], birthweight [57] and breastfeeding [55].

We did not find evidence for robust epigenome-wide significant associations in the total sample (1006 children, age 5–12), but we did observe associations in the younger age group (before 10 years) that did not appear in the group of children of 10–12 years old. This suggests that epigenetic alterations in certain genomic regions might be associated with nutritional differences in the early postnatal life that tend to fade across childhood. However, since the CpGs were not replicated in the small, buccal-cells replication NTR dataset and in the large blood-cells replication dataset from the ALSPAC, further studies are required to follow up on these findings. It also remains to be examined if the associations reflect a causal effect of breastfeeding on methylation and whether these methylation differences might influence developmental trajectories and later-life health of the child.

The observation that associations between breastfeeding and methylation at some CpGs are age-dependent may be explained by age-related changes in DNA methylation that have been reported in several studies [116,117], including children in the age range of our study [118–122]. Similarly, Sherwood et al. [55] observed that breastfeeding is associated with the DNA methylation of the *LEP* gene at age 10 but not at age 18. Previous studies have identified DNA methylation signatures of prenatal nutrition in peripheral tissues at various life stages, even in adulthood. DNA methylation signatures in many genomic regions have been identified in middle-aged individuals who were exposed to the 1944/45 Dutch hunger winter at the time of conception, and many of these sites have been found to be related to growth, developmental processes and metabolism [18,19]. It is unclear if the effects of early life postnatal exposures can have similar long-term effects to prenatal exposures in humans, as most studies of early life influences on the epigenome have focused on prenatal exposures or have not examined long-term effects. None of the genes reported in studies of prenatal malnutrition (*SMAD7, CDH23, INSR, RFTN1, CPT1A, KLF13* [19], *IGF2* [18], and *LEP* [123]) were present among the top CpGs associated with breastfeeding in our study. Several explanations can be proposed. First, postnatal nutrition and prenatal nutrition exposures might differently influence the DNA methylation. Second, DNA methylation signatures induced by early nutrition exposure can be different across examined tissues (buccal cells in our study versus peripheral blood in previous famine studies). Third, the prenatal famine study examined the effects of an extreme exposure during the prenatal period.

The presence of associations with breastfeeding initiation (breastfeeding never vs. ever), and the absence of findings with breastfeeding duration suggests that the association depends on the exposure to breast milk rather than its duration. This could potentially be in line with previous findings that have shown that effects of exposure on DNA methylation occur only when the individual is exposed in certain sensitive life periods [118]. Our finding of stronger epigenetic associations with breastfeeding ever vs. never than with the duration of breastfeeding is also in line with studies providing evidence that any breastfeeding has stronger biological effects than the duration of breastfeeding, e.g., the impact of first maternal milk (colostrum) on immunoglobulins and further neonatal health, especially for small for gestational age and low-birthweight infants [22,24].

We observed associations at a total of eight CpG sites: cg16279140, chromosome 14, intergenic; cg05823759, chr7, intergenic; cg27284194, chromosome 4, intergenic; cg03995300, chromosome 17, *ZNF232*; cg16387046, chromosome 12, *MUCL1*; cg11287055, chromosome 21, *VPS26C* (*DSCR3*); cg16704958, chromosome 21, *VPS26C* (*DSCR3*); and cg26479305, chromosome 12, *ATG10* (*C12orf44*). Methylation levels at these CpGs are potentially influenced by both environmental influences, such as breastfeeding, and by genetic variation, although an alternative interpretation could be that the genomic regions of these CpGs affect breastfeeding function. Unfortunately, no GWAS on breastfeeding is available to verify this suggestion. It remains to be examined whether methylation differences induced by breastfeeding have an effect on the aforementioned traits. Interestingly, associations with breastfeeding have been previously reported in epidemiological studies for bone mineral content and bone mineral density [124] and metabolite profiles [125]; outcomes that have been associated with SNPs in the regions detected in our study as differentially methylated between breastfed and non-breastfed children. It remains to be examined whether methylation differences induced by breastfeeding have an effect on these traits.

Since the role of nutrition is systemic, it has been assumed that biomarkers must be present in different tissues. To study the epigenetic mechanisms of breastfeeding, previous studies have examined DNA from peripheral blood [52–55,58] and also from tumor tissue [59]. Buccal epithelium is of interest because it offers a non-invasive way of biosample collection for an epigenetic analysis. A number of studies have demonstrated the potential of buccal cells to study DNA methylation [126]. We previously showed that, although there is some correlation between DNA methylation in buccal and blood cells ($n = 22$, age = 18 years), it is low for most CpGs interrogated by the Illumina 450k array [127]. The methylation levels of two of the CpG sites that were included in the ALSPAC replication study were highly correlated in buccal and blood cells: cg27284194 ($r = 0.864$) and cg03995300 ($r = 0.782$). In spite of this, the associations with breastfeeding observed in the NTR were not replicated in the ALSPAC. We observed some overlap with the study of Naumova et al. [53] in peripheral blood that used the EPIC array, and these sites had medium correlations between DNA methylation in buccal and blood cells (cg16387046 $r = 0.690$, cg11287055 $r = 0.413$, and cg16704958 $r = 0.328$).

We observed that breastfeeding-associated CpGs show strong correlations in MZ twins and larger correlations in MZ twins compared to DZ twins. As the large majority of twin pairs in our study were almost always concordant for breastfeeding, it is expected that twins of both types show resemblance for DNA methylation levels at these sites. The larger correlation in MZ compared to DZ twins in our study suggests that these sites are also subject to heritable influences. In line with this observation, some of these CpGs are associated with mQTLs. It should be noted that breastfeeding and lactation itself are heritable traits. In previous twin studies, the heritability of initiation of breastfeeding ranged from 49% [128] to 70% [129]. DNA-methylation profiles may be influenced by several early life factors. In our study, almost all early environmental factors of interest were shared by twins: SES, maternal age at birth, maternal pre-pregnancy BMI, and maternal smoking during pregnancy and gestational age.

Some CpGs that did not reach epigenome-wide significance can have potential for further epigenetic studies of breastfeeding. The CpG cg22491379, located in the *PTPN4* on chromosome 2, was discovered in total sample of children of 5–12 years old and, after outlier removal, had suggestive significance ($p = 5.78 \times 10^{-3}$). *PTPN4* was listed in suggestive regions associated with breast morphology (breast size) [130]. Some top CpGs in the discovery study (non-adjusted model) are associated with genes that are involved in growth and metabolism. The *PRLR* (prolactin receptor) gene, located on chromosome 5, is involved in prolactin receptor activity and the growth hormone receptor signaling pathway. Growth hormone binds to the prolactin receptor, this being the basis of induction of lactation by growth hormone [131]. The *FOXK2* gene, located on chromosome 17, is a member of forkhead box transcription factors and is involved in glucose metabolism, aerobic glycolysis and autophagy [132], thus playing a role in metabolic reprogramming towards aerobic glycolysis [133]. It is associated lean body mass [134] and has been found to be hypomethylated in CpG islands in obese patients' adipose tissues [135]. We observed a cluster of associations on chromosome 21, each individual association just below epigenome-wide significance. The *VPS26C* (*DSCR3*) gene is located on chromosome 21 and, as mentioned earlier, contains two CpGs previously associated with breastfeeding in blood [53].

The strengths of our study include the use of the buccal epithelium methylome to investigate breastfeeding for the first time, sample size, and the availability of replication data, including data from another tissue (blood). Furthermore, our exposure, breastfeeding, was assessed very shortly after it occurred, reducing the risk of measurement error and recall bias. Both the discovery and replication samples have been thoroughly phenotyped and extensively studied. Our study also has limitations. First, the findings in the discovery study were not replicated in the cohort of children with buccal cell DNA methylation of the same age, possibly due to the small size of this cohort (98 monozygotic twins). Second, the discovery sample was included in a study of aggressive behavior, and not primarily examined for the purposes of research on breastfeeding. Third, we did not have longitudinal DNA methylation data to measure the stability of effects; however, we examined the possible attenuation of breastfeeding effects through an age-stratified analysis. Fourth, there are currently no datasets available on gene expression in buccal cells; thus, we could not examine relationships between DNA methylation and transcription. A strength of the current analysis is that it used the Illumina EPIC array, which has much greater coverage than the 450k array. Importantly, some of the top CpGs identified in the discovery EWAS were all novel EPIC probes. The replication analysis in the ALSPAC on DNA methylation data from peripheral blood, however, used the 450k array and therefore did not permit look-up of the same CpGs. The findings of this study require further replication in cohorts with buccal epithelium and other tissues to improve our understanding of breastfeeding-associated methylation changes in different tissues, and the possible utility as a biomarker of early life nutrition. Finally, a difficulty in studies of breastfeeding is that breast milk composition is unique in each mother. Lactation is influenced not only by genetic variation but also by many environmental factors such as the mother's nutrition, lifestyle, level of stress, and attachment to the child [24,25,136–139]. Future epigenetic studies of breastfeeding could stratify the breastfeeding sample on the basis of criteria of breast milk composition. This might be more informative for predicting a child's outcome but might also be a better indicator of a mother's well-being. The value of our research is that it combined breastfeeding, prenatal characteristics, and methylation data. In the future, results from studies that will integrate epigenomic data with genomics, transcriptomics, and metabolomics may be used to develop prediction models of long-term outcomes in child development and health. Understanding of the mechanisms associated with breastfeeding will help to develop interventions to improve children's health and reduce risk of chronic disease by supporting breastfeeding or optimizing infant nutrition when breastfeeding is not possible.

5. Conclusions

Our study provided a first indication that breastfeeding as an early life environmental factor may be associated with epigenetic variation in buccal cells in children. The findings point at new candidate loci influenced by breastfeeding. Future studies are needed to investigate if the DNA methylation signatures are caused by breastfeeding or by other unmeasured confounders (including a genetic predisposition to give or receive breastfeeding and other aspects of prenatal or postnatal diet), whether they are influenced by percentage of breastfed meals, exclusive breastfeeding duration, breastmilk composition, etc., and what age-related mechanisms drive changes in the association between breastfeeding and methylation.

Supplementary Materials:
Table S1: Overview of previous EWAS of breastfeeding in humans, Table S2: EWAS Model Equations, Table S3: Associations of covariates with breastfeeding duration (six categories), Table S4: Discovery study subsample of children <10 years population characteristics, Table S5: Discovery study subsample of children >10 years population characteristics, Table S6: NTR replication sample population characteristics, Table S7: ALSPAC replication sample population characteristics, Table S8: Association of breastfeeding "never"/"ever" with CpG sites in basic Model 1 in total sample: top 100 and genomic annotation, Table S9: Association of breastfeeding duration (six categories) with CpG sites in basic Model 1 in total sample: top 100 and genomic annotation, Table S10: Association of breastfeeding "never"/"ever" with CpG sites in basic Model 1 in sub-sample <10 years: top 100 and genomic annotation, Table S11: Association of breastfeeding duration (six categories) with CpG sites in basic Model 1 in sub-sample <10 years: top 100 and genomic annotation, Table S12: Association of breastfeeding "never"/"ever" with CpG sites in adjusted Model 2 in total sample: top 100 and genomic annotation, Table S13: Association of breastfeeding duration (six categories) with CpG sites in adjusted Model 2 in total sample: top 100 and genomic annotation, Table S14: Association of breastfeeding "never"/"ever" with CpG sites in adjusted Model 2 in sub-sample <10 years: top 100 and genomic annotation, Table S15: Association of breastfeeding duration (six categories) with CpG sites in adjusted Model 2 in sub-sample <10 years: top 100 and genomic annotation, Table S16: Association of breastfeeding "never"/"ever" with CpG sites in adjusted Model 2 in sub-sample >10 years: top 100 and genomic annotation, Table S17: Follow-up of associations of breastfeeding with CpGs from literature in discovery total sample (n = 1006), Table S18: Follow-up of associations of breastfeeding with CpGs from literature in discovery sub-sample < 10 years old (n = 517), Table S19: Association of CpGs associated with breastfeeding in discovery study with mQTLs, Figure S1: QQ plots that shows epigenome-wide association study results of breastfeeding ever/never and breastfeeding duration (six categories) in total sample (n = 1006) and in sub-sample of children < 10 years (n = 517), Figure S2: Methylation level (beta) at significant CpGs in Model 1 in sub-sample of children <10 years (n = 517), Figure S3: Manhattan plot show the epigenome-wide association study results of breastfeeding 'never'/'ever' in discovery sample Model 2 (n = 1006), Figure S4: Methylation level (beta) at significant CpG in Model 2 in total sample (n = 1006), Figure S5: Methylation level (beta) at significant CpGs in Model 2 in sub-sample of children <10 years (n = 517) with outliers excluded from further replication, Figure S6: Methylation level (beta) at significant CpGs in Model 2 in sub-sample of children <10 years included in replication study, Figure S7: Methylation level (beta) at significant CpGs in Model 2 in NTR replication study (n = 98).

Author Contributions: Conceptualization, D.I.B., C.R., M.S., J.v.D.; Data curation, F.A.H., C.E.M.v.B. and J.v.D.; formal analysis, V.V.O. and J.v.D.; funding acquisition, D.I.B., M.B.,V.V.O.; investigation, F.A.H., C.E.M.v.B., E.A.E., N.A.K. and G.E.D.; methodology, D.I.B., M.S., J.v.D.; resources, E.A.E., G.E.D. and J.v.D.; software, V.V.O. and J.v.D.; supervision, D.I.B., C.R., M.B. and J.v.D.; visualization, V.V.O; validation, V.V.O., J.v.D., M.S., D.C. and C.R.; writing—original draft, V.V.O., M.S. and J.v.D.; writing—review & editing, F.A.H., C.E.M.v.B., D.C., G.T.S., V.F., D.I.B. and J.v.D.

Acknowledgments: We are very thankful to all NTR families for their participation in this study, which involved biosample collection and phenotyping. We are grateful to all the families who took part in the ALSPAC study, the midwives for their help in recruiting them, and the whole ALSPAC team, which includes interviewers, computer and laboratory technicians, clerical workers, research scientists, volunteers, managers, receptionists and nurses.

Abbreviations

CpG	cytosine-phosphate-guanine
EWAS	epigenome-wide association study
NTR	Netherlands Twin Register
ALSPAC	Avon Longitudinal Study of Parents and Children
SES	socio-economic status
GA	gestational age
BMI	body mass index

GEE	generalized estimating equations
mQTL	methylation quantitative trait locus
SNP	single nucleotide polymorphism
MZ	monozygotic
DZ	dizygotic

References

1. Godfrey, K.M.; Lillycrop, K.A.; Burdge, G.C.; Gluckman, P.D.; Hanson, M.A. Epigenetic Mechanisms and the Mismatch Concept of the Developmental Origins of Health and Disease. *Pediatr. Res.* **2007**, *61*, 5R–10R. [CrossRef]
2. Gluckman, P.D.; Hanson, M.A.; Low, F.M. The role of developmental plasticity and epigenetics in human health. *Birth Defects Res. Part C Embryo Today Rev.* **2011**, *93*, 12–18. [CrossRef]
3. Verduci, E.; Banderali, G.; Barberi, S.; Radaelli, G.; Lops, A.; Betti, F.; Riva, E.; Giovannini, M. Epigenetic Effects of Human Breast Milk. *Nutrients* **2014**, *6*, 1711–1724. [CrossRef]
4. Langley-Evans, S.C. Nutrition in Early Life and the Programming of Adult Disease: A Review. *J. Hum. Nutr. Diet.* **2015**, *28*, 1–14. [CrossRef]
5. Hochberg, Z.; Feil, R.; Constancia, M.; Fraga, M.; Junien, C.; Carel, J.-C.; Boileau, P.; Le Bouc, Y.; Deal, C.L.; Lillycrop, K.; et al. Child Health, Developmental Plasticity, and Epigenetic Programming. *Endocr. Rev.* **2011**, *32*, 159–224. [CrossRef]
6. Raghuraman, S.; Donkin, I.; Versteyhe, S.; Barrès, R.; Simar, D. The Emerging Role of Epigenetics in Inflammation and Immunometabolism. *Trends Endocrinol. Metab.* **2016**, *27*, 782–795. [CrossRef] [PubMed]
7. Paparo, L.; Di Costanzo, M.; Di Scala, C.; Cosenza, L.; Leone, L.; Nocerino, R.; Canani, R.B. The Influence of Early Life Nutrition on Epigenetic Regulatory Mechanisms of the Immune System. *Nutrients* **2014**, *6*, 4706–4719. [CrossRef] [PubMed]
8. Canani, R.B.; Di Costanzo, M.; Leone, L.; Bedogni, G.; Brambilla, P.; Cianfarani, S.; Nobili, V.; Pietrobelli, A.; Agostoni, C. Epigenetic mechanisms elicited by nutrition in early life. *Nutr. Res. Rev.* **2011**, *24*, 198–205. [CrossRef] [PubMed]
9. Wadhwa, P.D.; Buss, C.; Entringer, S.; Swanson, J.M. Developmental origins of health and disease: Brief history of the approach and current focus on epigenetic mechanisms. *Semin. Reprod. Med.* **2009**, *27*, 358–368. [CrossRef] [PubMed]
10. Gluckman, P.D.; Hanson, M.A.; Beedle, A.S. Early Life Events and Their Consequences for Later Disease: A Life History and Evolutionary Perspective. *Am. J. Hum. Biol.* **2007**, *19*, 1–19. [CrossRef]
11. Bateson, P.; Barker, D.; Clutton-Brock, T.; Deb, D.; D'Udine, B.; Foley, R.A.; Gluckman, P.; Godfrey, K.; Kirkwood, T.; Lahr, M.M.; et al. Developmental Plasticity and Human Health. *Nature* **2004**, *430*, 419–421. [CrossRef] [PubMed]
12. Choi, S.-W.; Friso, S. Epigenetics: A New Bridge between Nutrition and Health. *Adv. Nutr.* **2010**, *1*, 8–16. [CrossRef] [PubMed]
13. Peter, C.J.; Fischer, L.K.; Kundakovic, M.; Garg, P.; Jakovcevski, M.; Dincer, A.; Amaral, A.C.; Ginns, E.I.; Galdzicka, M.; Bryce, C.P.; et al. DNA Methylation Signatures of Early Childhood Malnutrition Associated With Impairments in Attention and Cognition. *Boil. Psychiatry* **2016**, *80*, 765–774. [CrossRef] [PubMed]
14. Waterland, R.A.; Michels, K.B. Epigenetic Epidemiology of the Developmental Origins Hypothesis. *Annu. Rev. Nutr.* **2007**, *27*, 363–388. [CrossRef]
15. Cutfield, W.S.; Hofman, P.L.; Mitchell, M.; Morison, I.M. Could Epigenetics Play a Role in the Developmental Origins of Health and Disease? *Pediatr. Res.* **2007**, *61*, 68R–75R. [CrossRef]
16. Tammen, S.A.; Friso, S.; Choi, S.-W. Epigenetics: The Link between Nature and Nurture. *Mol. Asp. Med.* **2013**, *34*, 753–764. [CrossRef]
17. Faa, G.; Manchia, M.; Pintus, R.; Gerosa, C.; Marcialis, M.A.; Fanos, V. Fetal programming of neuropsychiatric disorders. *Birth Defects Res. Part C Embryo Today Rev.* **2016**, *108*, 207–223. [CrossRef]
18. Heijmans, B.T.; Tobi, E.W.; Stein, A.D.; Putter, H.; Blauw, G.J.; Susser, E.S.; Slagboom, P.E.; Lumey, L.H. Persistent epigenetic differences associated with prenatal exposure to famine in humans. *Proc. Natl. Acad. Sci. USA* **2008**, *105*, 17046–17049. [CrossRef]

19. Tobi, E.W.; Goeman, J.J.; Monajemi, R.; Gu, H.; Putter, H.; Zhang, Y.; Slieker, R.C.; Stok, A.P.; Thijssen, P.E.; Müller, F.; et al. DNA methylation signatures link prenatal famine exposure to growth and metabolism. *Nat. Commun.* **2014**, *5*, 5592. [CrossRef]
20. Barker, D.J. The fetal and infant origins of adult disease. *BMJ* **1990**, *301*, 1111. [CrossRef]
21. Ruiz, L.; García-Carral, C.; Rodriguez, J.M. Unfolding the Human Milk Microbiome Landscape in the Omics Era. *Front. Microbiol.* **2019**, *10*, 1378. [CrossRef] [PubMed]
22. Fanos, V.; Reali, A.; Marcialis, M.A.; Bardanzellu, F. What You Have to Know about Human Milk Oligosaccharides. *J. Pediatr. Neonatal Individ. Med.* **2018**, *7*, e070137.
23. Hassiotou, F.; Beltran, A.; Chetwynd, E.; Stuebe, A.M.; Twigger, A.-J.; Metzger, P.; Trengove, N.; Lai, C.T.; Filgueira, L.; Blancafort, P.; et al. Breastmilk Is a Novel Source of Stem Cells with Multilineage Differentiation Potential. *Stem Cells* **2012**, *30*, 2164–2174. [CrossRef] [PubMed]
24. Bardanzellu, F.; Fanos, V.; Reali, A. "Omics" in Human Colostrum and Mature Milk: Looking to Old Data with New Eyes. *Nutrients* **2017**, *9*, 843. [CrossRef] [PubMed]
25. Dessì, A.; Briana, D.; Corbu, S.; Gavrili, S.; Marincola, F.C.; Georgantzi, S.; Pintus, R.; Fanos, V.; Malamitsi-Puchner, A. Metabolomics of Breast Milk: The Importance of Phenotypes. *Metabolites* **2018**, *8*, 79. [CrossRef]
26. Forsum, E.; Lonnerdal, B. Variation in the contents of nutrients of breast milk during one feeding. *Nutrients Rep. Int.* **1979**, *19*, 815–820.
27. Victora, C.G.; Bahl, R.; Barros, A.J.D.; França, G.V.A.; Horton, S.; Krasevec, J.; Murch, S.; Sankar, M.J.; Walker, N.; Rollins, N.C.; et al. Breastfeeding in the 21st Century: Epidemiology, Mechanisms, and Lifelong Effect. *Lancet* **2016**, *387*, 475–490. [CrossRef]
28. McInerny, T.K. Breastfeeding, Early Brain Development, and Epigenetics—Getting Children off to Their Best Start. *Breastfeed. Med.* **2014**, *9*, 333–334. [CrossRef]
29. Ip, S.; Chung, M.; Raman, G.; Chew, P.; Magula, N.; Devine, D.; Trikalinos, T.; Lau, J. Breastfeeding and maternal and infant health outcomes in developed countries. *Évid. Rep. Assess.* **2007**, *153*, 1–186.
30. Wisnieski, L.; Kerver, J.; Holzman, C.; Todem, D.; Margerison-Zilko, C. Breastfeeding and Risk of Metabolic Syndrome in Children and Adolescents: A Systematic Review. *J. Hum. Lact.* **2018**, *34*, 515–525. [CrossRef]
31. Chirico, G.; Marzollo, R.; Cortinovis, S.; Fonte, C.; Gasparoni, A. Antiinfective Properties of Human Milk. *J. Nutr.* **2008**, *138*, 1801S–1806S. [CrossRef] [PubMed]
32. Martin, C.R.; Ling, P.-R.; Blackburn, G.L. Review of Infant Feeding: Key Features of Breast Milk and Infant Formula. *Nutrients* **2016**, *8*, 279. [CrossRef] [PubMed]
33. Else-Quest, N.M.; Hyde, J.S.; Clark, R. *Breastfeeding, Bonding, and the Mother-Infant Relationship. Merrill-Palmer Quarterly*; Wayne State University Press: Detroit, MI, USA, 2003; pp. 495–517. [CrossRef]
34. WHO. *Protecting, Promoting, and Supporting Breastfeeding in Facilities Providing Maternity and Newborn Services: The Revised Baby-Friendly Hospital Initiative 2018*; WHO: Geneva, Switzerland, 2019.
35. Michaelsen, K.F.; Lauritzen, L.; Mortensen, E.L. Effects of Breast-Feeding on Cognitive Function. In *Breast-Feeding: Early Influences on Later Health*; Springer: Dordrecht, The Netherlands, 2009; Volume 639, pp. 199–215. [CrossRef]
36. Kramer, M.S.; Aboud, F.; Mironova, E.; Vanilovich, I.; Platt, R.W.; Matush, L.; Igumnov, S.; Fombonne, E.; Bogdanovich, N.; Ducruet, T.; et al. Breastfeeding and child cognitive development: New evidence from a large randomized trial. *Arch. Gen. Psychiatry* **2008**, *65*, 578–584. [CrossRef] [PubMed]
37. Horta, B.L.; De Mola, C.L.; Victora, C.G. Breastfeeding and intelligence: A systematic review and meta-analysis. *Acta Paediatr.* **2015**, *104*, 14–19. [CrossRef]
38. Blesa, M.; Sullivan, G.; Anblagan, D.; Telford, E.J.; Quigley, A.J.; Sparrow, S.A.; Serag, A.; Semple, S.I.; Bastin, M.E.; Boardman, J.P. Early breast milk exposure modifies brain connectivity in preterm infants. *NeuroImage* **2019**, *184*, 431–439. [CrossRef]
39. Bartels, M.; Van Beijsterveldt, C.E.M.; Boomsma, D.I. Breastfeeding, Maternal Education and Cognitive Function: A Prospective Study in Twins. *Behav. Genet.* **2009**, *39*, 616–622. [CrossRef]
40. Harder, T.; Bergmann, R.; Kallischnigg, G.; Plagemann, A. Duration of Breastfeeding and Risk of Overweight: A Meta-Analysis. *Am. J. Epidemiol.* **2005**, *162*, 397–403. [CrossRef]
41. Burke, V.; Beilin, L.J.; Simmer, K.; Oddy, W.H.; Blake, K.V.; Doherty, D.; Kendall, G.E.; Newnham, J.P.; Landau, L.I.; Stanley, F.J. Breastfeeding and Overweight: Longitudinal Analysis in an Australian Birth Cohort. *J. Pediatr.* **2005**, *147*, 56–61. [CrossRef]

42. Gillman, M.W.; Rifas-Shiman, S.L.; Camargo, J.C.A.; Berkey, C.S.; Frazier, A.L.; Rockett, H.R.H.; Field, A.E.; Colditz, G.A. Risk of Overweight Among Adolescents Who Were Breastfed as Infants. *JAMA* **2001**, *285*, 2461. [CrossRef]
43. Owen, C.G.; Whincup, P.H.; Odoki, K.; Gilg, J.A.; Cook, D.G. Infant feeding and blood cholesterol: A study in adolescents and a systematic review. *Pediatrics* **2002**, *110*, 597–608. [CrossRef]
44. Shoji, H.; Shimizu, T. Effect of Human Breast Milk on Biological Metabolism in Infants. *Pediatr. Int.* **2019**, *61*, 6–15. [CrossRef] [PubMed]
45. Klement, E.; Cohen, R.V.; Boxman, J.; Joseph, A.; Reif, S. Breastfeeding and risk of inflammatory bowel disease: A systematic review with meta-analysis. *Am. J. Clin. Nutr.* **2004**, *80*, 1342–1352. [CrossRef] [PubMed]
46. Amitay, E.L.; Keinan-Boker, L. Breastfeeding and childhood leukemia incidence: A meta-analysis and systematic review. *JAMA Pediatr.* **2015**, *169*, e151025. [CrossRef] [PubMed]
47. Horta, B.L.; Victora, C.G.; World Health Organization. *Short-Term Effects of Breastfeeding: A Systematic Review on the Benefits of Breastfeeding on Diarrhoea and Pneumonia Mortality*; World Health Organization: Geneva, Switzerland, 2013.
48. Horta, B.L.; De Mola, C.L.; Victora, C.G. Long-term consequences of breastfeeding on cholesterol, obesity, systolic blood pressure and type 2 diabetes: A systematic review and meta-analysis. *Acta Paediatr.* **2015**, *104*, 30–37. [CrossRef]
49. Lodge, C.; Tan, D.; Lau, M.; Dai, X.; Tham, R.; Lowe, A.; Bowatte, G.; Allen, K.; Dharmage, S.; Lodge, C. Breastfeeding and asthma and allergies: A systematic review and meta-analysis. *Acta Paediatr.* **2015**, *104*, 38–53. [CrossRef]
50. Fall, C.H.; Borja, J.B.; Osmond, C.; Richter, L.; Bhargava, S.K.; Martorell, R.; Stein, A.D.; Barros, F.C.; Victora, C.G.; COHORTS group. Infant-Feeding Patterns and Cardiovascular Risk Factors in Young Adulthood: Data from Five Cohorts in Low- and Middle-Income Countries. *Int. J. Epidemiol.* **2011**, *40*, 47–62. [CrossRef]
51. Hartwig, F.P.; Loret de Mola, C.; Davies, N.M.; Victora, C.G.; Relton, C.L. Breastfeeding Effects on DNA Methylation in the Offspring: A Systematic Literature Review. *PLoS ONE* **2017**, *12*, e0173070.
52. Obermann-Borst, S.A.; Eilers, P.H.; Tobi, E.W.; De Jong, F.H.; Slagboom, P.E.; Heijmans, B.T.; Steegers-Theunissen, R.P.; Slagboom, P. Duration of breastfeeding and gender are associated with methylation of the LEPTIN gene in very young children. *Pediatr. Res.* **2013**, *74*, 344–349. [CrossRef]
53. Naumova, O.Y.; Odintsova, V.V.; Arincina, I.A.; Rychkov, S.Y.; Muhamedrahimov, R.J.; Shneider, Y.V.; Grosheva, A.N.; Zhukova, O.V.; Grigorenko, E.L. A Study of the Association between Breastfeeding and DNA Methylation in Peripheral Blood Cells of Infants. *Russ. J. Genet.* **2019**, *55*, 749–755. [CrossRef]
54. Rossnerova, A.; Tulupova, E.; Tabashidze, N.; Schmuczerova, J.; Dostal, M.; Jr, P.R.; Gmuender, H.; Sram, R.J. Factors affecting the 27K DNA methylation pattern in asthmatic and healthy children from locations with various environments. *Mutat. Res. Mol. Mech. Mutagen.* **2013**, *741*, 18–26. [CrossRef]
55. Sherwood, W.B.; Bion, V.; Lockett, G.A.; Ziyab, A.H.; Soto-Ramírez, N.; Mukherjee, N.; Kurukulaaratchy, R.J.; Ewart, S.; Zhang, H.; Arshad, S.H.; et al. Duration of breastfeeding is associated with leptin (LEP) DNA methylation profiles and BMI in 10-year-old children. *Clin. Epigenet.* **2019**, *11*, 128. [CrossRef] [PubMed]
56. Joubert, B.R.; Felix, J.F.; Yousefi, P.; Bakulski, K.M.; Just, A.C.; Breton, C.; Reese, S.E.; Markunas, C.A.; Richmond, R.C.; Xu, C.-J.; et al. DNA Methylation in Newborns and Maternal Smoking in Pregnancy: Genome-wide Consortium Meta-analysis. *Am. J. Hum. Genet.* **2016**, *98*, 680–696. [CrossRef] [PubMed]
57. Küpers, L.K.; Monnereau, C.; Sharp, G.C.; Yousefi, P.; Salas, L.A.; Ghantous, A.; Page, C.M.; Reese, S.E.; Wilcox, A.J.; Czamara, D.; et al. Meta-analysis of epigenome-wide association studies in neonates reveals widespread differential DNA methylation associated with birthweight. *Nat. Commun.* **2019**, *10*, 1893. [CrossRef] [PubMed]
58. Soto-Ramírez, N.; Arshad, S.H.; Holloway, J.W.; Zhang, H.; Schauberger, E.; Ewart, S.; Patil, V.; Karmaus, W. The interaction of genetic variants and DNA methylation of the interleukin-4 receptor gene increase the risk of asthma at age 18 years. *Clin. Epigenet.* **2013**, *5*, 1. [CrossRef]
59. Tao, M.-H.; Marian, C.; Shields, P.G.; Potischman, N.; Nie, J.; Krishnan, S.S.; Berry, D.L.; Kallakury, B.V.; Ambrosone, C.; Edge, S.B.; et al. Exposures in early life: Associations with DNA promoter methylation in breast tumors. *J. Dev. Orig. Health Dis.* **2013**, *4*, 182–190. [CrossRef]

60. Hartwig, F.P.; Smith, G.D.; Simpkin, A.J.; Victora, C.G.; Relton, C.L.; Caramaschi, D. Association between Breastfeeding and DNA Methylation over the Life Course: Findings from the Avon Longitudinal Study of Parents and Children (ALSPAC). *bioRxiv* **2019**, 800722. [CrossRef]
61. Smith, A.K.; Kilaru, V.; Klengel, T.; Mercer, K.B.; Bradley, B.; Conneely, K.N.; Ressler, K.J.; Binder, E.B. DNA Extracted from Saliva for Methylation Studies of Psychiatric Traits: Evidence Tissue Specificity and Relatedness to Brain. *Am. J. Med. Genet. Part B Neuropsychiatr. Genet.* **2015**, *168*, 36–44. [CrossRef]
62. Papavassiliou, P.; York, T.P.; Gursoy, N.; Hill, G.; Nicely, L.V.; Sundaram, U.; McClain, A.; Aggen, S.H.; Eaves, L.; Riley, B.; et al. The phenotype of persons having mosaicism for trisomy 21/Down syndrome reflects the percentage of trisomic cells present in different tissues. *Am. J. Med. Genet. Part A* **2009**, *149*, 573–583. [CrossRef]
63. Van Dongen, J.; Ehli, E.A.; Jansen, R.; Van Beijsterveldt, C.E.M.; Willemsen, G.; Hottenga, J.J.; Kallsen, N.A.; Peyton, S.A.; Breeze, C.E.; Kluft, C.; et al. Genome-wide analysis of DNA methylation in buccal cells: A study of monozygotic twins and mQTLs. *Epigenet. Chromatin* **2018**, *11*, 54. [CrossRef]
64. Van Beijsterveldt, C.E.M.; Groen-Blokhuis, M.; Hottenga, J.J.; Franić, S.; Hudziak, J.J.; Lamb, D.; Huppertz, C.; de Zeeuw, E.; Nivard, M.; Schutte, N.; et al. The Young Netherlands Twin Register (YNTR): Longitudinal Twin and Family Studies in Over 70,000 Children. *Twin Res. Hum. Genet.* **2013**, *16*, 252–267. [CrossRef]
65. Boomsma, D.I.; Fanos Cagliari, V.; Mussap Genoa, M.; Del Vecchio Bari, A.; Sun Shanghai, B.; Faa Cagliari, G.; Giordano Philadelphia, A. Aggression in Children: Unravelling the Interplay of Genes and Environment through (Epi)Genetics and Metabolomics. *J. Pediatr. Neonatal Individ. Med.* **2015**, *4*. [CrossRef]
66. Bartels, M.; Hendriks, A.; Mauri, M.; Krapohl, E.; Whipp, A.; Bolhuis, K.; Conde, L.C.; Luningham, J.; Ip, H.F.; Hagenbeek, F.; et al. Childhood aggression and the co-occurrence of behavioural and emotional problems: Results across ages 3-16 years from multiple raters in six cohorts in the EU-ACTION project. *Eur. Child Adolesc. Psychiatry* **2018**, *27*, 1105–1121. [CrossRef] [PubMed]
67. Hagenbeek, F.A.; Roetman, P.J.; Pool, R.; Kluft, C.; Harms, A.C.; van Dongen, J.; Colins, O.F.; Talens, S.; Van Beijsterveldt, C.E.M.; de Zeeuw, E.L.; et al. Urinary Amine and Organic Acid Metabolites Evaluated as Markers for Childhood Aggression: The ACTION Biomarker Study. *Frontiers in Psychiatry* **2019**, submitted.
68. Van Dongen, J. Epigenome-Wide Association Study Meta-Analysis of Aggressive Behavior. In Proceedings of the ECS Workshop on Aggression, Nijmegen, The Netherlands, 31 October 2016.
69. Boyd, A.; Golding, J.; Macleod, J.; Lawlor, D.A.; Fraser, A.; Henderson, J.; Molloy, L.; Ness, A.; Ring, S.; Davey Smith, G. Cohort Profile: The 'Children of the 90s'—The Index Offspring of the Avon Longitudinal Study of Parents and Children. *Int. J. Epidemiol.* **2013**, *42*, 111–127. [CrossRef]
70. Fraser, A.; Macdonald-Wallis, C.; Tilling, K.; Boyd, A.; Golding, J.; Davey Smith, G.; Henderson, J.; Macleod, J.; Molloy, L.; Ness, A.; et al. Cohort Profile: The Avon Longitudinal Study of Parents and Children: ALSPAC Mothers Cohort. *Int. J. Epidemiol.* **2013**, *42*, 97–110. [CrossRef]
71. Relton, C.L.; Gaunt, T.; McArdle, W.; Ho, K.; Duggirala, A.; Shihab, H.; Woodward, G.; Lyttleton, O.; Evans, D.M.; Reik, W.; et al. Data Resource Profile: Accessible Resource for Integrated Epigenomic Studies (ARIES). *Int. J. Epidemiol.* **2015**, *44*, 1181–1190. [CrossRef]
72. CBS. *Standard Classification of Occupations*; Central Bureau of Statistics: Heerlen/Voorburg, The Netherlands, 2001.
73. Erikson, R.; Goldthorpe, J.H.; Portocarero, L. Intergenerational class mobility and the convergence thesis: England, France and Sweden. *Br. J. Sociol.* **2010**, *61*, 185–219. [CrossRef]
74. Dolan, C.V.; Geels, L.; Vink, J.M.; van Beijsterveldt, C.E.M.; Neale, M.C.; Bartels, M.; Boomsma, D.I. Testing Causal Effects of Maternal Smoking during Pregnancy on Offspring's Externalizing and Internalizing Behavior. *Behav. Genet.* **2016**, *46*, 378–388. [CrossRef]
75. Van Beijsterveldt, C.E.M.T.; Hoekstra, C.; Schats, R.; Montgomery, G.W.; Willemsen, G.; Boomsma, D.I. Mode of Conception of Twin Pregnancies: Willingness to Reply to Survey Items and Comparison of Survey Data to Hospital Records. *Twin Res. Hum. Genet.* **2008**, *11*, 349–351. [CrossRef]
76. Odintsova, V.V.; Dolan, C.V.; Van Beijsterveldt, C.E.M.; De Zeeuw, E.L.; Van Dongen, J.; Boomsma, D.I. Pre- and Perinatal Characteristics Associated with Apgar Scores in a Review and in a New Study of Dutch Twins. *Twin Res. Hum. Genet.* **2019**, *22*, 164–176. [CrossRef]
77. Meulenbelt, I.; Droog, S.; Trommelen, G.J.; Boomsma, D.I.; Slagboom, P.E. High-yield noninvasive human genomic DNA isolation method for genetic studies in geographically dispersed families and populations. *Am. J. Hum. Genet.* **1995**, *57*, 1252–1254. [PubMed]

78. Moran, S.; Arribas, C.; Esteller, M. Validation of a DNA methylation microarray for 850,000 CpG sites of the human genome enriched in enhancer sequences. *Epigenomics* **2016**, *8*, 389–399. [CrossRef] [PubMed]
79. Sinke, L.; van Iterson, M.; Cats, D.; Slieker, R.; Heijmans, B. DNAmArray: Streamlined Workflow for the Quality Control, Normalization, and Analysis of Illumina Methylation Array Data. *Zenodo* **2019**. [CrossRef]
80. Van Iterson, M.; Tobi, E.W.; Slieker, R.C.; Hollander, W.D.; Luijk, R.; Slagboom, P.; Heijmans, B.T. MethylAid: Visual and interactive quality control of large Illumina 450k datasets. *Bioinformatics* **2014**, *30*, 3435–3437. [CrossRef]
81. Van Iterson, M.; Cats, D.; Hop, P.; Heijmans, B.T.; BIOS Consortium. omicsPrint: Detection of data linkage errors in multiple omics studies. *Bioinformatics* **2018**, *34*, 2142–2143. [CrossRef]
82. Min, J.L.; Hemani, G.; Smith, G.D.; Relton, C.; Suderman, M. Meffil: Efficient normalization and analysis of very large DNA methylation datasets. *Bioinformatics* **2018**, *34*, 3983–3989. [CrossRef]
83. Pidsley, R.; Zotenko, E.; Peters, T.J.; Lawrence, M.G.; Risbridger, G.P.; Molloy, P.; Van Djik, S.; Muhlhausler, B.; Stirzaker, C.; Clark, S.J. Critical evaluation of the Illumina MethylationEPIC BeadChip microarray for whole-genome DNA methylation profiling. *Genome Boil.* **2016**, *17*, 208. [CrossRef]
84. Zheng, S.C.; Webster, A.P.; Dong, D.; Feber, A.; Graham, D.G.; Sullivan, R.; Jevons, S.; Lovat, L.B.; Beck, S.; Widschwendter, M.; et al. A novel cell-type deconvolution algorithm reveals substantial contamination by immune cells in saliva, buccal and cervix. *Epigenomics* **2018**, *10*, 925–940. [CrossRef]
85. Houseman, E.A.; Accomando, W.P.; Koestler, D.C.; Christensen, B.C.; Marsit, C.J.; Nelson, H.H.; Wiencke, J.K.; Kelsey, K.T. DNA methylation arrays as surrogate measures of cell mixture distribution. *BMC Bioinform.* **2012**, *13*, 86. [CrossRef]
86. Van Iterson, M.; Van Zwet, E.W.; BIOS Consortium; Heijmans, B.T. Controlling bias and inflation in epigenome- and transcriptome-wide association studies using the empirical null distribution. *Genome Boil.* **2017**, *18*, 19. [CrossRef]
87. Tukey, J.W. Exploratory Data Analysis. *Biom. J.* **1981**, *23*, 413–414.
88. Leek, J.T.; Storey, J.D. Capturing Heterogeneity in Gene Expression Studies by Surrogate Variable Analysis. *PLoS Genet.* **2007**, *3*, e161. [CrossRef] [PubMed]
89. Ritchie, M.E.; Phipson, B.; Wu, D.; Hu, Y.; Law, C.W.; Shi, W.; Smyth, G.K. limma powers differential expression analyses for RNA-sequencing and microarray studies. *Nucleic Acids Res.* **2015**, *43*, e47. [CrossRef] [PubMed]
90. Li, M.; Zou, D.; Li, Z.; Gao, R.; Sang, J.; Zhang, Y.; Li, R.; Xia, L.; Zhang, T.; Niu, G.; et al. EWAS Atlas: A Curated Knowledgebase of Epigenome-Wide Association Studies. *Nucleic Acids Res.* **2019**, *47*, D983–D988. [CrossRef]
91. Yousefi, P.; Huen, K.; Davé, V.; Barcellos, L.; Eskenazi, B.; Holland, N. Sex differences in DNA methylation assessed by 450 K BeadChip in newborns. *BMC Genom.* **2015**, *16*, 911. [CrossRef]
92. Husquin, L.T.; Rotival, M.; Fagny, M.; Quach, H.; Zidane, N.; McEwen, L.M.; MacIsaac, J.L.; Kobor, M.S.; Aschard, H.; Patin, E.; et al. Exploring the genetic basis of human population differences in DNA methylation and their causal impact on immune gene regulation. *Genome Boil.* **2018**, *19*, 222. [CrossRef]
93. Marioni, R.E.; Harris, S.E.; Zhang, Q.; McRae, A.F.; Hagenaars, S.P.; Hill, W.D.; Davies, G.; Ritchie, C.W.; Gale, C.R.; Starr, J.M.; et al. GWAS on family history of Alzheimer's disease. *Transl. Psychiatry* **2018**, *8*, 99. [CrossRef]
94. Xue, J.; Gharaibeh, R.Z.; Pietryk, E.W.; Brouwer, C.; Tarantino, L.M.; Valdar, W.; Ideraabdullah, F.Y. Impact of vitamin D depletion during development on mouse sperm DNA methylation. *Epigenetics* **2018**, *13*, 959–974. [CrossRef]
95. Sujit, K.M.; Sarkar, S.; Singh, V.; Pandey, R.; Agrawal, N.K.; Trivedi, S.; Singh, K.; Gupta, G.; Rajender, S. Genome-wide differential methylation analyses identifies methylation signatures of male infertility. *Hum. Reprod.* **2018**, *33*, 2256–2267. [CrossRef]
96. Kim, S.K. Identification of 613 new loci associated with heel bone mineral density and a polygenic risk score for bone mineral density, osteoporosis and fracture. *PLoS ONE* **2018**, *13*, e0200785. [CrossRef]
97. Morris, J.A.; Kemp, J.P.; Youlten, S.E.; Laurent, L.; Logan, J.G.; Chai, R.C.; Vulpescu, N.A.; Forgetta, V.; Kleinman, A.; Mohanty, S.T.; et al. An Atlas of Genetic Influences on Osteoporosis in Humans and Mice. *Nat. Genet.* **2019**, *51*, 258–266. [CrossRef] [PubMed]
98. Kemp, J.P.; Morris, J.A.; Medina-Gomez, C.; Forgetta, V.; Warrington, N.M.; Youlten, S.E.; Zheng, J.;

Gregson, C.L.; Grundberg, E.; Trajanoska, K.; et al. Identification of 153 new loci associated with heel bone mineral density and functional involvement of GPC6 in osteoporosis. *Nat. Genet.* **2017**, *49*, 1468–1475. [CrossRef] [PubMed]

99. Estrada, K.; Styrkarsdottir, U.; Evangelou, E.; Hsu, Y.-H.; Duncan, E.L.; Ntzani, E.E.; Oei, L.; Albagha, O.M.E.; Amin, N.; Kemp, J.P.; et al. Genome-wide meta-analysis identifies 56 bone mineral density loci and reveals 14 loci associated with risk of fracture. *Nat. Genet.* **2012**, *44*, 491–501. [CrossRef] [PubMed]
100. Medina-Gómez, C.; Kemp, J.P.; Trajanoska, K.; Luan, J.; Chesi, A.; Ahluwalia, T.S.; Mook-Kanamori, D.O.; Ham, A.; Hartwig, F.P.; Evans, D.S.; et al. Life-Course Genome-wide Association Study Meta-analysis of Total Body BMD and Assessment of Age-Specific Effects. *Am. J. Hum. Genet.* **2018**, *102*, 88–102. [CrossRef] [PubMed]
101. Emilsson, V.; Ilkov, M.; Lamb, J.R.; Finkel, N.; Gudmundsson, E.F.; Pitts, R.; Hoover, H.; Gudmundsdottir, V.; Horman, S.R.; Aspelund, T.; et al. Co-regulatory networks of human serum proteins link genetics to disease. *Science* **2018**, *361*, 769–773. [CrossRef] [PubMed]
102. Sun, B.B.; Maranville, J.C.; Peters, J.E.; Stacey, D.; Staley, J.R.; Blackshaw, J.; Burgess, S.; Jiang, T.; Paige, E.; Surendran, P.; et al. Genomic atlas of the human plasma proteome. *Nature* **2018**, *558*, 73–79. [CrossRef] [PubMed]
103. De Vries, P.S.; Brown, M.R.; Bentley, A.R.; Sung, Y.J.; Winkler, T.W.; Ntalla, I.; Schwander, K.; Kraja, A.T.; Guo, X.; Franceschini, N.; et al. Multiancestry Genome-Wide Association Study of Lipid Levels Incorporating Gene-Alcohol Interactions. *Am. J. Epidemiol.* **2019**, *188*, 1033–1054. [CrossRef]
104. Imaizumi, A.; Adachi, Y.; Kawaguchi, T.; Higasa, K.; Tabara, Y.; Sonomura, K.; Sato, T.-A.; Takahashi, M.; Mizukoshi, T.; Yoshida, H.-O.; et al. Genetic basis for plasma amino acid concentrations based on absolute quantification: A genome-wide association study in the Japanese population. *Eur. J. Hum. Genet.* **2019**, *27*, 621–630. [CrossRef]
105. Shin, S.-Y.; The Multiple Tissue Human Expression Resource (MuTHER) Consortium; Fauman, E.B.; Petersen, A.-K.; Krumsiek, J.; Santos, R.; Huang, J.; Arnold, M.; Erte, I.; Forgetta, V.; et al. An atlas of genetic influences on human blood metabolites. *Nat. Genet.* **2014**, *46*, 543–550. [CrossRef]
106. Johnston, K.J.A.; Adams, M.J.; Nicholl, B.I.; Ward, J.; Strawbridge, R.J.; Ferguson, A.; McIntosh, A.M.; Bailey, M.E.S.; Smith, D.J. Genome-wide association study of multisite chronic pain in UK Biobank. *PLoS Genet.* **2019**, *15*, e1008164. [CrossRef]
107. Li, Y.; Sekula, P.; Wuttke, M.; Wahrheit, J.; Hausknecht, B.; Schultheiss, U.T.; Gronwald, W.; Schlosser, P.; Tucci, S.; Ekici, A.B.; et al. Genome-Wide Association Studies of Metabolites in Patients with CKD Identify Multiple Loci and Illuminate Tubular Transport Mechanisms. *J. Am. Soc. Nephrol.* **2018**, *29*, 1513–1524. [CrossRef] [PubMed]
108. Wellcome Trust Case Control Consortium. Genome-Wide Association Study of 14,000 Cases of Seven Common Diseases and 3000 Shared Controls. *Nature* **2007**, *447*, 661–678. [CrossRef] [PubMed]
109. Liu, M.; Jiang, Y.; Wedow, R.; Li, Y.; Brazel, D.M.; Chen, F.; Datta, G.; Davila-Velderrain, J.; McGuire, D.; Tian, C.; et al. Association studies of up to 1.2 million individuals yield new insights into the genetic etiology of tobacco and alcohol use. *Nat. Genet.* **2019**, *51*, 237–244. [CrossRef] [PubMed]
110. Linnér, R.K.; Biroli, P.; Kong, E.; Meddens, S.F.W.; Wedow, R.; Fontana, M.A.; Lebreton, M.; Tino, S.P.; Abdellaoui, A.; Hammerschlag, A.R.; et al. Genome-wide association analyses of risk tolerance and risky behaviors in over 1 million individuals identify hundreds of loci and shared genetic influences. *Nat. Genet.* **2019**, *51*, 245–257. [CrossRef]
111. Hosokawa, N.; Sasaki, T.; Iemura, S.; Natsume, T.; Hara, T.; Mizushima, N. Atg101, a Novel Mammalian Autophagy Protein Interacting with Atg13. *Autophagy* **2009**, *5*, 973–979. [CrossRef]
112. Ahola-Olli, A.V.; Würtz, P.; Havulinna, A.S.; Aalto, K.; Pitkänen, N.; Lehtimäki, T.; Kähönen, M.; Lyytikäinen, L.-P.; Raitoharju, E.; Seppälä, I.; et al. Genome-Wide Association Study Identifies 27 Loci Influencing Concentrations of Circulating Cytokines and Growth Factors. *Am. J. Hum. Genet.* **2017**, *100*, 40–50. [CrossRef]
113. Astle, W.J.; Elding, H.; Jiang, T.; Allen, D.; Ruklisa, D.; Mann, A.L.; Mead, D.; Bouman, H.; Riveros-McKay, F.; Kostadima, M.A.; et al. The Allelic Landscape of Human Blood Cell Trait Variation and Links to Common Complex Disease. *Cell* **2016**, *167*, 1415–1429. [CrossRef]
114. Rojas, D.; Rager, J.E.; Smeester, L.; Bailey, K.A.; Drobná, Z.; Rubio-Andrade, M.; Stýblo, M.; García-Vargas, G.; Fry, R.C. Prenatal Arsenic Exposure and the Epigenome: Identifying Sites of 5-Methylcytosine Alterations

That Predict Functional Changes in Gene Expression in Newborn Cord Blood and Subsequent Birth Outcomes. *Toxicol. Sci.* **2015**, *143*, 97–106. [CrossRef]

115. McNally, K.E.; Faulkner, R.; Steinberg, F.; Gallon, M.; Ghai, R.; Pim, D.; Langton, P.; Pearson, N.; Danson, C.M.; Nägele, H.; et al. Retriever is a multiprotein complex for retromer-independent endosomal cargo recycling. *Nature* **2017**, *19*, 1214–1225. [CrossRef]
116. Johansson, Å.; Enroth, S.; Gyllensten, U. Continuous Aging of the Human DNA Methylome Throughout the Human Lifespan. *PLoS ONE* **2013**, *8*, e67378. [CrossRef]
117. Gervin, K.; Andreassen, B.K.; Hjorthaug, H.S.; Carlsen, K.C.L.; Carlsen, K.-H.; Undlien, D.E.; Lyle, R.; Munthe-Kaas, M.C. Intra-individual changes in DNA methylation not mediated by cell-type composition are correlated with aging during childhood. *Clin. Epigenet.* **2016**, *8*, 110. [CrossRef] [PubMed]
118. Dunn, E.C.; Soare, T.W.; Simpkin, A.J.; Suderman, M.J.; Zhu, Y.; Klengel, T.; Smith, A.D.A.C.; Ressler, K.; Relton, C.L. Sensitive Periods for the Effect of Childhood Adversity on DNA Methylation: Results from a Prospective, Longitudinal Study. *bioRxiv* **2018**. [CrossRef] [PubMed]
119. Simpkin, A.J.; Suderman, M.; Gaunt, T.R.; Lyttleton, O.; McArdle, W.L.; Ring, S.M.; Tilling, K.; Smith, G.D.; Relton, C.L. Longitudinal analysis of DNA methylation associated with birth weight and gestational age. *Hum. Mol. Genet.* **2015**, *24*, 3752–3763. [CrossRef] [PubMed]
120. Agha, G.; Hajj, H.; Rifas-Shiman, S.L.; Just, A.C.; Hivert, M.-F.; Burris, H.H.; Lin, X.; Litonjua, A.A.; Oken, E.; DeMeo, D.L.; et al. Birth weight-for-gestational age is associated with DNA methylation at birth and in childhood. *Clin. Epigenet.* **2016**, *8*, 118. [CrossRef] [PubMed]
121. Alfano, R.; Guida, F.; Galobardes, B.; Chadeau-Hyam, M.; Delpierre, C.; Ghantous, A.; Henderson, J.; Herceg, Z.; Jain, P.; Nawrot, T.S.; et al. Socioeconomic position during pregnancy and DNA methylation signatures at three stages across early life: Epigenome-wide association studies in the ALSPAC birth cohort. *Int. J. Epidemiol.* **2019**, *48*, 30–44. [CrossRef] [PubMed]
122. Richmond, R.C.; Simpkin, A.J.; Woodward, G.; Gaunt, T.R.; Lyttleton, O.; McArdle, W.L.; Ring, S.M.; Smith, A.D.A.C.; Timpson, N.J.; Tilling, K.; et al. Prenatal Exposure to Maternal Smoking and Offspring DNA Methylation across the Lifecourse: Findings from the Avon Longitudinal Study of Parents and Children (ALSPAC). *Hum. Mol. Genet.* **2015**, *24*, 2201–2217. [CrossRef]
123. Tobi, E.W.; Lumey, L.H.; Talens, R.P.; Kremer, D.; Putter, H.; Stein, A.D.; Slagboom, P.E.; Heijmans, B.T. DNA methylation differences after exposure to prenatal famine are common and timing- and sex-specific. *Hum. Mol. Genet.* **2009**, *18*, 4046–4053. [CrossRef]
124. Muniz, L.C.; Menezes, A.M.B.; Buffarini, R.; Wehrmeister, F.C.; Assunção, M.C.F. Effect of Breastfeeding on Bone Mass from Childhood to Adulthood: A Systematic Review of the Literature. *Int. Breastfeed. J.* **2015**, *10*, 31. [CrossRef]
125. Dessì, A.; Murgia, A.; Agostino, R.; Pattumelli, M.G.; Schirru, A.; Scano, P.; Fanos, V.; Caboni, P. Exploring the Role of Different Neonatal Nutrition Regimens during the First Week of Life by Urinary GC-MS Metabolomics. *Int. J. Mol. Sci.* **2016**, *17*, 265. [CrossRef]
126. San-Cristobal, R.; Navas-Carretero, S.; Milagro, F.I.; Riezu-Boj, J.I.; Guruceaga, E.; Celis-Morales, C.; Livingstone, K.M.; Brennan, L.; Lovegrove, J.A.; Daniel, H.; et al. Gene methylation parallelisms between peripheral blood cells and oral mucosa samples in relation to overweight. *J. Physiol. Biochem.* **2016**, *73*, 465–474. [CrossRef]
127. Van Dongen, J.; Nivard, M.G.; Willemsen, G.; Hottenga, J.-J.; Helmer, Q.; Dolan, C.V.; Ehli, E.A.; Davies, G.E.; Van Iterson, M.; Breeze, C.E.; et al. Genetic and environmental influences interact with age and sex in shaping the human methylome. *Nat. Commun.* **2016**, *7*, 11115. [CrossRef] [PubMed]
128. Colodro-Conde, L.; Sánchez-Romera, J.F.; Ordoñana, J.R. Heritability of Initiation and Duration of Breastfeeding Behavior. *Twin Res. Hum. Genet.* **2013**, *16*, 575–580. [CrossRef] [PubMed]
129. Merjonen, P.; Dolan, C.V.; Bartels, M.; Boomsma, D.I. Does Breastfeeding Behavior Run in Families? Evidence from Twins, Their Sisters and Their Mothers in the Netherlands. *Twin Res. Hum. Genet.* **2015**, *18*, 179–187. [CrossRef] [PubMed]
130. Eriksson, N.; Benton, G.M.; Do, C.B.; Kiefer, A.K.; Mountain, J.L.; Hinds, D.A.; Francke, U.; Tung, J.Y. Genetic variants associated with breast size also influence breast cancer risk. *BMC Med. Genet.* **2012**, *13*, 53. [CrossRef] [PubMed]
131. Cunningham, B.; Bass, S.; Fuh, G.; Wells, J. Zinc mediation of the binding of human growth hormone to the human prolactin receptor. *Science* **1990**, *250*, 1709–1712. [CrossRef]

132. Sukonina, V.; Ma, H.; Zhang, W.; Bartesaghi, S.; Subhash, S.; Heglind, M.; Foyn, H.; Betz, M.J.; Nilsson, D.; Lidell, M.E.; et al. FOXK1 and FOXK2 regulate aerobic glycolysis. *Nature* **2019**, *566*, 279–283. [CrossRef]
133. Hannenhalli, S.; Kaestner, K.H. The evolution of Fox genes and their role in development and disease. *Nat. Rev. Genet.* **2009**, *10*, 233–240. [CrossRef]
134. Tachmazidou, I.; Süveges, D.; Min, J.L.; Ritchie, G.R.; Steinberg, J.; Walter, K.; Iotchkova, V.; Schwartzentruber, J.; Huang, J.; Memari, Y.; et al. Whole-Genome Sequencing Coupled to Imputation Discovers Genetic Signals for Anthropometric Traits. *Am. J. Hum. Genet.* **2017**, *100*, 865–884. [CrossRef]
135. Crujeiras, A.B.; Pissios, P.; Moreno-Navarrete, J.M.; Díaz-Lagares, A.; Sandoval, J.; Gómez, A.; Ricart, W.; Esteller, M.; Casanueva, F.F.; Fernandez-Real, J.M. An Epigenetic Signature in Adipose Tissue Is Linked to Nicotinamide N-Methyltransferase Gene Expression. *Mol. Nutr. Food Res.* **2018**, *62*, 1700933. [CrossRef]
136. Bardanzellu, F.; Fanos, V.; Strigini, F.A.L.; Artini, P.G.; Peroni, D.G. Human Breast Milk: Exploring the Linking Ring Among Emerging Components. *Front. Pediatr.* **2018**, *6*, 215. [CrossRef]
137. Lehmann, G.M.; LaKind, J.S.; Davis, M.H.; Hines, E.P.; Marchitti, S.A.; Alcala, C.; Lorber, M. Environmental Chemicals in Breast Milk and Formula: Exposure and Risk Assessment Implications. *Environ. Health Perspect.* **2018**, *126*, 096001. [CrossRef] [PubMed]
138. Gómez-Gallego, C.; Morales, J.M.; Monleón, D.; Du Toit, E.; Kumar, H.; Linderborg, K.M.; Zhang, Y.; Yang, B.; Isolauri, E.; Salminen, S.; et al. Human Breast Milk NMR Metabolomic Profile across Specific Geographical Locations and Its Association with the Milk Microbiota. *Nutrients* **2018**, *10*, 1355. [CrossRef] [PubMed]
139. Hermansson, H.; Kumar, H.; Collado, M.C.; Salminen, S.; Isolauri, E.; Rautava, S. Breast Milk Microbiota Is Shaped by Mode of Delivery and Intrapartum Antibiotic Exposure. *Front. Nutr.* **2019**, *6*, 4. [CrossRef] [PubMed]

6

Validation and Application of Biocrates Absolute*IDQ*® p180 Targeted Metabolomics Kit Using Human Milk

Daniela Hampel [1,2,*], Setareh Shahab-Ferdows [1], Muttaquina Hossain [3], M. Munirul Islam [3], Tahmeed Ahmed [3] and Lindsay H. Allen [1,2]

1 USDA/ARS Western Human Nutrition Research Center, 430 West Health Sciences Drive, Davis, CA 95616, USA
2 Department of Nutrition, University of California, One Shields Ave, Davis, CA 95616, USA
3 Nutrition and Clinical Services Division, International Centre for Diarrhoeal Disease Research, 68 Shaheed Tajuddin Ahmed Sarani, Mohakhali, Dhaka 1212, Bangladesh
* Correspondence: daniela.hampel@usda.gov or dhampel@ucdavis.edu

Abstract: Human-milk-targeted metabolomics analysis offers novel insights into milk composition and relationships with maternal and infant phenotypes and nutritional status. The Biocrates Absolute*IDQ*® p180 kit, targeting 40 acylcarnitines, 42 amino acids/biogenic amines, 91 phospholipids, 15 sphingolipids, and sum of hexoses, was evaluated for human milk using the AB Sciex 5500 QTRAP mass-spectrometer in liquid chromatography-tandem mass-spectrometry (LC-MS/MS) and flow-injection analysis (FIA) mode. Milk (<6 months lactation) from (A) Bangladeshi apparently healthy mothers (body mass index (BMI) > 18.5; n = 12) and (B) Bangladeshi mothers of stunted infants (height-for-age Z (HAZ)-score <−2; n = 13) was analyzed. Overall, 123 of the possible 188 metabolites were detected in milk. New internal standards and adjusted calibrator levels were used for improved precision and concentration ranges for milk metabolites. Recoveries ranged between 43% and 120% (coefficient of variation (CV): 2.4%–24.1%, 6 replicates). Milk consumed by stunted infants vs. that from mothers with BMI > 18.5 was lower in 6 amino acids/biogenic amines but higher in isovalerylcarnitine, two phospholipids, and one sphingomyelin ($p < 0.05$ for all). Associations between milk metabolites differed between groups. The Absolute*IDQ*® p180 kit is a rapid analysis tool suitable for human milk analysis and reduces analytical bias by allowing the same technique for different specimens. More research is needed to examine milk metabolite relationships with maternal and infant phenotypes.

Keywords: human milk; targeted metabolomics; amino acids; lipid metabolites; LC-MS; flow injection analysis

---

1. Introduction

The postnatal period is a critical stage for infant's physiology, accompanied by rapid changes in brain development, and in metabolic, immunologic, intestinal, and physiological systems [1]. Human milk undergoes dynamic changes in composition during lactation to provide all nutrients and other bioactive substrates for optimal infant growth and development, and exclusive breastfeeding (EBF) is recommended during the first 6 months of life [2]. Even beyond the EBF period, it remains a vital dietary source of nutrients; however, the mechanisms behind its ability to drive and affect infant metabolism, health, development, and long-term outcomes are not fully understood. The recent resurgent interest in human milk composition triggered the development of state-of-the-art methods for analyzing micronutrients [3–10], peptides and oligosaccharides (HMOs) [11,12], the human milk microbiome [13,14], and milk lipids [15,16]. Within this scope, metabolomics provides novel insight into the complexity of the milk metabolome and its influence on infant metabolism and physiology via intestinal enzymes [17,18].

The effects of human milk bioactives on early infant physiology and development are diverse; effects may reach the insulin signaling cascade, the hepatic mitochondrial system, and possibly the mechanistic target of rapamycin (mTOR) signaling pathway, vital to cell growth, protein and lipid synthesis, or lipid and adiposity accumulation and adipogenesis [1,19–22]. On the other hand, associations of human milk metabolites were also found with maternal phenotype and diet [22,23]. The observed relationships of milk metabolites and maternal and infant status and phenotypes demand further investigation and analyzing the human milk metabolome as the interface between mother and infant can provide key information for maternal and infant health. Moreover, milk metabolites are not only derived from maternal blood but also from *de novo* synthesis in the mammary gland [23,24]. Consequently, obtaining the metabolic profile of the mothers as well as their milk may offer important insights into the contributions of the maternal metabolic state to the milk metabolome compared to the mammary-gland-derived compounds. Using the same analytical technique on different matrices reduces method bias and produces more robust results.

The Absolute*IDQ*® p180 kit (https://www.biocrates.com/images/p180_Folder_HP_v01-2018.pdf) from Biocrates Life Science AG covers multiple compound classes (acylcarnitines, amino acids, biogenic amines, sphingolipids, phospholipids, and sum of hexoses) which are involved in various central metabolic processes, such as immune regulation, fatty acid oxidation, membrane composition, cell cycle control, insulin resistance, or nutritional status. While this assay has been validated for various species and matrices, the human milk matrix has not yet been evaluated. Therefore, the purpose of this study was to assess application of this kit for the analysis of human milk metabolites. The validated assay was then used in a feasibility plate to analyze milk samples from (A) apparently healthy Bangladeshi mothers ("BMI > 18.5 mothers" (BMI—body mass index), < 6 months lactation) and (B) mothers of stunted infants ("stunted infants", height-for-age Z (HAZ)-score <−2) as proof of concept.

2. Materials and Methods

2.1. Chemicals and Materials

All reagents, internal and calibration standards, quality controls, test mix, and a patented 96-well filter plate required for the Absolute*IDQ*®p180 analysis were included in the kit or provided by Biocrates Life Science AG (Innsbruck, Austria).

2.2. AbsoluteIDQ® p180 Assay and Sample Preparation

The Absolute*IDQ*® p180 kit is a fully automated assay based on phenylisothiocyanate (PITC) derivatization of the target analytes in bodily fluids (e.g., plasma, serum, urine) using internal standards for quantitation. Amino acids and biogenic amines are determined in LC-MS mode, acylcarnitines, phospholipids (lyso-phosphatidylcholines with acyl residue at CXX:X, phosphatidylcholine with diacyl residue sum CXX:X (PC aa), and phosphatidylcholine with acyl-alkyl residue sum CXX:X (PC ae)), sphingomyelins, and the sum of hexoses are analyzed in flow injection analysis (FIA). Human milk sample preparation was carried out according to the manufacturer's protocol. Briefly, 2 to 10 μL of human milk was transferred to the upper 96-well plate and dried under a nitrogen stream. Thereafter, 50 μL of a 5% PITC solution was added to derivatize amino acids and biogenic amines. After incubation, the filter spots were dried again before the metabolites were extracted using 5 mM ammonium acetate in methanol (300 μL) into the lower 96-well plate for analysis after further dilution using the MS running solvent A. Quantification was carried out using internal standards and a calibration curve (Cal 1 to Cal 7). The experimental metabolomics measurement technique is described in detail by patents EP1897014B1 and EP1875401B1 [25,26]. See Supplementary Materials (Table S1) for the full list of metabolites and their abbreviations.

2.3. LC-MS

The LC-MS/MS system was comprised of an ACQUITY UPLC-system (Waters, Milford, MA, USA) coupled to a QTRAP 5500 mass spectrometer (AB Sciex, Redwood City, CA, USA) in electrospray ionization (ESI) mode. Amino acids and biogenic amines were analyzed via LC-MS in positive mode. Two microliters of the sample extract were injected onto an ACQUITY UPLC BEH C18 column, 2.1 × 7.5 mm, 1.7 μm protected by an ACQUITY BEH C18, 1.7 μm VanGuard pre-column (Waters, Milford, MA, USA) at 50 °C using a 7.3 min solvent gradient employing 0.2% formic acid in water (solvent A) and 0.2% formic acid in acetonitrile (solvent B).

Twenty microliters of the sample extract were used in the flow injection analysis (FIA) in positive mode to capture acylcarnitines, glycerophospholipids, and sphingolipids, while hexoses were monitored in a subsequent run in negative mode. All FIA injections were carried out using the Biocrates MS Running Solvent. Additional LC and MS settings for LC-MS and FIA mode are described in Table 1. All metabolites were identified and quantified using isotopically-labeled internal standards and multiple reaction monitoring (MRM) as optimized and provided by Biocrates Life Sciences AG (Innsbruck, Austria).

Table 1. LC and MS parameters [1].

Instrument	Parameter	LC-MS	FIA (MS Only)
5500 QTRAP MS	CUR	45	20
	IS	5500	5500
	TEM	500	200
	GS1	60	40
	GS2	70	50
	CAD	9	9
	EP	10	10
	CXP	15	15
ACQUITY UPLC	**Time [min]**	**Flow rate [mL/min]**	**Solvent A [%]**
LC-MS	0	0.8	100
	0.45	0.8	100
	3.3	0.8	85
	5.9	0.8	30
	6.05	0.8	0
	6.2	0.9	0
	6.42	0.9	0
	6.52	0.8	0
	6.7	0.8	100
	7.3	0.8	100
FIA	0	0.03	Biocrates Solvent I MS running buffer in isocratic mode
	1.6	0.03	
	2.4	0.2	
	2.8	0.2	
	3.0	0.03	

[1] CUR—curtain gas; IS—ion spray voltage (V);—temperature (°C); GS1/GS2—ion source gas 1 and 2 (psi); CAD—CAD gas (psi); EP—entrance potential (V); CXP—collision cell exit potential (V); LC-MS—liquid chromatography—mass spectrometry; FIA—flow injection analysis.

2.4. Method Validation

Pooled milk was used to evaluate matrix effects and metabolite recovery. The samples were diluted in phosphate buffered saline solution (PBS) 1:2 and 1:5 to assess ion suppression due to the matrix. A 3-level analyte recovery was carried out using Cal 2, 3, and 5 in half, normal, and double concentrations, covering up to 230-fold of the endogenous milk concentrations. All experiments were conducted in replicates of six. Individual milk samples (n = 25) from Bangladeshi women were prepared according to the manufacturer's protocol and analyzed at 3 different sample volumes (2, 5, and 10 μL).

Analyte recovery was calculated using the following equation:

$$\text{Recovery } [\%] = (C_{\text{measured}} - C_{\text{endogenous}}) \times 100/C_{\text{added}} \quad (1)$$

where $C_{measured}$ is the measured concentrations of the spiked sample, $C_{endogenous}$ the measured concentration of the non-spiked sample, and C_{added} the theoretically added concentration by spiking.

Relative recovery in the diluted samples was calculated as follows:

$$\text{Relative recovery } [\%] = C_{X/dF} \times dF \times 100/C_X \quad (2)$$

where $C_{X/dF}$ is the concentration measured in the diluted sample, dF the dilution factor (2 or 5), and C_X the concentrations measured in the non-diluted milk samples.

2.5. Human Milk Samples

To determine recovery rates and evaluate matrix effects, a human milk pool, obtained from milk samples provided by apparently healthy women in the Vancouver, BC, Canada area, was used. Individual milk samples, available in the laboratory but not collected for the purpose of this validation, were analyzed in the feasibility plate. These convenient samples were collected during the first 6 months of lactation from apparently healthy Bangladeshi lactating women ("BMI > 18.5 mothers", body mass index (BMI) > 18.5, n = 12) whose infants' anthropometry was unknown, and Bangladeshi mothers with stunted infants ("stunted infants", HAZ-score < −2, n = 13), to try to obtain a wide range of metabolite concentrations in the milk. All milk samples were shipped from the United States Department of Agriculture – Agricultural Research Service (USDA/ARS) Western Human Nutrition Research Center in Davis, CA, USA on dry ice to Biocrates Life Science AG in Innsbruck, Austria for testing. Upon arrival, samples were stored at −80 °C until analysis.

2.6. Statistical Analysis

Raw data was computed in Met*IDQ*™ version Carbon (Biocrates Life Science AG, Innsbruck, Austria). Mean, standard deviation, and coefficient of variation (CV) for the validation were calculated in Excel 2016 (Microsoft Corporation, Redmond, WA, USA). R statistical software (3.5.2, R Foundation for Statistical Computing) was used for statistical analysis and visualization of the results for the feasibility study. The Wilcoxon rank sum test was used to explore differences in analyte concentrations based on group assignment (BMI > 18.5 mothers vs. stunted infants), and metabolite associations were assessed using Spearman's rank correlation. p-values < 0.05 were considered significant.

3. Results

3.1. Validation Using Pooled Human Milk

3.1.1. LC-MS (Amino Acids and Biogenic Amines)

Since the development of the assay, new internal standards became available for lysine, acetyl-ornithine, alpha-aminoadipic acid, cis-4-OH-proline, histamine, kynurenine, nitro-tyrosine, phenylethylamine (PEA), symmetric dimethylarginine (SDMA), and trans-4-OH-proline. Using these new internal standards, mean CVs (range) were reduced from 11.3% (3.6%–26.6%) to 6.6% (2.3%–11.5%; $p = 0.017$, Student's paired t-test). The quantification of glutamate and taurine required additional calibrators (Cal 8 and 9), which was also true for putrescine (Cal 8). Saturation effects were observed for proline, tryptophan, and valine at Cal 5 and Cal 6 levels. The sensitivity of the 5500 QTRAP MS-system allowed the extension to calibrators (Cal 0.5 and 0.25) for most of the metabolites and was needed for asparagine, methionine, ornithine, tryptophan, asymmetric dimethylarginine (ADMA), kynurenine, methionine-sulfoxide, sarcosine, and SDMA. However, alanine, spermidine, spermine, and ADMA could not be accurately measured at the Cal 0.25 level.

All 21 amino acids and 12 biogenic amines were detectable in the pooled human milk sample. Overall recovery across three spiking levels ranged between 79%–106% (CV: 4.5%–19.2%) for amino acids, and 81%–108% (CV: 2.4%–11.0%) for biogenic amines, as shown in Figure 1a and Supplementary Table S2. Compared to the non-diluted milk samples, the diluted pooled milk revealed a relative concentration range for amino acids of (1:2/1:5 dilution) 70%–100%/67%–104% (CV: 2.4%–15.7%/2.7%–11.0%) and 87%–119%/80%–102% (CV: 0.8%–13.5%/10.8%–14.6%) for biogenic amines, as shown in Figure 1b and Supplementary Table S3. Ornithine relative concentration was in good agreement with the non-diluted milk samples for the 1:2 dilutions (96.7%) but revealed a higher variation of CV = 25.3%. However, some of the amino acids and biogenic amines, including ornithine, were only observed in very low concentrations in the non-diluted pooled milk samples.

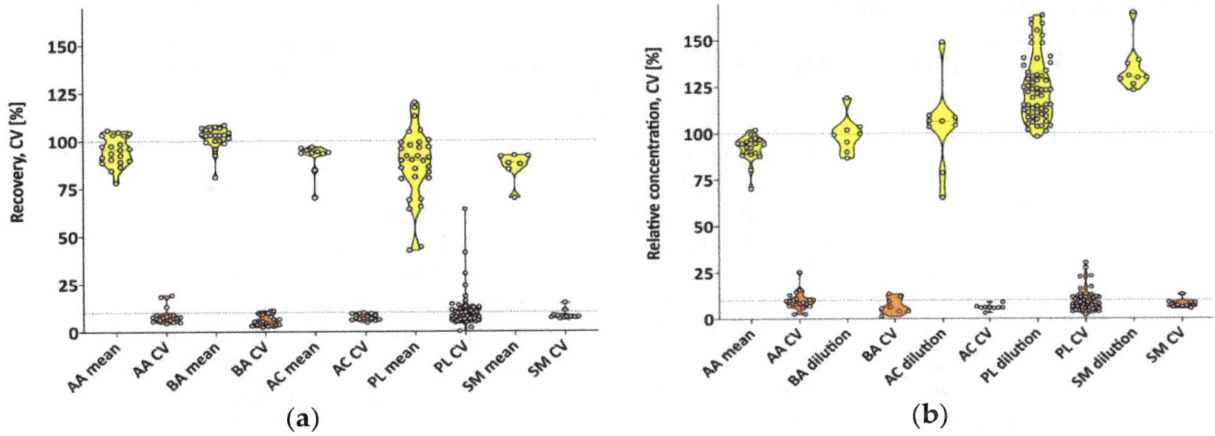

Figure 1. (**a**) Violin plots of mean milk metabolite recovery and coefficients of variation (CVs) determined by 3-level spiking experiments (n = 6); (**b**) relative milk metabolite recovery and CVs of the diluted milk samples. AA—amino acids; BA—biogenic amines; AC—acylcarnitines; PL—phospholipids; SM—sphingomyelins.

3.1.2. FIA (Acylcarnitines, Phospholipids, Sphingomyelins, Hexoses)

Sample extracts were diluted 1:20 for analysis using the 5500 QTRAP mass spectrometer. A relatively low recovery (CV) for PC aa C32:1 (42.6% (41.3%)) and to a lesser extent for PC aa C42:1 (44.4% (15.0%)) were observed. Overall, 89 (11 acylcarnitines, 63 phospholipids, 15 sphingomyelins) out of 146 FIA-analytes were quantifiable, with five additional metabolites detectable above (LOD) with no measurable carry-over effects. Overall recovery across the three spiking levels ranged between 70%–97% (CV: 5.8%–9.6%; acylcarnitines), 70%–92% (CV: 6.4%–8.6%; sphingomyelins), and 91.4% (CV: 7.1%) for the sum of hexoses. Excluding the above mentioned phospholipids, the recovery ranges between 64%–120% (CV: 3.9%–15.9%). PC ae C30:1 showed a good recovery of 85.7% but high variation (CV: 24.1%), as shown in Figure 1a and Supplementary Table S4.

Compared to the concentrations measured in the non-diluted pooled milk samples, acylcarnitines revealed relative concentration ranges (1:2/1:5 dilution) of 70%–134%/60%–164% (CV: 3.0%–7.0%/6.7%–10.7%), sphingomyelins ranged between 110%–167%/135%–228% (CV: 4.1%–13.0%/6.1%–20.5%), and hexoses 111%/143% (CV: 6.0%/10.5%). Phospholipids relative concentrations spanned between 97%–158%/95%–173% (CV: 1.8%–19.3%/2.3%–28.5%). Only five of the metabolites had a CV > 20% at the higher dilution. PC aa C32:1 and PC ae C30:1 experienced higher variations (CVs: 27% to 36.3%). PC aa C 38:1 was not detectable at a higher dilution and showed extreme variations at the lower dilution level with a mean relative concentration of 157% and CV = 55.7%, as shown in Figure 1b and Supplementary Table S5.

3.2. Feasibility Plate

Across all analyzed milk samples (BMI > 18.5 mothers and stunted infants), all 21 amino acids, 15 sphingomyelins, and the sum of hexoses were quantifiable. In addition, 10 biogenic amines, 11 acylcarnitines, and 54 phospholipids were observed, as shown in Supplementary Table S6.

Milk from BMI > 18.5 mothers had significantly higher concentrations of the amino acids and biogenic amines citrulline, glutamate, glycine, phenylalanine, serine, and the biogenic amine sarcosine (all $p < 0.045$), and lower concentrations of isovalerylcarnitine, phosphatidylcholine with diacyl residue sum C36:6 (PC aa), phosphatidylcholine with acyl-alkyl residue sum C30:2 (PC ae), and sphingomyelin with acyl residue sum C22:3 (all $p < 0.048$), as shown in Table 2, when compared to milk fed to stunted infants.

Table 2. Median concentrations and interquartile range (IQR) for milk metabolites affected by group (BMI > 18.5 mothers vs. stunted infants).

Metabolite [1]	BMI > 18.5 Mothers	Stunted Infants	*p*-Value [2]
	[μmol/L]		
C 5	0.13 (0.12, 0.14)	0.19 (0.17, 0.37)	0.011
PC aa C36:6	0.028 (0.025, 0.028)	0.031 (0.028, 0.035)	0.044
PC ae C30:2	0.011 (0.01, 0.011)	0.012 (0.012, 0.013)	0.047
SM C22:3	0.017 (0.014, 0.019)	0.022 (0.018, 0.037)	0.014
Citrulline	18.5 (12.2, 22.3)	10.6 (8.7, 16.3)	0.021
Glutamate	1825 (1477, 1977)	1181 (976, 1472)	0.002
Glycine	116 (103, 147)	96.0 (79.5, 104)	0.017
Phenylalanine	12.5 (11.7, 16.1)	11.2 (10.3, 12.0)	0.012
Serine	142 (94.2, 184)	85.0 (79.4, 108)	0.026
Sarcosine	0.61 (0.52, 0.72)	0.46 (0.38, 0.51)	0.044

[1] C 5—isovalerylcarnitine/2-methylbutyrylcarnitine/valerylcarnitine; PC aa C36:6—phosphatidylcholine with diacyl residue sum C36:6; PC ae C30:2—phosphatidylcholine with acyl-alkyl residue sum C30:2; SM C22:3—sphingomyelin with acyl residue sum C22:3. [2] *p*-values by Wilcoxon rank sum test.

While milk metabolites were significantly associated ($p < 0.05$) in both groups, the correlation profile differed considerably. These significant relationships were found not only among metabolites that were significantly different in concentration between the two groups but also among metabolites that had similar concentrations in all milk samples across groups, as shown in Figure 2.

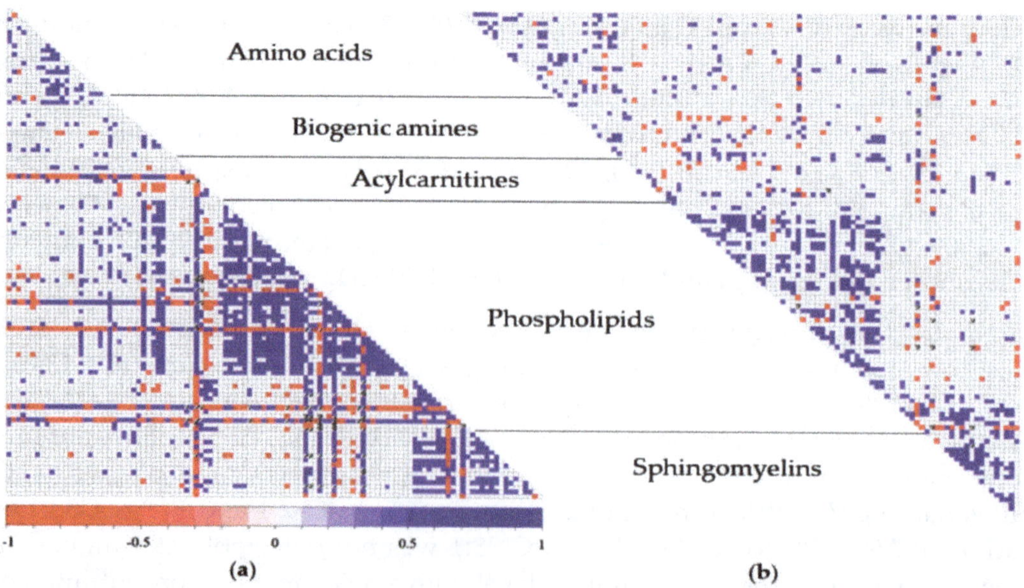

Figure 2. Spearman rank correlation map of milk metabolites in (**a**) BMI > 18.5 mothers and (**b**) stunted infants groups. Only significant correlations are shown ($p < 0.05$).

4. Discussion

4.1. Validation Using Pooled Human Milk

LC-MS: The new internal standards for amino acids and biogenic amines, and the extension of the calibrator curve allowed a more accurate analysis of the milk metabolites. While proline, tryptophan, and valine revealed saturation effects at mid calibrator levels, the measured milk concentrations of these amino acids, however, were well within the linear calibrator curve and the high level calibrators were not needed. While the low range of the calibrator curve was also extended to Cal 0.5 and 0.25, alanine, spermidine, spermine, and ADMA were not quantifiable at the lowest calibrator. Given that these metabolites were present in milk above Cal 0.5, the low accuracy at Cal 0.25 concentrations was not problematic. Some of the amino acids and biogenic amines, including ornithine, were found already in very low concentrations in the non-diluted pooled milk sample; consequently, their concentrations in the diluted samples were around or below the limit of detection (LOD) and reliable data could not be obtained. For metabolites within the calibrator curve, the diluted samples were mostly within 80%–120%, indicating some but not serious effects for quantification due to the matrix. The lower ion spray voltage (IS) intensity found for milk samples when compared to plasma further confirmed effects due to the milk matrix. To reduce matrix interferences due to early eluting matrix components (e.g., lactose), results for creatinine, the first eluting metabolite in LC-MS mode could be sacrificed to maintain MS-integrity and accuracy over time.

FIA: Phospholipids showed the greatest variation in metabolite recovery, and also represented the largest compound class of metabolites analyzed. Some of the variation could be explained by low abundance of metabolites at the edges of the calibrator range, or standard additions possibly to levels of saturation and therefore loss of linearity and accuracy. However, selectivity issues by milk-specific interferences cannot be excluded. No extended calibrator curve was necessary in FIA mode. The relative concentration of the analytes in the diluted samples compared to the non-diluted samples of generally above 100%, and often above 150% at higher dilutions, suggested some ion suppression due to the matrix which can be overcome by sample dilution. However, no metabolite was affected by the matrix to a degree that would not allow quantitation. However, given the abundance of lactose in the sample (~7%), a greater dilution would be preferable to reduce contamination of the MS by matrix constituents in FIA mode.

We found all detectable amino acids, sphingomyelins, and the sum of hexoses in human milk, but only 25% of the acylcarnitines, 50% of the biogenic amines, and 68% of the phospholipids. A recent study on plasma metabolites of healthy men and women (18–80 years) using the Absolute*IDQ*® p180 kit reported fewer of the amino acids, biogenic amines, acylcarnitines, and sphingomyelins in plasma, but more phospholipids [27], illustrating the variations in metabolite profile depending on specimen analyzed. Moreover, that study reported that the metabolic profile of plasma and urine can predict sex with >90% accuracy, as well as age (based on gender), and within females the menopausal status could be predicted with >80% accuracy. Other studies showed that differences in plasma metabolite profiles could be a useful diagnostic tool for Alzheimer's disease and cognitive impairment, or type 2 diabetes [28,29], further indicating the importance and relevance of the information than can be derived from the milk metabolome to the phenotype and status [27].

4.2. Feasibility Plate

Differences by Group Assignment

Overall, the metabolites detected in the feasibility plate using milk from Bangladeshi women were similar to those in the pooled human milk sample. The observed higher concentrations in milk from BMI > 18.5 mothers for selected amino amides and biogenic amines and lower concentrations of phospholipids, acylcarnitines, and sphingomyelins are consistent with alterations found in the serum metabolome of stunted compared to non-stunted children (1 to 5 years of age) in Malawi by Semba et al., using the same Absolute*IDQ*® p180 kit [30]. Stunting can be caused by intrauterine growth retardation, inadequate nutrition for optimal infant growth and development, or repeated infections early in life, and usually originates in utero [31]. Thus, the reported low circulating amino acids and other metabolome alterations in the blood of stunted children in Malawi may stem from challenges in utero and early infancy, including possible effects derived from the lower supply of amino acids in human milk as reported here. This hypothesis is supported by the fact that human growth is regulated by the mechanistic target of rapamycin complex C1 (mTORC1), a major growth regulating pathway, which suppresses protein and lipid synthesis and cellular growth when intake of specific amino acids is insufficient [30,32]. However, since we do not have the full information about maternal and infant characteristics, including exact stage of lactation for each sample, we cannot exclude that additional maternal or infant factors possibly affect the milk metabolome. Nonetheless, correlation patterns changed in milk fed to stunted infants, indicating alterations of the milk metabolome and its pattern could be related to the infant phenotype. Since the alterations in the metabolome correlation profile were not limited to metabolites showing significant differences in concentrations, these relationships may be also affected by maternal or infant status. However, our sample size was very small, the anthropometric status of infants in the group of BMI > 18.5 mothers was unknown, and further research is needed to confirm and explore the results found in this feasibility study.

5. Conclusions

This is the first study to validate the commercially available Absolute*IDQ*® p180 assay for targeted metabolomics in the human milk matrix. A greater range of calibrators is needed to accommodate the wide range of milk metabolite concentrations; new available internal standards improved accuracy of the results. While the primary purpose of this study was the validation of the Absolute*IDQ*® p180 assay for the human milk matrix, and it was not our intention to draw conclusions about group differences in metabolites from the feasibility plate, the observed differences in concentrations and metabolome profiles in the two groups warrant further investigation of the mother–infant relationship and the importance of milk metabolome for infant optimal growth and development, which is now possible using identical targeted metabolomics assays for blood and milk samples.

Supplementary Materials:
Table S1: List and abbreviations of metabolites, Table S2: Metabolite concentrations (mean ± SD) and recovery rates (CV) of pooled milk in LC-MS mode, Table S3: Relative recovery (mean ± SD) of milk metabolites in diluted pooled human milk based on non-diluted samples in LC-MS mode, Table S4: Metabolite concentrations (mean ± SD) and recovery rates (CV) of pooled milk in FIA mode, Table S5: Relative recovery (mean ± SD) of milk metabolites in diluted pooled human milk based on non-diluted samples in FIA mode, Table S6: Median concentrations and interquartile ranges (IQR) of milk metabolites in the BMI > 18.5 mothers and the stunted infants groups.

Author Contributions: Conceptualization and Study Design and Validation, D.H., S.S.-F., and L.H.A.; Field Study: M.H., M.M.I., and T.A.; Formal Analysis, D.H.; Writing—Original Draft Preparation, D.H.; Writing—Review and Editing, D.H. and L.H.A.; Funding Acquisition, L.H.A. All authors read and approved the final version of the manuscript.

Acknowledgments: The authors thank Denise Sonntag and Cornelia Roehring at Biocrates Life Science AG for support in data interpretation, and Excel Que for statistical analysis. USDA is an equal opportunity employer and provider.

References

1. Slupsky, C. Metabolomics in Human Milk Research. In *Human Milk: Composition, Clinical Benefits and Future Opportunities*; Donovan, S.M., German, B.J., Lonnerdal, B., Lucas, A., Eds.; Karger AG: Basel, Switzerland, 2019; Volume 90, pp. 179–190.
2. World Health Organization. *The Optimal Duration of Exclusive Breastfeeding*; Report of an Expert Consultation; WHO: Geneva, Switzerland, 2001.
3. Hampel, D.; York, E.R.; Allen, L.H. Ultra-performance liquid chromatography tandem mass-spectrometry (UPLC-MS/MS) for the rapid, simultaneous analysis of thiamin, riboflavin, flavin adenine dinucleotide,

nicotinamide and pyridoxal in human milk. *J. Chromatrogr. B Anal. Technol. Biomed. Life Sci.* **2012**, *903*, 7–13. [CrossRef] [PubMed]

4. Hampel, D.; Shahab-Ferdows, S.; Domek, J.M.; Siddiqua, T.; Raqib, R.; Allen, L.H. Competitive chemiluminescent enzyme immunoassay for vitamin B12 analysis in human milk. *Food Chem.* **2014**, *153*, 60–65. [CrossRef] [PubMed]
5. Hampel, D.; Shahab-Ferdows, S.; Adair, L.S.; Bentley, M.E.; Flax, V.L.; Jamieson, D.J.; Ellington, S.R.; Tegha, G.; Chasela, C.S.; Kamwendo, D.; et al. Thiamin and Riboflavin in Human Milk: Effects of Lipid-Based Nutrient Supplementation and Stage of Lactation on Vitamer Secretion and Contributions to Total Vitamin Content. *PLoS ONE* **2016**, *11*, e0149479. [CrossRef] [PubMed]
6. Redeuil, K.; Bénet, S.; Affolter, M.; Thakkar, S.; Campos-Giménez, E. A Novel Methodology for the Quantification of B-Vitamers in Breast Milk. *J. Anal. Bioanal. Tech.* **2017**, *8*. [CrossRef]
7. Ren, X.N.; Yin, S.A.; Yang, Z.Y.; Yang, X.G.; Bing, S.; Ren, Y.P.; Zhang, J. Application of UPLC-MS/MS Method for Analyzing B-vitamins in Human Milk. *Biomed. Environ. Sci.* **2015**, *28*, 738–750. [PubMed]
8. Lildballe, D.L.; Hardlei, T.F.; Allen, L.H.; Nexo, E. High concentrations of haptocorrin interfere with routine measurement of cobalamins in human serum and milk. A problem and its solution. *Clin. Chem. Lab. Med.* **2009**, *47*, 182–187. [CrossRef] [PubMed]
9. Hampel, D.; Shahab-Ferdows, S.; Gertz, E.; Flax, V.L.; Adair, L.S.; Bentley, M.E.; Jamieson, D.J.; Tegha, G.; Chasela, C.S.; Kamwendo, D.; et al. The effects of a lipid-based nutrient supplement and antiretroviral therapy in a randomized controlled trial on iron, copper, and zinc in milk from HIV-infected Malawian mothers and associations with maternal and infant biomarkers. *Matern. Child. Nutr.* **2017**, *14*. [CrossRef]
10. Redeuil, K.; Vulcano, J.; Prencipe, F.P.; Bénet, S.; Campos-Giménez, E.; Meschiari, M. First quantification of nicotinamide riboside with B3 vitamers and coenzymes secreted in human milk by liquid chromatography-tandem-mass spectrometry. *J. Chrom. B Analyt. Technol. Biomed. Life Sci.* **2019**, *1110–1111*, 74–80. [CrossRef]
11. Huang, J.; Kailemia, M.J.; Goonatilleke, E.; Parker, E.A.; Hong, Q.; Sabia, R.; Smilowitz, J.T.; German, J.B.; Lebrilla, C.B. Quantitation of human milk proteins and their glycoforms using multiple reaction monitoring (MRM). *Anal Bioanal. Chem.* **2017**, *409*, 589–606. [CrossRef]
12. Wu, S.; Tao, N.; German, J.B.; Grimm, R.; Lebrilla, C.B. Development of an annotated library of neutral human milk oligosaccharides. *J. Proteome Res.* **2010**, *9*, 4138–4151. [CrossRef]
13. Fernández, L.; Langa, S.; Martín, V.; Maldonado, A.; Jiménez, E.; Martín, R.; Rodríguez, J.M. The human milk microbiota: Origin and potential roles in health and disease. *Pharmacol. Res.* **2013**, *69*, 1–10. [CrossRef] [PubMed]
14. McGuire, M.K.; McGuire, M.A. Got bacteria? The astounding, yet not-so-surprising, microbiome of human milk. *Cur. Opin. Biotechnol.* **2017**, *44*, 63–68. [CrossRef] [PubMed]
15. Sokol, E.; Ulven, T.; Færgeman, N.J.; Ejsing, C.S. Comprehensive and quantitative profiling of lipid species in human milk, cow milk and a phospholipid-enriched milk formula by GC and MS/MSALL. *Eur. J. Lipid Sci. Technol.* **2015**, *117*, 751–759. [CrossRef] [PubMed]
16. Sinanoglou, V.J.; Cavouras, D.; Boutsikou, T.; Briana, D.D.; Lantzouraki, D.Z.; Paliatsiou, S.; Volaki, P.; Bratakos, S.; Malamitsi-Puchner, A.; Zoumpoulakis, P. Factors affecting human colostrum fatty acid profile: A case study. *PLoS ONE* **2017**, *12*, e0175817. [CrossRef] [PubMed]
17. Marincola, F.C.; Dessì, A.; Corbu, S.; Reali, A.; Fanos, V. Clinical impact of human breast milk metabolomics. *Clin. Chim. Acta* **2015**, *451*, 103–106. [CrossRef] [PubMed]
18. Gay, M.; Koleva, P.; Slupsky, C.; Toit, E.; Eggesbo, M.; Johnson, C.; Wegienka, G.; Shimojo, N.; Campbell, D.; Prescott, S.; et al. Worldwide Variation in Human Milk Metabolome: Indicators of Breast Physiology and Maternal Lifestyle? *Nutrients* **2018**, *10*, 1151. [CrossRef] [PubMed]
19. Melnik, B. Milk—A nutrient system of mammalian evolution promoting mTORC1-dependent translation. *Int. J. Mol. Sci.* **2015**, *16*, 17048–17087. [CrossRef] [PubMed]
20. Russell, H.; Taylor, P.M.; Hundal, H.S. Amino acid transporters: Roles in amino acid sensing and signalling in animal cells. *Biochem. J.* **2003**, *373*, 1–18.
21. Moran-Ramos, S.; Ocampo-Medina, E.; Gutierrez-Aguilar, R.; Macías-Kauffer, L.; Villamil-Ramírez, H.; López-Contreras, B.E.; León-Mimila, P.; Vega-Badillo, J.; Gutierrez-Vidal, R.; Villarruel-Vazquez, R.; et al. An amino acid signature associated with obesity predicts 2-year risk of hypertriglyceridemia in school-age children. *Sci. Rep.* **2017**, *7*, 5607. [CrossRef]

22. Isganaitis, E.; Venditti, S.; Matthews, T.J.; Lerin, C.; Demerath, E.W.; Fields, D.A. Maternal obesity and the human milk metabolome: Associations with infant body composition and postnatal weight gain. *Am. J. Clin. Nutr.* **2019**, *110*, 111–120. [CrossRef]
23. Smilowitz, J.T.; O'Sullivan, A.; Barile, D.; German, J.B.; Lönnerdal, B.; Slupsky, C.M. The human milk metabolome reveals diverse oligosaccharide profiles. *J. Nutr.* **2013**, *143*, 1709–1718. [CrossRef] [PubMed]
24. Anderson, S.M.; Rudolph, M.C.; McManaman, J.L.; Neville, M.C. Key stages in mammary gland development. Secretory activation in the mammary gland: It's not just about milk protein synthesis! *Breast Cancer Res.* **2007**, *9*, 204. [CrossRef] [PubMed]
25. Ramsay, S.L.; Stoeggl, W.M.; Weinberger, K.M.; Graber, A.; Guggenbichler, W. Apparatus and method for analyzing a metabolite profile. Google Patents US8265877 B2, 11 September 2012.
26. Ramsay, S.L.; Guggenbichler, W.; Weinberger, K.M.; Graber, A.; Stoeggl, W.M. Device for Quantitative Analysis of a Drug or Metabolite Profile. Google Patents US8116983 B2, 14 February 2012.
27. Rist, M.J.; Roth, A.; Frommherz, L.; Weinert, C.H.; Krüger, R.; Merz, B.; Bunzel, D.; Mack, C.; Egert, B.; Bub, A.; et al. Metabolite patterns predicting sex and age in participants of the Karlsruhe Metabolomics and Nutrition (KarMeN) study. *PLoS ONE* **2017**, *12*, e0183228. [CrossRef] [PubMed]
28. Klavins, K.; Koal, T.; Dallmann, G.; Marksteiner, J.; Kemmler, G.; Humpel, C. The ratio of phosphatidylcholines to lysophosphatidylcholines in plasma differentiates healthy controls from patients with Alzheimer's disease and mild cognitive impairment. *Alzheimers Dement* **2015**, *1*, 295–302. [CrossRef] [PubMed]
29. Floegel, A.; Stefan, N.; Yu, Z.; Mühlenbruch, K.; Drogan, D.; Joost, H.G.; Fritsche, A.; Häring, H.U.; de Angelis, M.H.; Peters, A.; et al. Identification of serum metabolites associated with risk of type 2 diabetes using a targeted metabolomic approach. *Diabetes* **2013**, *62*, 639–648. [CrossRef] [PubMed]
30. Semba, R.D.; Shardell, M.; Ashour, F.A.S.; Moaddel, R.; Trehan, I.; Maleta, K.M.; Ordiz, M.I.; Kraemer, K.; Khadeer, M.A.; Ferrucci, L.; et al. Child stunting is associated with low circulating essential amino acids. *EBioMedicine* **2016**, *6*, 246–252. [CrossRef] [PubMed]
31. Dewey, K.G.; Begum, K. Long-term consequences of stunting in early life. *Matern. Child. Nutr.* **2011**, *7*, 5–18. [CrossRef] [PubMed]
32. Laplante, M.; Sabatini, D.M. mTOR signaling in growth control and disease. *Cell* **2012**, *149*, 274–293. [CrossRef] [PubMed]

7

Preterm Infant Feeding: A Mechanistic Comparison between a Vacuum Triggered Novel Teat and Breastfeeding

Donna Geddes [1,*], Chooi Kok [2,3], Kathryn Nancarrow [2,3], Anna Hepworth [1] and Karen Simmer [2,3]

1 School of Molecular Sciences, Faculty of Science, The University of Western Australia, Perth, WA 6009, Australia; arhepworth@westnet.com.au
2 Centre for Neonatal Research and Education, School of Medicine, Faculty of Health and Medical Sciences, The University of Western Australia, Perth, WA 6009, Australia; Chooi.Kok@health.wa.gov.au (C.K.); Nancarrow.Kathryn@health.wa.gov.au (K.N.); Karen.Simmer@health.wa.gov.au (K.S.)
3 The Neonatal Directorate, King Edward Memorial Hospital, Perth, WA 6008, Australia
* Correspondence: donna.geddes@uwa.edu.au

Abstract: The goal for preterm infants is to achieve full oral feeds quickly and ultimately progress to full breastfeeding. Supplementary oral feeds are often given when the mother is not available to breastfeed. Bottles typically deliver milk in a different fashion compared to breastfeeding, which is thought to hamper transition to full breastfeeding. The aim of this study was to compare the sucking dynamics of preterm infants fed at the breast to feeding with an experimental novel teat (NT) designed to release milk only upon the application of vacuum. Simultaneous ultrasound imaging of the infant oral cavity and measurement of intra-oral vacuum was performed during a breastfeed and a feed with the NT. Test weighs were used to measure milk intake. Linear mixed effects models were performed to investigate differences by feed type, and simultaneous linear regression was performed to investigate individual patterns. Tongue movement was not different between breastfeeding and the NT. Intra-oral vacuums (median (interquartile range: IQR)) were significantly lower with the NT (Baseline vacuum: −5.8 mmHg (−11.0, 0.1); Peak: 40.0 mmHg (−54.6, −27.1)) compared to breastfeeding (Baseline: −31.1 mmHg (−60.0, −12.7); Peak: −106.2 mmHg (−153.0, −65.5)). Milk intake was significantly higher with the NT (33 mL (22.5, 42.5)) compared to the breastfeed (12 mL (3, 15.5)). The novel teat encouraged a similar tongue action to breastfeeding, and infants transferred a greater volume of milk with the novel teat. Intra-oral vacuums were lower in strength with the novel teat compared to the breast. Use of the novel teat for the training of sucking dynamics in preterm infants has the potential to improve breastfeeding success and requires further investigation.

Keywords: infant; feeding; preterm; premature; bottle; human milk; breastfeeding; nipple shield; infant feeding

1. Introduction

The importance of human milk (HM) for the preterm infant cannot be understated. In addition to protecting the infant from infection, which can often be life threatening for these infants, and providing nutrients for growth, several studies have linked HM with improved long-term health outcomes. Most recently, donor HM–fed preterm infants have been shown to have better cardiac morphology in adulthood compared to those fed high protein formulas, and these differences potentially increase the likelihood of better cardiopulmonary outcomes later in life [1]. Further, improved neurodevelopment [2,3] later in life has been documented in this population despite predominantly HM-fed preterm infants having slower growth rates than those that are formula-fed [4]. Predominant HM feeds in the first 28 days of life has been linked to a greater volume of deep gray matter volume at term along with higher IQ, working memory, academic achievement, and motor function at seven years of age in infants born less than 30 weeks gestation [5].

These important benefits of HM often overshadow the development of the oro-facial structures due to the necessity for provision of adequate infant nutrition. Preterm infant nutrition is a tenuous balance of type of nutrition, fortification, mode of delivery, and volume of feeds the infant can tolerate. As such, the mechanics of feeding or the delivery of milk are unfortunately largely underemphasized. The bones of the skull and face are malleable in early life, and stresses or lack of stress impacts bone growth [6]. Indeed, there are suggestions that extrinsic factors such as changes in head shape due to infant position and orotracheal intubation [7,8] can alter both palate size and shape, with the potential to affect the entire nasomaxillary complex, particularly in the preterm infant. Further, intrinsic factors such as under nutrition, endocrine anomalies, central nervous system impairments, metabolic dysfunction, and particular medications may impact development of the nasomaxillary complex [9].

Thus, the positive associations of HM and breastfeeding with both short- and long-term health outcomes as well as better development of infant structure and form [10] underpins the goal of the Neonatal Intensive Care Unit (NICU) to facilitate full breastfeeding. Unfortunately, achievement of this goal is hampered by the immaturity of the infant as well as infant co-morbidities such as bronchopulmonary dysplasia, gastrointestinal surgeries, sepsis, neurological impairment, and growth [11], which is further compounded by a range of feed competence between infants [12]. Since discharge of the infant home is also a major goal of the NICU due to evidence suggesting preterm infant health is improved [13], achievement of full oral feeds that are both safe and efficient is imperative. Independent oral feeding is a requirement for discharge home, and often, this may be the last milestone the infant met prior to discharge [14]. More rapid discharge can be achieved by supplementing infants with expressed HM milk via a bottle whilst breastfeeding is being established [12], and this strategy is commonly employed in many units due to infant health, availability of the mother to breastfeed, and economic constraints.

In the pursuit of full breastfeeding in the preterm infant, one must recognise that marked differences in the delivery of milk exist between breastfeeding and bottle-feeding. During bottle-feeding, milk is constantly available to the infant. However, during breastfeeding, milk is only available at milk ejection, and during this transient period, milk flow rates vary markedly. Milk flow rates are important as preterm infants may not be mature enough to regulate milk flow and co-ordinate sucking, swallowing, and breathing at the same time [15]. High flow rates require the infant to swallow frequently to clear the milk from the oral cavity and increase the risk of aspiration [16]. A bottle designed for term infants to release milk only when the infant sucks (applies vacuum; Calma, Medela AG, Baar, Switzerland) has been shown to have a similar tongue action, suck-swallow-breathe patterns, and equivalent heart rate and oxygen saturation to breastfeeding [17]. It was speculated that a similar bottle design for preterm infants would encourage a similar tongue action to breastfeeding when intra-oral vacuum was applied.

The aim of this study was to compare the sucking dynamics of preterm infants fed at the breast and with an experimental novel teat (NT) designed to release milk only upon the application of vacuum and stimulate a tongue movement similar to that of breast feeding.

2. Materials and Methods

2.1. Participants

A convenience sample of 17 mothers and infants (birth gestation age: 23.6–33.3 weeks; post menstrual age (PMA) 32.7–39.9 weeks) whose mothers intended to breastfeed were examined in the special care nurseries of King Edward Memorial Hospital for Women (KEMH), Perth between 1 August 2011 and 30 June 2012. These participants were part of a randomized controlled trial [18] to assess the efficacy of a novel teat designed compared to a conventional teat to meet the needs of the developing preterm infant (Australian New Zealand Clinical Trials Registry, ACTRN12614000875606 [19]).

Inclusion criteria were infants of gestational age (GA) 25 to 34 weeks whose mothers intended to breastfeed and who required 75% enteral feeds by intragastric tube with the remainder provided by intravenous fluids. Exclusion criteria were congenital anomalies, grade 4 intra-cerebral hemorrhage, and periventricular leukomalacia and oral anomalies (for example, ankyloglossia, cleft palate) [18].

The study period was from 1 August 2011 to 30 June 2012. Breastfeeds were timed when the mother was available to feed and the infant could attach to the breast. 15/17 infants therefore were monitored during a breastfeed prior to the NT as it is policy not to introduce bottle feeds until after an infant has demonstrated the ability to attach and suckle at the breast. Monitored sessions were one day apart for eight infants and the same day for two infants, with the remainder ranging between two and seven days. Infant sucking dynamics has previously been shown to be similar to feeding without a nipple shield in a cross-sectional study [20].

For this sub analysis, due to limited resources, only the NT was assessed to determine if the incorporated features encouraged a suck mechanism was similar to breastfeeding. As per standard clinical practice of the study hospital, a nipple shield was used for all breastfeeds where the infant was unable to sustain attachment at the breast. Typically, mothers regularly attempted attachment without a nipple shield and proceeded with a nipple shield if the infant was unable to achieve and/or sustain attachment.

Exclusion criteria included oro-facial anomalies with the potential to affect feeding, grade IV intra-cranial haemorrhage, and other congenital anomalies. All infants were latching and sucking at the breast before participating.

Mothers supplied written, informed consent to participate in the study, which was approved by the Scientific Research Ethics Committee of King Edward Memorial Hospital.

2.2. *Experimental Novel Teat*

The infants were fed with a novel teat (Medela AG, Baar, Switzerland) that was designed to integrate oral feeding skills known to improve outcomes: development of vacuum [21] and self-paced feeding [22]. A shut-off valve ensured milk flowed only when the infant created a vacuum, and venting ensured the NT did not collapse. All infants fed with the valve threshold level of -10 ± 5 mmHg [18].

2.3. *Ultrasound Imaging and Measurement of Intra-Oral Pressure*

Submental ultrasound scans of the midline of the infant's oral cavity as described previously [23–25] were acquired with a Sonsite TITAN system and an endocavity convex transducer ICT 8-5 MHz (SonoSite Inc., Bothell, WA, USA). Infant intra-oral pressures were measured via a small Silastic tube filled with sterile water and taped alongside the nipple and attached to a disposable pressure transducer (Cobe Laboratories, Frenchs Forest, NSW, Australia). The transducer was connected to the amp bridge (ADInstruments, Castle Hill, NSW, Australia), and the output was recorded using MacLab (ADInstruments) and software package Chart v5.0.2 (ADInstruments) on a laptop computer (Mac OS X v10.3.8, Apple Inc., Kupatino, CA, USA). Signals from the ultrasound machine and pressure transducer were recorded simultaneously with a Video Capture Module (ADInstruments) for the entire feed.

2.4. *Ultrasound and Intra-Oral Vacuum Measurement*

The first three well-visualized nutritive suck cycles were selected from each feed. Tongue and nipple movement were measured from two images of each suck cycle when the mid tongue was at its highest (TU) and lowest point (TD) [26] using Screen Calipers v 3.2 (Iconico Inc., New York, NY, USA). Measurements made included nipple to hard–soft palate junction (N-HSPJ), intra-oral depth (IOD; vertical measurement of the mid tongue lowering creating the space accommodating the milk bolus), and nipple diameter at 2, 5, 10, 15, and 20 mm from the tip of the nipple.

Measures of suck bursts included mean minimum pressure (peak vacuum) and mean maximum pressure (baseline vacuum), mean pressure, maximum and minimum pressure, suck rate, and duration of the burst. Mean pressure and pause duration were also measured.

2.5. *Infant Milk Intake*

Milk intake was measured by test weights made before and after the breastfeed [27] (Baby Weigh Scale, Medela AG, Baar, Switzerland). Milk transfer (mL/min) was calculated by dividing the volume of milk consumed by the duration of the feed (minutes).

2.6. *Bradycardia and Desaturation Events*

Bradycardia was defined as <90 bpm and desaturation episodes defined as <91% were recorded during each of the monitored feeds.

2.7. *Statistical Analysis*

Data analysis was run in R v3.0.3 for Mac OS X (Apple Inc., Cupertino, CA, USA), with additional packages nlme and lattice. Unless otherwise specified, summary statistics are presented as mean ± SD (range), while model parameters are presented as estimate (95% confidence interval (95% CI)). Model parameters are not presented for transformed data.

Summary variables presented in Table 1 were compared using either paired *t*-tests or paired Wilcoxon signed rank tests. Comparison of infants included in this study with those omitted used either independent samples *t*-tests or Fisher's Exact test. All other analyses used linear mixed effects models to investigate differences by feed type, and simultaneous linear regression to investigate individual patterns, using the same fixed effects as the final mixed effects model. Model fit was assessed with residual plots. Where more than one random effects grouping was considered, models were compared using likelihood ratio tests. Multiple comparisons used Tukey's all pair comparisons.

Table 1. Infant and monitored feed characteristics for breastfeeding and the novel teat.

Infant and Feed Characteristics	Breast	Novel Teat	Difference	*p*-Value
Feed duration (min)	10.6 (9.0, 20.3)	12.3 (9.1, 16.6)	1.9 (−4.0, 9.4)	0.28
Time sucking (min)	3.4 (2.4, 7.8)	2.7 (1.8, 3.7)	1.4 (0.0, 4.6)	0.027
Time Pausing (min)	7.9 (5.2, 11.7)	9.5 (5.8, 11.4)	0.3 (−3.6, 2.4)	0.078
Mean vacuum (mmHg)	−30.7 (−50.0, −21.2)	−6.0 (−14.0, −3.4)	−24.6 (−46.4, −9.2)	<0.001
Proportion of feed spent sucking	0.36 ± 0.16	0.27 ± 0.15	0.14 (−0.07, 0.09)	0.072
Number of suck bursts	35 (29, 66)	34 (25, 51)	6 (−5, 29)	0.28
Prescribed volume (mL)	46.1 ± 8.2	45.7 ± 7.1	0 (0, 0)	0.36
Milk intake (mL)	12 (3, 15.5)	33 (22.5, 42.5)	−19 (−35, −4)	0.007
Milk transfer (mL/min)	2.2 (1.2, 3.2)	9.2 (7.0, 13.2)	−7.9 (−12.6, −3.4)	<0.001
Age at monitored feed PMA (weeks)	36.3 ± 1.8	36.4 ± 1.5	−0.14 (−0.3, 0)	0.74
Post-natal (weeks)	7.1 ± 4.2	7.2 ± 3.9		
Weight at monitored feed (g)	2120 ± 421.7	2146 ± 294.8	−65 (−129, 0)	0.50

Intra-oral vacuum data consisted of 1641 suck burst and 1607 pause records. Single sucks (102 breast, 193 NT) were omitted from vacuum analyses (other than mean pressure) as these measures cannot be made on single sucks. Five records (three breast, two NT) with a sucking rate ≥ 200 sucks/min were omitted as this indicates measurement artifacts. Missing data included tongue movement for two NT feeds; nipple diameters at 15 mm in 37 records, as insufficient nipple was drawn into the mouth to make the measurement and milk intakes for four feeds in three infants.

2.8. *Tongue Movement*

Linear mixed effects models were used to investigate relationships between feed type and N-HSPJ, IOD, and nipple diameter after accounting for tongue position and measurement location. Main effect, two-way interaction involving feed, and three way interaction models investigated whether there was differing movement patterns between feed types. For each fixed effects model, four random intercept groupings were compared, allowing for differences between infants, amount of tongue movement between infants, and between feed types between infants, in the amount of tongue movement by feed type within the infant.

2.9. Intra-Oral Vacuum

All vacuum and sucking measures were analysed with linear mixed effects models. Minimal random effects considered were random intercepts by feed type within infant. Random slopes by time (linear or second order polynomial), burst type, and suck burst vacuum were also considered as random effects when included in the fixed effects; groupings were by infant or by feed within infant. Fixed effects are detailed for each analysis. Models, which did not converge, were considered to be misspecified, and alternate fixed and/or random effects were considered. Suck burst/pause duration and sucking events data were log transformed before analysis. Measurements of vacuum strength were square root transformed.

Effect of feed type on suck burst/pause durations considered both main effects of and interactions between feed type and burst type. Effect of feed type on changes over the course of the feed for suck bursts, for duration, sucking rate, and number of sucking events per burst, were analysed with either main effects or interaction models, with feed type and time since the beginning of the feed (linear or second order polynomial) as the fixed effects of interest. Effect of baseline and peak suck burst vacuum on overall sucking rate was analysed with either main effects or interaction models for feed type and vacuum. Number of sucks per burst was grouped as 'single' (1 suck), 'immature' (2–9 sucks), and 'mature' (10+ sucks). Number and proportion of suck bursts in the 'single' and 'mature' categories were compared using paired Wilcoxon signed rank tests.

Variability of vacuum within a feed was characterised by calculating the width of the inter-quartile range across all suck bursts for each of the pressures and compared with fixed effects of measure type and feed type, and random intercepts for feed type within infant.

2.10. Milk Intake

The association between milk intake and feed type was tested using a linear mixed effects model with random intercepts by infant and a fixed effect of feed type. Covariates are listed in Table 1, and vacuum variability measures; main effect and interactions with feed type were considered separately for each covariate. Milk intake data was square root transformed prior to analysis.

3. Results

3.1. Participant Characteristics

Seventeen mothers and infants participated in this study. These infants were more likely than the others in the NT group of the larger study to be discharged home rather than back transferred ($p = 0.002$) and had spent longer on continuous positive airway pressure (CPAP) ($p = 0.004$).

Infant (11 female, 6 male; 8 singletons, 9 twins from 5 twin pairs) characteristics were birth gestation 29.2 ± 3.0 weeks (23.6–33.1 weeks), birth weight 1218 ± 43 g (540–1940 g), post-menstrual age (PMA) 33.6 ± 0.8 weeks (31.9–35.3 weeks)/post-natal age 4.4 ± 2.8 weeks (1.0–10.6 weeks) at introduction of full oral feeds, post-menstrual age 37.1 ± 1.2 weeks (35.9–40.1 weeks)/post-natal age 7.9 ± 3.6 weeks (2.7–16.6 weeks) at achievement of full oral feeds. Fifteen infants had been on respiratory support (CPAP: 3 infants for <1 week, 12 for longer; ventilation: 7 for <48 h, 4 for longer; oxygen: 13 for 1 h or longer).

3.2. Characteristics of Monitored Feeds

Characteristics of the monitored feeds are presented in Table 1. Monitored feeds occurred 2.7 ± 1.7 (0, 5.9) weeks after introduction of suck feeds and −0.8 ± 1.0 (−2.7, 1.1) weeks after achievement of full suck feeds. Nipple shields were used during 15/17 breastfeeds.

3.3. Tongue Movement

Nipple diameters for the breastfeed and the NT are documented in Table 2.

Table 2. Measures of ultrasound images during breastfeeding and feeding with the novel teat. N-HSPJ: nipple-hard soft palate junction.

Infant Intra-Oral and Nipple Diameter Measures	Breast		Novel Teat	
	Tongue Up	Tongue Down	Tongue Up	Tongue Down
N-HSPJ distance (mm)	7.1 ± 2.9	5.2 ± 2.6	5.6 ± 1.4	4.7 ± 1.4
Intra-oral depth (mm)	0.3 ± 0.5	4.2 ± 2.0	0.1 ± 0.2	4.1 ± 1.3
Nipple diameters (mm)				
2 mm	10.0 ± 3.0	11.3 ± 2.3	8.0 ± 1.1	8.8 ± 1.1
5 mm	11.4 ± 2.6	12.8 ± 2.5	9.2 ± 0.9	9.6 ± 1.3
10 mm	12.2 ± 2.5	13.2 ± 2.4	9.8 ± 1.0	10.3 ± 1.3
15 mm	12.5 ± 2.7	13.5 ± 2.6	10.0 ± 1.0	10.2 ± 1.5

Effect sizes (95% CI, associated *p*-value) for the main effects models and models with interactions involving feed type are presented in Table 3. No associations were seen between feed type and either N-HSPJ distance or intra-oral depth ($p > 0.21$). The amount of inferior movement (IOD) was between −2.4 ± 0.8 and 3.4 ± 0.8 mm greater during NT feeds.

Nipple diameters were on average 2.3 mm (1.0, 3.6) smaller during NT feeds (Table 3; $p = 0.002$). The amount of change between tongue up and tongue down was on average 0.6 (−0.1, 1.3) mm greater during NT feeds. Overall, the pattern of nipple diameter measurements did not differ by feed, except at 2 mm from the tip of the nipple, where larger values were seen during NT feeds (Figure 1). The three-way interaction between measurement location, tongue position, and feed type was not significant ($p = 0.80$). Individual differences were seen in the relative patterns between NT and breastfeeds.

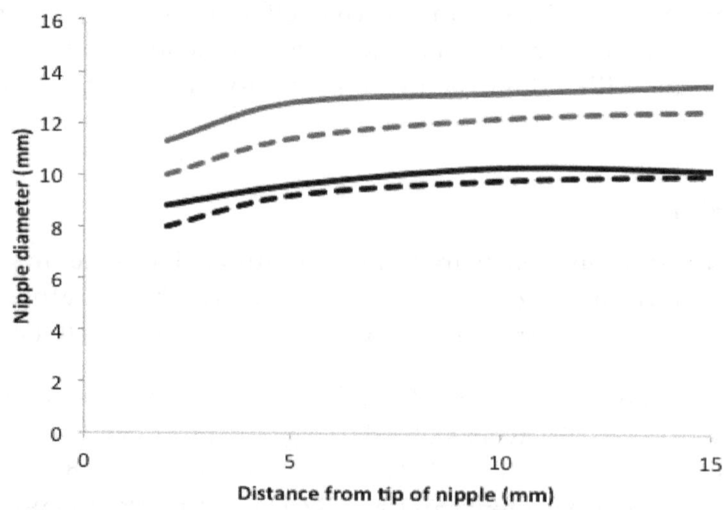

Figure 1. The movement of the infant tongue from its uppermost point to its lowest point for a breastfeed and feed with the novel teat. Solid grey line: breastfeed tongue down; dashed grey line: breastfeed tongue up; solid black line: novel teat tongue down; dashed black line: novel teat tongue up.

Table 3. Effect (parameter ± SE) of tongue position (tongue down) and feed type (NT) on N-HSPJ distance, and intra oral depth; and tongue position, feed type, and measurement location (location) on nipple diameters. Reference levels are tongue position is up, feed type is breastfeed, and location is 5 mm from the nipple tip. Random effects indicates the sub-groups of the data for which random intercepts were fitted, allowing for individual (infant) differences between measurements. The main effects models include all considered terms; interaction models consider only interactions, which include feed type.

Random Effects	N-HSPJ		IOD		Nipple Diameters	
	Coeff (95% CI)	*p*-Value	Coeff (95% CI)	*p*-Value	Coeff (95% CI)	*p*-Value
	Feed within Infant		Tongue Position within Feed within Infant		Tongue Position within Feed within Infant	
Main effects models						
Reference [a]	5.2 (4.1, 6.2)	-	0.3 (−0.2, 0.7)	0.30	11.2 (10.3, 12.2)	-
Tongue down	1.6 (1.3, 1.8)	<0.001	3.9 (3.4, 4.5)	<0.001	1.0 (0.7, 1.4)	<0.001
Novel Teat	−0.5 (−1.9, 0.8)	0.42	−0.1 (−0.7, 0.5)	0.72	−2.3 (−3.6, −1.0)	0.002
Location						<0.001 [b]
2 mm	-	-	-	-	−1.2 (−1.4, −1.0)	<0.001
10 mm	-	-	-	-	0.6 (0.4, 0.8)	<0.001
15 mm	-	-	-	-	0.8 (0.6, 1.0)	<0.001
Interaction models						
Reference [a]	5.1 (4.0, 6.1)	-	0.3 (−0.5, 0.8)	0.28	11.1 (10.1, 12.1)	
Tongue down	1.7 (1.3, 2.1)	<0.001	3.8 (3.1, 4.6)	<0.001	1.3 (0.9, 1.8)	<0.0001
Novel Teat feed	−0.4 (−1.8, 1.1)	0.60	−0.2 (−1.0, 0.6)	0.61	−2.0 (−3.4, −0.6)	0.007
Location						<0.0001 [b]
2	-	-	-	-	−1.4 (−1.7, −1.1)	<0.0001
10	-	-	-	-	0.6 (0.3, 0.9)	<0.0001
15	-	-	-	-	0.9 (0.6, 1.2)	<0.0001
Tongue down Teat	−0.4 (−0.9, 0.2)	0.21	0.2 (−0.9, 1.3)	0.72	−0.6 (−1.3, 0.1)	0.069
Location Teat						0.010 [b]
2 mm	-	-	-	-	0.4 (0.002, 0.8)	0.039
10 mm	-	-	-	-	−0.1 (−0.5, 0.3)	0.56
15 mm	-	-	-	-	0.3 (−0.7, 0.2)	0.26

[a] *p*-Values not included for reference levels except models for IOD, as the question 'is this significantly different from zero' is not meaningful for other analyses. [b] Omnibus *p*-values, indicating the overall chance that there is at least measurement points with significantly different measurements. *p*-Values for each of the measurement locations show significance of difference with respect to measurement made at 5 mm from nipple tip.

3.4. Intra-Oral Vacuum

Summary statistics for intra-oral vacuum are presented in Table 4.

Changes in vacuum and sucking measures over the feed differed between infants ($p < 0.001$, all), with effects of feed on the pattern of change differing between infants ($p < 0.001$). Effect of feed type on burst (suck vs. pause) duration differed by infant ($p < 0.001$). Effect of suck burst vacuums on sucking rate differed by infant ($p \leq 0.001$).

Mean suck burst vacuums, mean pause vacuums, baseline suck burst vacuums, and peak suck burst vacuums were all stronger during breastfeeding ($p < 0.001$, $p = 0.003$, $p < 0.001$, $p < 0.001$, respectively). Mean suck burst vacuums varied over the course of breast ($p = 0.011$) but not NT ($p = 0.68$) feeds. Mean pause vacuums and peak suck burst vacuums did not display consistent patterns of change over the feed ($p = 0.12$, $p = 0.22$, respectively). Baseline suck burst vacuums showed consistent patterns over the feed, which differed by feed type ($p = 0.043$; Figure 2). Variability of all three measures was greater during breastfeeds ($p < 0.008$). Peak suck burst vacuums are more variable than baseline or mean suck burst vacuums ($p < 0.001$). The difference was smaller in NT feeds than breastfeeds but only significant for the comparison between peak and baseline suck burst vacuums ($p = 0.021$).

Table 4. Summary statistics for infant intra-oral vacuum measures, separated by feed and burst type. Data is presented as median (IQR) (range).

	Breast		Novel Teat	
	Sucks (n = 912)	**Pauses (n = 895)**	**Sucks (n = 729)**	**Pauses (n = 712)**
Duration * (s)	4.5 (2.7, 7.4) (0.5, 52.4)	5.4 (2.7, 9.0) (0.5, 712.6)	2.4 (1.3, 4.6) (0.4, 132.8)	5.2 (2.4, 11.6) (0.6, 379.7)
Sucking Events * (n)	6 (3.8, 9) (1, 54)	-	3 (1, 5) (1, 147)	-
Sucking Rate (n/min)	88.0 (73.7, 102.6) (19.0, 194.4)	-	77.6 (62.4, 96.6) (14.2, 191.2)	-
		Vacuum (mmHg)		
Baseline	−31.1 (−60.0, −12.7) (−181.0, 12.4)	-	−5.8 (−11.0, 0.1) (−53.3, 14.3)	-
Mean *	−53.6 (−89.3, −31.5) (−199.3, 0.4)	−23.9 (−48.8, −11.7) (−185.1, 1.9)	−15.5 (−21.8, −8.9) (−77.6, 2.2)	−5.1 (−11.0, −0.6) (−79.6, 5.3)
Peak	−106.2 (−153.0, −65.5) (−325.7, −9.6)	-	−40.0 (−54.6, −27.1) (−116.7, −3.1)	-
		Vacuum variability		
Baseline	23.4 (17.3, 37.0) (5.3, 47.3)	-	5.5 (4.4, 6.1) (1.4, 12.0)	-
Mean *	26.2 (25.0, 41.6) (11.2, 73.9)	-	9.3 (7.8, 10.5) (3.6, 18.9)	-
Peak	50.0 (33.0, 60.7) (18.9, 154.3)	-	25.4 (20.6, 29.3) (3.9, 39.4)	-

* includes single sucks.

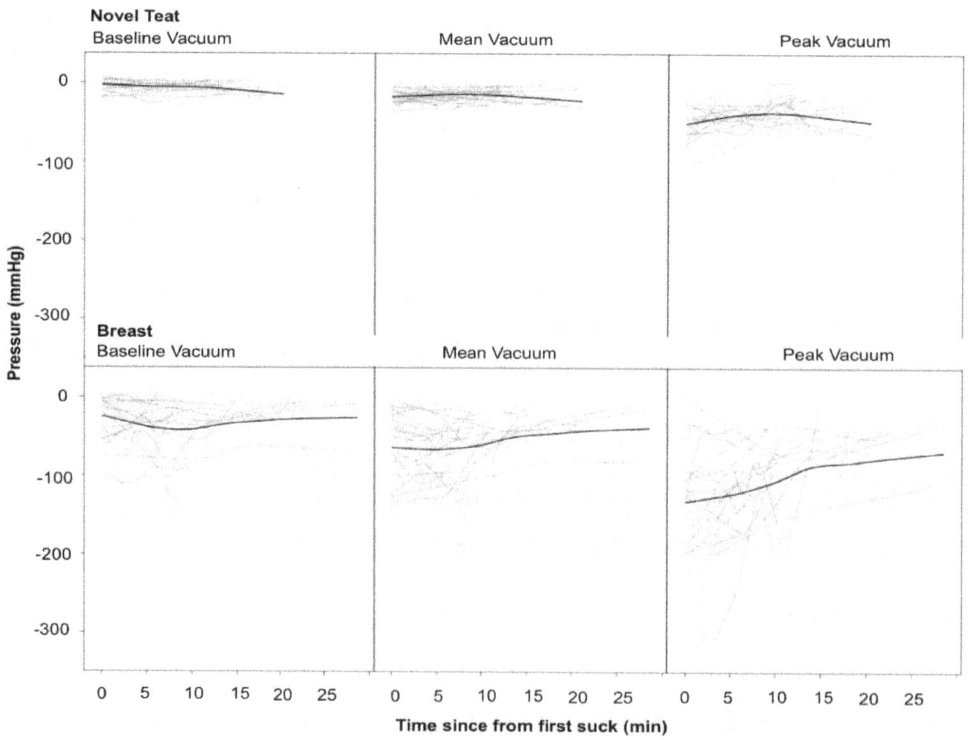

Figure 2. Sucking vacuums over the course of both the breastfeed and novel teat feed. Black lines are local regression smoothers for the full data set; grey lines are local regression smoothers indicating individual infant patterns.

Suck bursts were shorter than pauses ($p < 0.001$), and no overall association with feed type was seen ($p > 0.13$). Suck burst durations did not change over the course of the feed ($p = 0.29$). At the beginning of the feeds, pause durations did not differ significantly by feed type ($p = 0.063$). Pause durations decreased over the course of NT feeds ($p = 0.017$), but no change was seen during breastfeeds ($p = 0.37$). Breastfeeds had more sucks per burst ($p = 0.001$) and higher sucking rates (10.4 (2.1, 18.6) sucks/minute, $p = 0.001$) than NT feeds; neither showed a consistent pattern of change over the feed ($p = 0.32$, $p = 0.93$, respectively). Higher sucking rates were associated with few sucks per burst ($p = 0.004$), but this association did not differ by feed type ($p = 0.88$). No association was seen between suck burst vacuums and sucking rate (peak, $p > 0.54$; baseline, $p > 0.082$).

Suck bursts of $\geq$10 sucks occurred during all breast and 15 of the 17 NT feeds; single sucks occurred during 15/17 of the breast and NT feeds. The number ($p = 0.002$) and proportion ($p = 0.017$) of suck bursts with $\geq$10 sucks were higher in breastfeeds 9 (6, 12) (22.2% (15.8, 31.0)) than NT feeds 3 (1, 7) (8.8% (3.3, 12.5)). The number ($p = 0.031$) and proportion ($p = 0.008$) of single sucks were higher during NT feeds: 6 (3, 8) (10.0% (6.7, 15.2)) than during breastfeeds; 10 (4, 14) (24.1% (15.8, 32.9)). Proportion of bursts with 2–9 sucks did not differ ($p = 0.78$), being 64.0% (58.8, 69.5) and 63.3% (56.2, 68.2) of NT and breastfeed suck bursts respectively.

3.5. *Bradycardia and Desaturation Events*

Desaturation events were reported for 4 infants for 6 of the 32 feeds. The breast:NT incidence for the four infants with desaturations was 3:3, 1:3, 0:1, and 1:0. Bradycardia events were recorded for three infants only during breastfeeding; one infant had two episodes, and two infants had one episode. Data was not recorded for two feeds.

3.6. *Milk Intake*

No measureable milk intake occurred for one breastfeed; three breastfeeds had milk intakes of 4 mL or less, whereas milk intake from the NT feeds was never this low. Milk intakes were larger during NT feeds ($p = 0.003$) and for longer feeds ($p = 0.011$), when a greater proportion of the feed was spent sucking ($p = 0.023$) and/or had a greater number of suck bursts ($p = 0.007$). The association between milk intake and feed type remained significant after accounting for each of the covariates ($p < 0.004$); no significant interactions were seen ($p > 0.10$). No association was seen between milk intake and any of the vacuum variability measures ($p > 0.32$).

4. Discussion

This study has found that movement of the tongue to create a vacuum with the NT was similar to that of breastfeeding. Whilst infants were required to exert a vacuum to remove milk from the NT, the intra-oral vacuums were weaker compared to the breast. Infants, however, consistently removed more milk from the NT than the breast.

4.1. *Tongue Movement*

The introduction of bottles during the establishment of breastfeeding in the term infant is considered detrimental due to the potential of nipple confusion, where the infant refuses the breast [28,29]. Whilst there is little evidence of nipple confusion, the infant has been shown to be highly adaptable. Infants will elect to use compression of the tongue to remove milk from a teat if it is easier than using vacuum. However, if the teat is designed to minimise or exclude the compression effect [30], the infant will employ vacuum to remove milk. Healthy preterm infants fed with an NT that only released milk with the application of vacuum moved their tongue in a similar fashion to breastfeeding (Figure 1). During a breast or NT feed, the infant drew their tongue downward, the nipple/NT expanded evenly, and intra-oral vacuum strength increased to peak vacuum (minimum pressure). Milk flowed into the cavity bounded by the hard and soft palate, the nipple, and the tongue surface. As the tongue was raised, intra-oral vacuum strength reduced to baseline vacuum (maximum pressure), milk was cleared under the soft palate to the phalangeal area and the nipple/NT diameter decreased (Figure 1). The only difference was that the tip of the NT was larger than the nipple (Figure 1) due to its shape and being less compressible than the human nipple. The absence of peristaltic tongue action with the NT compared to other teats [31,32] can be attributed greater thickness of silicone at the base of the NT, which minimised infant tongue compression. While the pattern of tongue movement was similar to breastfeeding, the degree of movement was greater during the breastfeed (Figure 1), which was likely due to the difference in elasticity between the nipple and the NT. Further, whilst most of the infants in this study used a nipple shield to feed, we have shown previously that tongue movement with a nipple shield is not different to tongue movement without [20].

Nipple shields are often used in our NICU to facilitate breastfeeding in preterm infants, enabling them to remain attached to the breast. Evidence shows that for the hospitalised preterm infant, nipple shield (NS) use is associated with improved milk removal [33]. There is limited evidence regarding the impact of NS on breastfeeding exclusivity and duration beyond discharge from hospital. The absence of a relationship between nipple shield use and age at achievement of exclusive breastfeeding [34] has been reported, while lower rates of exclusive breastfeeding have been reported in infants that have used a shield (49% with nipple shield use and 66% without) [35]. Indeed, several factors impact the achievement of exclusive breastfeeding in preterm infants [35]. Complicating factors such as low maternal milk production and/or low infant intraoral vacuum with subsequent insufficient milk transfer are rarely measured. Thus there is a critical need to understand the mechanisms by which nipple shields function to enhance transfer of milk from the breast in the context complicating maternal and infant factors.

The tongue movements of the preterm infants studied are also comparable to that documented in term breastfeeding infants [26,36–38] as well as a larger cohort of breastfeeding preterm infants also recruited from this study [20]. The absence of any marked peristaltic tongue action during breastfeeding or feeding with the NT is in contrast to other studies of bottle-feeding, implying the design of the teat influences tongue movement [31,39]. The unique stresses of tongue movement during feeding likely impact the development of the form and structure of facial structures, particularly the palate [40,41], evidenced by a 68% reduction of malocclusion if infants are breastfed [42]. Further, anthropological observations of prehistoric skulls show broader flatter palates suggesting the forces exerted during breastfeeding influences developing structures [43]. Given the malleability of preterm infants' facial structure and immaturity of muscular control and strength, it could be potentially beneficial to emulate the tongue motion of breastfeeding in the event of the unavailability of the mother to breastfeed.

Positioning of the teat/nipple in the oral cavity is important in order to avoid gagging, which may progress to oral aversion and also to ensure optimal placement of the milk bolus so that it can be easy cleared in co-ordination with breathing and swallowing [44]. We found no difference in the positioning of the nipple and NT in relation to the N-HSPJ (Table 2), indicating good positioning [45]. The infants, however, drew their tongue down more (IOD) during the NT feed, which may be due to not having to apply as much vacuum to obtain a bolus. Thus, greater volumes of milk were transferred during the NT feeds.

4.2. Intra-Oral Vacuum

Preterm infants are recognised to have individual trajectories to attainment of feeding milestones that are complicated by immaturity and associated co-morbidities [28,46]. Commensurate with this notion, measures of preterm intra-oral vacuum were variable across the course of a feed, and patterns were different between individual infants in this study.

One of the factors implicated in more effective and efficient bottle-feeding is increased strength of vacuum [47]. The breastfeeding preterm infants in this study displayed vacuums approximately a half to two-thirds that applied by term infants [36,48] (Table 4). This is consistent with our larger descriptive study of preterm breastfeed infants [20] and also the low milk transfer from the breast

(Table 1). Peak vacuums were also weaker when infants fed at the NT likely due the threshold set for milk flow from the NT while peak vacuums at the breast are due to the greater flexibility of the human nipple. With the NT the infant may also adjust vacuums applied to modulate milk flow rate so that suck-swallow-breathe co-ordination is not compromised.

To suck effectively, infants latch to the breast or the teat, and this is measured as the baseline vacuum. It is important to form a seal to the breast/teat to stretch and position the nipple/teat optimally in the oral cavity in relation to the N-HSPJ to remove milk [49]. If this is not possible, the infant may compensate by allowing milk to spill out of the mouth [50]. The baseline seal to the NT increased in strength over the feed and weakened during the breastfeed (Figure 2), perhaps reflecting fatigue due to the stronger applied vacuums. In contrast, term breastfed infants increase their baseline vacuums over a feed [49]. These changes might be due to changes in breast elasticity due to the drainage of milk, whereas preterm infants remove small volumes from the breast (Table 1).

Mature sucking patterns are frequently described as the ability to extend suck bursts and reduce the lengths of pauses [21]. In contrast, our preterm infants exhibited suck bursts that were shorter than the pauses for both the breast and NT feeds. This apparent reversal suggests a lack of feeding maturity and is further reflected by low milk transfer along with the low proportion of suck bursts comprised of >10 sucks, which is also considered a marker of feed progression. Single sucks were also frequently identified in nearly all breast and NT feeds which is rarely seen during a term breastfeed and itself perhaps a gauge of immaturity of oral feeding. Interestingly, the frequency and proportion of 'mature' suck bursts was higher in breastfeeds (nine per feed; 22.2%) than NT feeds (three per feed; 8.8%), yet milk transfer was more effective in the NT feeds.

Often, clinical observations of slowing of sucking rate are interpreted as a change from non-nutritive to nutritive sucking [17]. Infants in this study did not change their suck frequency across a feed but sucked more rapidly during breastfeeding. Conversely, sucking rates increase across a breastfeed in term infants [49]. This absence of change across a feed makes sucking rate an unreliable indicator of milk intake particularly during breastfeeding. Further, suck rate is not indicative of vacuum strength, with no relationships demonstrated with either peak or baseline vacuum.

Little attention is paid to the length of time a preterm infant pauses at the breast/teat, and long pauses are considered to be due to fatigue or state. We found that pause durations decreased over the course of NT feeds whilst remaining constant during breastfeeds. This may be a congruent with better suck-swallow-breathe co-ordination as the NT feed progressed. Further studies identifying the nutritive and non-nutritive portions of the feed as well as measurement of swallowing and breathing would serve to clarify these differences.

Cardiorespiratory stability is a major concern during oral feeding of the preterm infant. It is well documented that bottle-feeding is associated with more episodes of desaturation and bradycardias compared to breastfeeding [51]. Due to the design of the NT, we expected that the cardiorespiratory stability of the infant fed with the NT would be similar to breastfeeding due to the infant having the opportunity to self regulate their intake from the NT as they would from the breast. However, desaturation occurred overall in only six of 32 feeds (20%), and these were in only four infants. Similarly, bradycardia events were rare and occurred in three infants where one had two episodes and two had one episode during breastfeeding only. Although the numbers are too small to conduct meaningful statistical analysis, there did not appear to be more desaturations during NT feeds.

Good growth is critical for the preterm infant as under nutrition is associated deficits in neurodevelopment and increased risk of sepsis and necrotizing enterocolitis [52]. Thus, the ingestion of adequate volumes of milk from every oral feed is imperative. We have demonstrated in a previous study that intakes range from 0 to 40 mL in preterm breastfed infants [18], which is consistent with Meier et al. [33], who showed intakes from 2–62 mL, and this study. Typically, infants are supplemented to achieve the prescribed volume but without objective measures of the volume of milk ingested at a breastfeed. Overall, infants received significantly greater volumes from the NT that were much closer to the prescribed volume by the neonatologist. As aforementioned, the small volumes of milk removed from the breast is likely due to the low strength of vacuum generated, as [36,49] (Figure 2) this has been associated positively associated with milk intake in term breastfed infants [53]. Longer breastfeeds and a greater proportion of the breastfeed spent sucking usually resulted in increased milk intake, which is in contrast to the NT, where any suck resulted in milk transfer. Clearly, more research is required to identify factors that would improve milk intakes from the breast.

Clinically encouragement of a sucking action similar to breastfeeding during bottle-feeding is likely to confer immediate advantages such as increased infant feed regulation without reduction in feed volume and potentially less nipple 'confusion'. In the longer term, it may also impact development of the oro-facial development by reducing the incidence of conditions such as malocclusion, which is higher in preterm infants [54,55], and sleep disordered breathing where factors such as palate shape, hypotonia, and bottle-feeding appear to contribute [56].

The limitations of the study include the small numbers of participants that were not using a nipple shield to feed; thus, we were not able to directly compare breastfeeding without a shield and with the NT. A more extensive study is required to assess the sucking dynamics with and without a nipple shield. Further, these infants represent a relatively 'healthy' population that began oral feeding at approximately 34 to 35 weeks post menstrual age therefore the results are not applicable to younger infants or those with co-morbidities that are known to adversely affect feeding trajectories. It is anticipated that future studies will investigate suck, swallow, breathe co-ordination, and sucking during breastfeeding and feeding with the NT and conventional teat.

5. Conclusions

The novel teat, which only released milk when the preterm infant applied vacuum, encouraged a similar tongue action to breastfeeding and infants transferred a greater volume of milk compared to breastfeeding. Intra-oral vacuums were lower in strength with the novel teat compared to the breast. Further research is required to compare suck-swallow-breathe patterns with the novel teat and breastfeeding and improve transfer volumes at the breast.

Acknowledgments: This study was supported by an unrestricted research grant from Medela AG (Switzerland). Zoya Gridneva was supported by an Australian Postgraduate Award from the University of Western Australia (Australia). Many thanks are extended to all mothers who participated in this study.

Author Contributions: D.G. designed the study, conducted experiments and data analysis and interpretation, and wrote the manuscript; C.K. designed the study, collected the data and provided input to the manuscript; K.N. designed the study, collected the data and provided input to the manuscript; A.H. provided consultation for research design, conducted data analysis and interpretation, and critically reviewed the manuscript, K.S. designed the study, interpreted results, and critically reviewed the manuscript. All authors read and approved the final manuscript.

References

1. Lewandowski, A.J.; Lamata, P.; Francis, J.M.; Piechnik, S.K.; Ferreira, V.M.; Boardman, H.; Neubauer, S.; Singhal, A.; Leeson, P.; Lucas, A. Breast milk consumption in preterm neonates and cardiac shape in adulthood. *Pediatrics* **2016**, *138*, e20160050. [CrossRef] [PubMed]
2. Isaacs, E.B.; Gadian, D.G.; Sabatini, S.; Chong, W.K.; Quinn, B.T.; Fischl, B.R.; Lucas, A. The effect of early human diet on caudate volumes and IQ. *Pediatr. Res.* **2008**, *63*, 308–314. [CrossRef] [PubMed]
3. Isaacs, E.B.; Fischl, B.R.; Quinn, B.T.; Chong, W.K.; Gadian, D.G.; Lucas, A. Impact of breast milk on intelligence quotient, brain size, and white matter development. *Pediatr. Res.* **2010**, *67*, 357–362. [CrossRef] [PubMed]

4. O'Connor, D.L.; Jacobs, J.; Hall, R.; Adamkin, D.; Auestad, N.; Castillo, M.; Connor, W.E.; Connor, S.L.; Fitzgerald, K. Growth and development of premature infants fed predominantly human milk, predominantly premature infant formula, or a combination of human milk and premature formula. *J. Pediatr. Gastroenterol. Nutr.* **2003**, *37*, 437–446. [CrossRef] [PubMed]
5. Belfort, M.B.; Anderson, P.J.; Nowak, V.A.; Lee, K.J.; Molesworth, C.; Thompson, D.K.; Doyle, L.W.; Inder, T.E. Breast milk feeding, brain development, and neurocognitive outcomes: A 7-year longitudinal study in infants born at less than 30 weeks' gestation. *J. Pediatr.* **2016**, *177*, 133–139. [CrossRef] [PubMed]
6. Bronfin, D.R. Misshapen heads in babies: Position or pathology? *Ochsner J.* **2001**, *3*, 191–199. [PubMed]
7. Morris, K.M.; Burns, Y.R. Reduction of craniofacial and palatal narrowing in very low birthweight infants. *J. Paediatr. Child Health* **1994**, *30*, 518–522. [CrossRef] [PubMed]
8. Ash, S.P.; Moss, J.P. An investigation of the features of the preterm infant palate and the effect of prolonged orotracheal intubation with and without protective appliances. *Br. J. Orthod.* **1987**, *14*, 253–261. [CrossRef] [PubMed]
9. De Curtis, M.; Rigo, J. Extrauterine growth restriction in very low-birthweight infants. *Acta Paediatr.* **2004**, *93*, 1563–1568. [CrossRef] [PubMed]
10. Geddes, D.T.; Prescott, S.L. Developmental origins of health and disease: The role of human milk in preventing disease in the 21st century. *J. Hum. Lact.* **2013**, *29*, 123–127. [CrossRef] [PubMed]
11. Callen, J.; Pinelli, J. A review of the literature examining the benefits and challenges, incidence and duration, and barriers to breastfeeding in preterm infants. *Adv. Neonatal Care* **2005**, *5*, 72–88. [CrossRef] [PubMed]
12. Garber, J. Oral-motor function and feeding intervention. *Phys. Occup. Ther. Pediatr.* **2013**, *33*, 111–138. [CrossRef] [PubMed]
13. Casiro, O.G.; McKenzie, M.E.; McFadyen, L.; Shapiro, C.; Seshia, M.M.; MacDonald, N.; Moffatt, M.; Cheang, M.S. Earlier discharge with community-based intervention for low birth weight infants: A randomized trial. *Pediatrics* **1993**, *92*, 128–134. [PubMed]
14. Bertoncelli, N.; Cuomo, G.; Cattani, S.; Mazzi, C.; Pugliese, M.; Coccolini, E.; Zagni, P.; Mordini, B.; Ferrari, F. Oral feeding competences of healthy preterm infants: A review. *Int. J. Pediatr.* **2012**, *2012*, 896257. [CrossRef] [PubMed]
15. Mathew, O.P. Breathing patterns of preterm infants during bottle feeding: Role of milk flow. *J. Pediatr.* **1991**, *119*, 960–965. [CrossRef]
16. Al-Sayed, L.E.; Schrank, W.I.; Thach, B.T. Ventilatory sparing strategies and swallowing pattern during bottle feeding in human infants. *J. Appl. Physiol.* **1994**, *77*, 78–83. [CrossRef] [PubMed]
17. Sakalidis, V.S.; McClellan, H.L.; Hepworth, A.R.; Kent, J.C.; Lai, C.T.; Hartmann, P.E.; Geddes, D.T. Oxygen saturation and suck-swallow-breathe coordination of term infants during breastfeeding and feeding from a teat releasing milk only with vacuum. *Int. J. Pediatr.* **2012**. [CrossRef] [PubMed]
18. Simmer, K.; Kok, C.; Nancarrow, K.; Hepworth, A.R.; Geddes, D.T. Novel feeding system to promote establishment of breastfeeds after preterm birth: A randomized controlled trial. *J. Perinatol.* **2016**, *36*, 210–215. [CrossRef] [PubMed]
19. Trial Registered on ANZCTR. Available online: http://www.ANZCTR.org.au/ACTRN12614000875606.aspx (accessed on 19 March 2018).
20. Geddes, D.T.; Chooi, K.; Nancarrow, K.; Hepworth, A.R.; Gardner, H.; Simmer, K. Characterisation of sucking dynamics of breastfeeding preterm infants: A cross sectional study. *BMC* **2017**, *17*, 386. [CrossRef] [PubMed]
21. Lau, C.; Alagugurusamy, R.; Schanler, R.J.; Smith, E.O.; Shulman, R.J. Characterization of the developmental stages of sucking in preterm infants during bottle feeding. *Acta Paediatr.* **2000**, *89*, 846–852. [CrossRef] [PubMed]
22. Lau, C.; Schanler, R.J. Oral feeding in premature infants: Advantage of a self-paced milk flow. *Acta Paediatr.* **2000**, *89*, 453–459. [CrossRef] [PubMed]
23. Weber, F.; Woolridge, M.; Baum, J. An ultrasonographic study of the organisation of sucking and swallowing by newborn infants. *Dev. Med. Child Neurol.* **1986**, *28*, 19–24. [CrossRef] [PubMed]
24. Ardran, G.; Kemp, F. A correlation between suckling pressures and the movements of the tongue. *Acta Paediatr.* **1959**, *48*, 261–272. [PubMed]
25. Prieto, C.; Cárdenas, H.; Salvatierra, A.; Boza, C.; Montes, C.; Croxatto, H. Sucking pressure and its relationship to milk transfer during breastfeeding in humans. *J. Reprod. Fertil.* **1996**, *108*, 69–74. [CrossRef] [PubMed]

26. McClellan, H.L.; Sakalidis, V.S.; Hepworth, A.R.; Hartmann, P.E.; Geddes, D.T. Validation of nipple diameter and tongue movement measurements with B-mode ultrasound during breastfeeding. *Ultrasound Med. Biol.* **2010**, *36*, 1797–1807. [CrossRef] [PubMed]
27. Kent, J.C.; Mitoulas, L.R.; Cregan, M.D.; Ramsay, D.T.; Doherty, D.A.; Hartmann, P.E. Volume and frequency of breastfeedings and fat content of breast milk throughout the day. *Pediatrics* **2006**, *117*, e387–e395. [CrossRef] [PubMed]
28. Bagnall, A. Feeding problems. In *Feeding and Nutrition in the Preterm Infant*; Jones, E., King, C., Eds.; Elsevier Churchill Livingstone: Edinburgh, UK, 2005; pp. 165–183.
29. Zimmerman, E.; Thompson, K. Clarifying nipple confusion. *J. Perinatol.* **2015**, *35*, 895–899. [CrossRef] [PubMed]
30. Geddes, D.T.; Sakalidis, V.S.; Hepworth, A.R.; McClellan, H.L.; Kent, J.C.; Lai, C.T.; Hartmann, P.E. Tongue movement and intra-oral vacuum of term infants during breastfeeding and feeding from an experimental teat that released milk under vacuum only. *Early Hum. Dev.* **2012**, *88*, 443–449. [CrossRef] [PubMed]
31. Miller, J.L.; Kang, S.M. Preliminary ultrasound observation of lingual movement patterns during nutritive versus non-nutritive sucking in a premature infant. *Dysphagia* **2007**, *22*, 150–160. [CrossRef] [PubMed]
32. Eishima, K. The analysis of sucking behaviour in newborn infants. *Early Hum. Dev.* **1991**, *27*, 163–173. [CrossRef]
33. Meier, P.P.; Brown, L.P.; Hurst, N.M.; Spatz, D.L.; Engstrom, J.L.; Borucki, L.C.; Krouse, A.M. Nipple shields for preterm infants: Effect on milk transfer and duration of breastfeeding. *J. Hum. Lact.* **2000**, *16*, 106–114. [CrossRef] [PubMed]
34. Maastrup, R.; Hansen, B.M.; Kronborg, H.; Bojesen, S.N.; Hallum, K.; Frandsen, A.; Kyhnaeb, A.; Svarer, I.; Hallström, I. Breastfeeding progression in preterm infants is influenced by factors in infants, mothers and clinical practice: The results of a national cohort study with high breastfeeding initiation rates. *PLoS ONE* **2014**, *9*, e108208. [CrossRef] [PubMed]
35. Maastrup, R.; Hansen, B.M.; Kronborg, H.; Bojesen, S.N.; Hallum, K.; Frandsen, A.; Kyhnaeb, A.; Svarer, I.; Hallström, I. Factors associated with exclusive breastfeeding of preterm infants. Results from a prospective national cohort study. *PLoS ONE* **2014**, *9*, e89077. [CrossRef] [PubMed]
36. Geddes, D.T.; Kent, J.C.; Mitoulas, L.R.; Hartmann, P.E. Tongue movement and intra-oral vacuum in breastfeeding infants. *Early Hum. Dev.* **2008**, *84*, 471–477. [CrossRef] [PubMed]
37. Sakalidis, V.S.; Williams, T.M.; Garbin, C.P.; Hepworth, A.R.; Hartmann, P.E.; Paech, M.J.; Geddes, D.T. Ultrasound imaging of infant sucking dynamics during the establishment of lactation. *J. Hum. Lact.* **2013**, *29*, 205–213. [CrossRef] [PubMed]
38. Elad, D.; Kozlovsky, P.; Blum, O.; Laine, A.F.; Po, M.J.; Botzer, E.; Dollberg, S.; Zelicovich, M.; Ben Sira, L. Biomechanics of milk extraction during breast-feeding. *Proc. Natl. Acad. Sci. USA* **2014**, *111*, 5230–5235. [CrossRef] [PubMed]
39. Nowak, A.J.; Smith, W.L.; Erenberg, A. Imaging evaluation of breast-feeding and bottle-feeding systems. *J. Pediatr.* **1995**, *126*, S130–S134. [CrossRef]
40. Hohoff, A.; Rabe, H.; Ehmer, U.; Harms, E. Palatal development of preterm and low birthweight infants compared to term infants—What do we know? Part 1: The palate of the term newborn. *Head Face Med.* **2005**, *1*, 8. [CrossRef] [PubMed]
41. Hohoff, A.; Rabe, H.; Ehmer, U.; Harms, E. Palatal development of preterm and low birthweight infants compared to term infants—What do we know? Part 2: The palate of the preterm/low birthweight infant. *Head Face Med.* **2005**, *1*, 9. [CrossRef] [PubMed]
42. Victora, C.G.; Bahl, R.; Barros, A.J.; França, G.V.; Horton, S.; Krasevec, J.; Murch, S.; Sankar, M.J.; Walker, N.; Rollins, N.C.; et al. Breastfeeding in the 21st century: Epidemiology, mechanisms, and lifelong effect. *Lancet* **2016**, *387*, 475–490. [CrossRef]
43. Palmer, B. The influence of breastfeeding on the development of the oral cavity: A commentary. *J. Hum. Lact.* **1998**, *14*, 93–98. [CrossRef] [PubMed]
44. Arvedson, J.C. Assessment of pediatric dysphagia and feeding disorders: Clinical and instrumental approaches. *Dev. Disabil. Res. Rev.* **2008**, *14*, 118–127. [CrossRef] [PubMed]
45. Delaney, A.; Arvedson, J.C. Development of swallowing and feeding: Prenatal through first year of life. *Dev. Disabil. Res. Rev.* **2008**, *14*, 105–117. [CrossRef] [PubMed]

46. Barlow, S.M. Oral and respiratory control for preterm feeding. *Curr. Opin. Otolaryngol. Head Neck Surg.* **2009**, *17*, 179–186. [CrossRef] [PubMed]
47. Lau, C. Development of suck and swallow mechanisms in infants. *Ann. Nutr. Metab.* **2015**, *66*, 7–14. [CrossRef] [PubMed]
48. McClellan, H.; Geddes, D.; Kent, J.; Garbin, C.; Mitoulas, L.; Hartmann, P. Infants of mothers with persistent nipple pain exert strong sucking vacuums. *Acta Paediatr.* **2008**, *97*, 1205–1209. [CrossRef] [PubMed]
49. Sakalidis, V.S.; Kent, J.C.; Garbin, C.P.; Hepworth, A.R.; Hartmann, P.E.; Geddes, D.T. Longitudinal changes in suck-swallow-breathe, oxygen saturation, and heart rate patterns in term breastfeeding infants. *J. Hum. Lact.* **2013**, *29*, 236–245. [CrossRef] [PubMed]
50. Schrank, W.; Al-Sayed, L.E.; Beahm, P.H.; Thach, B.T. Feeding responses to free-flow formula in term and preterm infants. *J. Pediatr.* **1998**, *132*, 426–430. [CrossRef]
51. Chen, C.H.; Wang, T.M.; Chang, H.M.; Chi, C.S. The effect of breast- and bottle-feeding on oxygen saturation and body temperature in preterm infants. *J. Hum. Lact.* **2000**, *16*, 21–27. [CrossRef] [PubMed]
52. Hsiao, C.C.; Tsai, M.L.; Chen, C.C.; Lin, H.C. Early optimal nutrition improves neurodevelopmental outcomes for very preterm infants. *Nutr. Rev.* **2014**, *72*, 532–540. [CrossRef] [PubMed]
53. Cannon, A.M.; Sakalidis, V.S.; Lai, C.T.; Perrella, S.L.; Geddes, D.T. Vacuum characteristics of the sucking cycle and relationships with milk removal from the breast in term infants. *Early Hum. Dev.* **2016**, *96*, 1–6. [CrossRef] [PubMed]
54. Paulsson, L.; Soderfeldt, B.; Bondemark, L. Malocclusion traits and orthodontic treatment needs in prematurely born children. *Angle Orthod.* **2008**, *78*, 786–792. [CrossRef] [PubMed]
55. Zaidi, I.; Thayath, M.N.; Singh, S.; Sinha, A. Preterm birth: A primary etiological factor for delayed oral growth and development. *Int. J. Clin. Pediatr. Dent.* **2015**, *8*, 215–219. [CrossRef] [PubMed]
56. Huang, Y.S.; Guilleminault, C. Pediatric obstructive sleep apnea and the critical role of oral-facial growth: Evidences. *Front. Neurol.* **2012**, *3*, 184. [CrossRef] [PubMed]

8

Role of Vitamin A in Mammary Gland Development and Lactation

M. Teresa Cabezuelo [1,2], Rosa Zaragozá [3,*], Teresa Barber [4] and Juan R. Viña [4]

1 Department of Physiology, Universitat de València, Avda. Blasco Ibañez, 15, 46010 Valencia, Spain; tecabar@alumni.uv.es
2 University Hospital Doctor Peset, Gaspar Aguilar, 90, 46017 Valencia, Spain
3 Department of Human Anatomy and Embryology-INCLIVA Biomedical Research Institute, Universitat de València, 46010 Valencia, Spain
4 Department of Biochemistry and Molecular Biology-INCLIVA Biomedical Research Institute, Universitat de València, 46010 Valencia, Spain; teresa.barber@uv.es (T.B.); juan.r.vina@uv.es (J.R.V.)
* Correspondence: rosa.zaragoza@uv.es

Abstract: Vitamin A (all-*trans*-retinol), its active derivatives retinal and retinoic acid, and their synthetic analogues constitute the group of retinoids. It is obtained from diet either as preformed vitamin A or as carotenoids. Retinal plays a biological role in vision, but most of the effects of vitamin A are exerted by retinoic acid, which binds to nuclear receptors and regulates gene transcription. Vitamin A deficiency is an important nutritional problem, particularly in the developing world. Retinol and carotenoids from diet during pregnancy and lactation influence their concentration in breast milk, which is important in the long term, not only for the offspring, but also for maternal health. In this study, we review the role of vitamin A in mammary gland metabolism, where retinoid signaling is required not only for morphogenesis and development of the gland and for adequate milk production, but also during the weaning process, when epithelial cell death is coupled with tissue remodeling.

Keywords: vitamin A; retinoic acid; vitamin A deficiency; lactating mammary gland; weaning; involution

---

1. Introduction

Vitamin A, an isoprenic-derived micronutrient, strictly refers to the alcoholic form all-*trans*-retinol, although in a broad sense includes both its active derivatives as well as other synthetic analogues that exhibit its biological actions. All of these molecules constitute the group of retinoids [1]. Their important role has been demonstrated through many scientific approaches and clinical observations. Retinoids are required for embryonic development and exert important effects on postnatal physiological events, including cell differentiation and proliferation, immunity, ocular function, and reproduction, and are also important antioxidants [2–9]; however, it must also be considered that treatment with retinoic acid (RA) can increase oxidative stress [10].

Retinol is a liposoluble micronutrient essential in our diet. It is available in foods either as preformed vitamin A; as retinyl ester (RE), abundant in some animal-derived sources such as liver, eggs, dairy products, and fatty fish; or as provitamin A carotenoids, mainly β-carotene, abundant in dark colored fruits and vegetables such as green leaves, carrots, ripe mangos, and other orange–yellow vegetables. This heterogeneous group of carotenoids presents other healthy effects as well, including antioxidant, anti-inflammatory, and immunomodulatory properties [11]. Dietary vitamin A is absorbed in the small intestine in the form of retinol and transported in blood attached to retinol-binding protein (RBP). Inside the cells, retinol is oxidized into its main biologically active derivatives, first retinaldehyde (retinal), which plays a role in vision, and then retinoic acid (RA), which regulates the expression of multiple target genes. Most functions of vitamin A are mediated through the RA activation of two types of transcription factors, retinoic acid receptors (RARs) and retinoid X receptors (RXRs), each with three subtypes (α, β, and γ) and each of those with different isoforms [12]. All-*trans*-RA (atRA) is a high-affinity ligand for RARs, while 9-*cis*-RA binds to RARs and RXRs. Upon binding to RA, RAR–RXR heterodimers bind to the RA response element (RARE) in the promoter regions of target genes and stimulate their transcription. Moreover, RA also has extranuclear, nontranscriptional effects, which directly influence the expression of several genes through phosphorylation processes. Different transcriptional effects of retinol and retinal have also been extensively described [12–15].

According to the World Health Organization (WHO), vitamin A deficiency (VAD) is a public health problem in 50% of countries; it is the most common nutritional disorder in the world, along with protein malnutrition. The leading cause of VAD in humans is deficient dietary intake, which occurs particularly in developing countries and may be exacerbated by high rates of infection, especially diarrhea and measles. In low- and middle-income countries, where intake of animal-based foods is low, dietary provitamin A carotenoids are the main source of vitamin A, and higher amounts are needed to meet the requirements of this vitamin. VAD might be aggravated during the stages of life in which nutritional demands are greater, such as pregnancy, lactation, and early childhood [16]. Dietary deficiency can start early in life, with the colostrum being discarded or with inadequate breastfeeding, which means that babies are deprived of their first important source of vitamin A. Mothers from poorer populations, where intake of vitamin A and carotenoids is marginal, have a much lower content of these micronutrients in their milk compared to mothers from developed countries. It is important to consider that nutrients provided through maternal milk derive not only from the diet during pregnancy and lactation, but also from maternal reserves. In this sense, the potential long-term effects of nutrient depletion during any of these periods are important not only to fetal and child development, but also to maternal health [11,16–19].

This review focuses on the role of vitamin A in the mammary gland along each developmental stage. First, it covers the importance of retinoids in the morphogenesis and development of the gland. Next, we note that during lactation, it is essential to meet the requirements to fulfill an adequate milk production. Finally, we also consider the role of this micronutrient in the weaning process, when extensive tissue remodeling occurs and epithelial tissue regresses to return the gland to a structure similar to the pre-pregnant state, thus the tissue is prepared for the next pregnancy and lactation. We also cover the impact of vitamin A deficiency on both the mother and her offspring's health during the period of pregnancy and lactation, when the most important stages of development in human life occur.

2. Vitamin A Dietary Sources, Availability, and Requirements

Dietary vitamin A is obtained in mainly two forms, as preformed vitamin A or as provitamin A carotenoids. Preformed vitamin A is mainly found as long-chain fatty acid esters of retinol, particularly retinyl esters (REs), which are easily hydrolyzed endogenously to form retinol. Preformed vitamin A is found in animal sources such as eggs, fish oils, organ meats, and dairy products and their derivatives, although liver is considered the source with the greatest quantitative importance. On the other hand, the provitamin A carotenoids, polyisoprenoid pigments of vegetable origin, are partially converted to vitamin A in the intestinal mucosa. To date, more than 750 carotenoids have been identified, although only about 40 of them are consumed in substantial amounts in the human diet, the most abundant being β-carotene, lycopene, lutein, β-cryptoxanthin, α-carotene, and zeaxanthin [20]. Not all carotenoids exhibit provitamin A properties; only 10% of natural carotenoids can be metabolically cleaved to produce at least one molecule of retinol. The main structural requirement of a carotenoid for its provitamin A activity is the presence of at least one ring of unsubstituted β-ionone with a polyene chain of 11 or more carbon atoms [21,22]. As previously mentioned, only a few of these precursors with provitamin A activity are found in significant amounts in the human diet, mainly β-carotene, with minor contributions from α-carotene, β-cryptoxanthin, β-canthaxanthin, and β-echinenone.

The dietary sources of these carotenoids are colored fruits (orange, apricot, mango, etc.) and some vegetables and their formulations (carrot, tomato, sweet potato, pumpkin, broccoli, cabbage, spinach, red palm oil, etc.) [23–25]. Other carotenoids commonly found in foods, such as lycopene, lutein, and zeaxanthin, do not meet these structural requirements and are not precursors of vitamin A.

Dietary sources of vitamin A differ among countries, due to not only economic but also cultural factors. In Western countries, approximately 75% of vitamin A is ingested as preformed REs and comes mainly from dairy products, or fortified products such as breakfast cereals, butter or margarine, and infant formula. On the other hand, in developing countries, 70–90% of vitamin A is consumed as provitamin A carotenoids. Therefore, in populations in low-income countries where vitamin A is mainly consumed in the form of carotenoids, the risk of VAD increases [16,26]. Moreover, in low-income countries with a rice-based diet, VAD is aggravated, since rice lacks this vitamin. Consequently, in some developing countries, vitamin A is added to certain products, such as sugar, thus improving the vitamin A status in the global population. Several successful efforts have been made to improve the provitamin A content in major crops such as wheat, rice, and potato, which are poor in β-carotene (e.g., "golden" rice or "golden" potato tubers that overexpress three bacterial genes for β-carotene synthesis) [27–30]. In spite of these modifications, the prevalence of subclinical deficiency is increasing [25]. However, it also has to be taken into account that VAD is not exclusive to developing countries, as it can also occur in Western societies depending on different factors such as a highly restrictive diet [16,31–36].

The bioavailability of vitamin A in food is defined as the ingested fraction available for use and storage, and depends on the capacity of the digestive process to release it from its original matrix in the food and on the fraction, which, once absorbed, is converted into retinol. Vitamin A bioavailability is higher in foods of animal origin (retinyl esters, preformed vitamin A) compared to vegetable origin (provitamin A carotenoids), although some of the latter group are considered good sources of vitamin A. Based on the efficiency of absorption and conversion into vitamin A, 1 μg of all-*trans*-retinol is equivalent to 12 μg of β-carotene and 24 μg of α-carotene or β-cryptoxanthin. However, the efficiency of β-carotene to be converted into retinoids is probably worse than previously thought, particularly in developing countries where vitamin A status and several other factors can reduce its conversion efficiency [31,36]. Accordingly, the use of a 21:1 ratio for mixed diets (12:1 for fruits and 26:1 for vegetables) has been suggested [25,36]. Thus, compared with preformed vitamin A, provitamin A carotenoids are relatively poor but important sources of vitamin A for the global population, as a higher amount is needed to meet vitamin A needs. On the other hand, it is important to consider for all groups of populations that several factors can influence the bioavailability of vitamin A from the diet, including the presence and severity of infections and parasites, intestinal or liver disease, iron and zinc status, xenobiotics, levels of dietary fat, protein malnutrition, alcohol intake, dietary source (preformed or provitamin A carotenoids), and food processing [11,16,31,35,37–40].

The requirements for vitamin A are expressed in retinol activity equivalent (RAE): 1 μg of RAE is equal to 1 μg of all-*trans*-retinol. In terms of international units (IUs), 1 IU is equal to 0.3 μg of all-*trans*-retinol or 0.3 μg of RAE. The recommended dietary allowances (RDAs) for children, men, and women are 300–600, 900, and 700 mg of RAE/day, respectively. However, the demand for micronutrients increases to 750 mg of RAE/day during pregnancy and 1300 mg of RAE/day during lactation. The gestational period is nutritionally relevant for maternal, fetal, and infant health. During the breastfeeding period, lactating mothers are susceptible to vitamin deficiency as the neonate feeds on her stores through the milk. Vitamin A is one of the most critical micronutrients in this period, affecting lung function and maturation, and thus susceptibility to infection. Inadequate maternal intake of vitamin A translates to an inadequate supply to the fetus during pregnancy and to the neonate during lactation through breast milk [37,41–44]. It is noteworthy that this deficiency during embryogenesis and the early months of life cannot be compensated in the postnatal period. Furthermore, in humans, an insufficient supply of vitamin A to the fetus is associated with organ malformations, preterm birth, and low neonatal stores, which increase the risk of infectious diseases and could exert a negative effect on health later in life [36,45–47]. Pregnant and breastfeeding women are considered to be at risk due to their higher demand for micronutrients, and should be advised to consume enriched products with β-carotene or, even better, vitamin A plus β-carotene, in order to avoid nutritional deficits [16,19,25,31–34,48].

In contrast to what was established in the case of vitamin A, there is no dietary intake recommendation for carotenoids for any population group. The average intake of β-carotene in Western societies is 3.9 mg/day and the total intake of provitamin A carotenoids is approximately 5.2 mg/day, higher in woman than men. The maximum daily amount of β-carotene that the adult intestine can cleave is approximately 2.5 mg, and the minimum amount of fat required for optimal absorption of carotenoids is about 3–5 g per meal [31,34,41,45].

3. Intertissue Flux and Metabolic Transformations of Vitamin A

Vitamin A, mainly found in the diet as REs, is hydrolyzed in the lumen of the small intestine into retinol molecules. This free retinol enters the enterocytes by a carrier-mediated process and by passive diffusion. On the other hand, vitamin A precursors, carotenoids, cross the epithelial cells by membrane-bound transporters and are metabolized within the cells to retinal, which can then be converted to retinol. Absorption of vitamin A appears to be fairly high and more significant than that of carotenoids. However, due to their hydrophobic nature, the absorption of both preformed and vitamin A precursors depends on micellar solubilization and thus on the fat content of the diet [25].

After absorption, retinol is re-esterified to REs, incorporated into chylomicrons together with a small fraction of carotenoids, and transported for a short time in plasma. Finally, the action of lipoprotein lipase (LPL) in different tissues affects chylomicron remnants that contain REs. Those chylomicron remnants are directed mainly to the liver in a receptor-mediated process (low-density lipoprotein (LDL) receptor, or via LDL-related protein, LRP). REs are then hydrolyzed back to retinol in the liver, which is secreted into plasma associated with retinol binding protein (RBP4), oxidized to RA, or transferred to stellate cells for storage mainly as esters of palmitic acid. Thus, the liver serves as the main pool for vitamin A (Figure 1) [23,40,49–52]. When needed, the vitamin A reserve is mobilized and secreted as the all-*trans*-retinol–RBP (holo-RBP4) complex to circulating blood. This complex associates with transthyretin (1:1) in plasma, reducing the glomerular filtration of retinol in the kidneys.

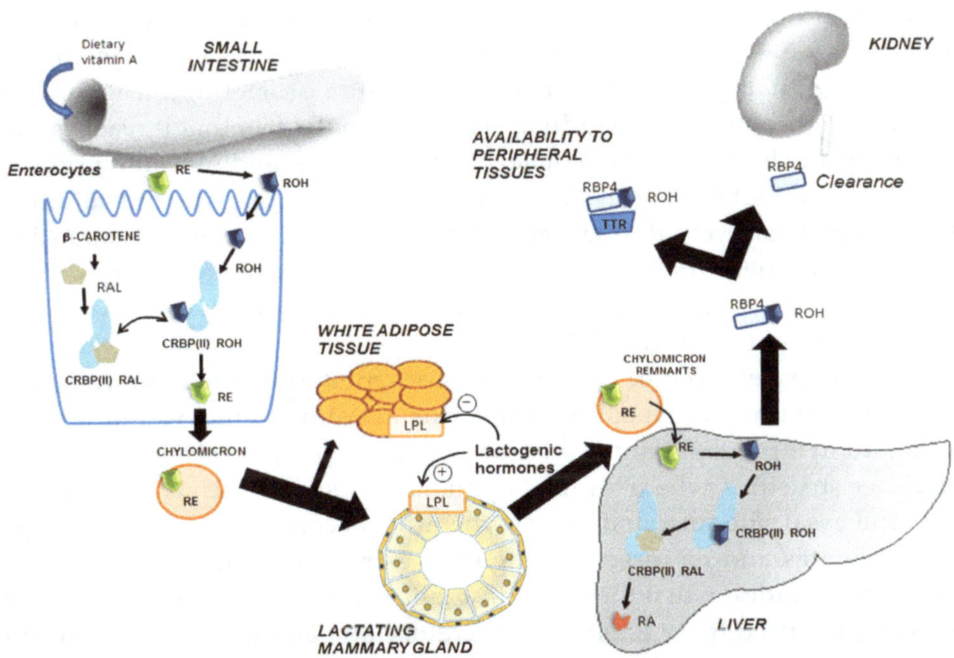

Figure 1. Intertissue flux of vitamin A during lactation. Dietary intake of vitamin A occurs mainly in

the form of precursor β-carotene from vegetables and fruits, or retinyl esters (REs) from sources of animal origin. Both molecules are absorbed by enterocytes in the small intestine, although REs must be hydrolyzed into retinol (ROH) within the intestinal lumen by means of hydrolases. Within enterocytes, ROH and β-carotene are metabolized into REs, which in turn are secreted into the lymph in chylomicrons. Circulating chylomicrons, before reaching the liver, are hydrolyzed in tissues with lipoprotein lipase (LPL) activity and REs released into these extrahepatic tissues. During lactation, increased levels of lactogenic hormones regulate LPL activity, inducing it in the mammary tissue, whereas it is reduced in white adipose tissue. The effect of these hormones redirects REs into the mammary epithelial cells during lactation. Finally, chylomicron remnants are taken up by hepatocytes, where REs are hydrolyzed into ROH, stored, or oxidized to retinoic acid (RA). When needed, ROH is released from hepatic cells into plasma bound to retinol-binding protein (RBP4). Once in plasma, it associates with the stabilizing protein transthyretin (TTR), which decreases the renal clearance of vitamin A [49–55].

Retinol is delivered from plasma to extrahepatic cells by free diffusion or a receptor-mediated process (stimulated by RA 6, STRA6) [56]. Once inside the cells, retinol is reversibly oxidized to retinal by enzymes of the retinol dehydrogenase complex and short-chain dehydrogenase/reductase (SDR/RDH) families. Retinal is irreversibly oxidized to RA by cytosolic aldehyde dehydrogenase 1 (ALDH1) isoenzymes. RA regulates gene transcription by binding to nuclear retinoid receptors (RARs and RXRs), which act as transcription factors and can be further oxidized for excretion, catalyzed by mono-oxygenases of the CYP family. There are cellular binding proteins for retinol and retinal (CRBP) and RA (CRABP), which enable their metabolism and action [25,40,49,56].

4. Role of Vitamin A during Development and Regression of the Mammary Gland

Vitamin A has several pleiotropic effects in cell differentiation, embryogenesis, apoptosis, etc. Retinoic acid and its precursor retinol are known to be involved in the maintenance, differentiation, and function of many epithelial tissues, among which the mammary gland is included.

4.1. An Overview of Mammary Gland Development

The mammary gland structure consists of a compound tubulo-alveolar gland embedded within irregular connective tissue. This complex organ undergoes a series of changes from conception to senescence, which are regulated by hormonal activity, mainly prolactin, estrogen, and progesterone. The peculiarity of this highly dynamic glandular tissue lies in the fact that it reaches full development only after birth. During the lifetime of the female, the mammary gland will suffer profound changes in structure and function to adapt to the physiological processes of pregnancy, lactation, and involution. Moreover, with each menstrual cycle, the mammary gland undergoes a round of expansion, proliferation, and regression under the influence of sexual hormones. Along these different stages, the subpopulations of cells that form mammary tissue will proliferate, differentiate, or even die, giving rise to significant remodeling of the glandular architecture [57].

At birth, a rudimentary embryonic ductal tree is present and will remain quiescent until puberty. At this point, under the control of sexual hormones, ductal epithelium develops and grows, invading the mammary fat pad in a process known as branching morphogenesis. Finally, the gland reaches a bilayered ductal tree structure, where luminal epithelial cells form the alveoli, with their apical side toward the lumen and basal side surrounded by myoepithelial contractile cells. Throughout adulthood, the epithelium proliferates and regresses during each estrous/menstrual cycle [58]. However, it is during pregnancy and lactation when the most dramatic changes occur: Proliferation of the alveolar epithelium concomitant with differentiation into secretory alveoli capable of producing milk. During lactation, oxytocin released by suckling stimuli will trigger the contraction of myoepithelial basal cells, and thus milk ejection toward the nipple. Then, after weaning, secretory epithelial cells are no longer needed and there is regression of the epithelial compartment, together with re-differentiation of adipocytes. This process, termed involution, includes programmed cell death and remodeling of the mammary gland and extracellular matrix (ECM), mainly driven by metalloproteases, returning the gland to the pre-pregnant state. Finally, during the postmenopausal period, the breast undergoes a second process of involution, characterized by atrophy of the parenchymal structures [59].

The mammary gland is a unique experimental model to study all of the physiological changes that occur along the different developmental stages: Proliferation, branching morphogenesis, differentiation, cell death, regression, and adipocyte differentiation. In this sense, several murine models have been extensively used to decipher the underlying mechanisms controlling all of these processes [60–70].

4.2. Retinoids and Mammary Gland Development

RA is an important regulator of cell differentiation and plays a major role in embryonic development and tissue remodeling [71]. The biological action of RA is mediated by three nuclear receptors, RARα, β, and γ, which are ubiquitously expressed in the breast. Moreover, several in vivo and in vitro studies have shown that RA is required for mammary gland morphogenesis. RA signaling is involved in initiating mammary gland formation, and precise levels of RA are crucial for normal mammary epithelium development during embryogenesis. Indeed, the expression of several genes involved in RA signaling, such as retinaldehyde dehydrogenase 2 (*Raldh2*) or RARβ, has been detected in mouse embryos at day 10.5. In cultured mouse flanks, the expression of genes involved in mammary gland development could be modulated by retinoic acid signaling. It is interesting to point out that during embryonic development, the mammary epithelium was inhibited by both increased and decreased levels of RA, reinforcing the importance of a narrow range for this molecule to exert its physiological function [60].

Nevertheless, the role of retinoids within the mammary gland is not restricted to the early embryonic stages when rudimentary mammary gland is formed. On the contrary, retinoid signaling regulates almost all developmental stages of the mammary tissue. Several studies have shown that retinoic acid signaling is required for development of the mammary gland after birth. The effects of retinoids are mediated through RARs and RXRs, which are differently expressed in distinct phases of mammary gland development [61]. Indeed, RARα controls mammary development before and during puberty, and loss of this nuclear receptor has a major effect on expansion of the neonatal ductal tree and branching morphogenesis in pubertal mice [61,62]. Similarly, in adult human breast tissue, RARα is also ubiquitously expressed in the nuclei of mammary epithelial cells, and the effects of RA seem to be controlled by the expression of *Raldh1*, which converts retinol to RA. In fact, in primary cultures from human mammary epithelial cells, when this gene was knocked down, mammosphere formation was significantly reduced. This effect could be rescued by treating the cells with RA, suggesting that the retinoic acid pathway is essential for mammosphere formation and thus for branching morphogenesis [63].

Analogous results were obtained in murine models of pregnancy and lactation. Abrogation of the RA signaling pathway in transgenic mouse models led to mammary gland hyperplasia [61,64] and excessive branching morphogenesis, and these mice displayed lactational deficiency. These effects of VAD deficiency could be reverted by RA supplementation, confirming that vitamin A is essential for mammary gland development at both nulliparous and pregnancy/lactation stages [61]. Further reinforcing these results, it was shown that RA induced lumen formation in vitro in a two-dimensional (2D) model where mammary epithelial cells were grown in collagen gels [65], and treatment of MCF-10A cells with RA induced re-differentiation of these cells [66]. The role of vitamin A in lumen morphogenesis is by mediation through the RARα signaling pathway, extending beyond the intracellular effects, since extracellular matrix remodeling is required for lumen formation. Moreover, RA deficiency in mice shows stromal hypercellularity and increased collagen, altering homeostasis in the ECM [64]. All of these findings therefore indicate that retinoids play an important role in the development and maintenance of glandular epithelial structures.

4.3. Retinoid Signaling During Mammary Gland Involution

At the end of lactation, following weaning of the offspring, the mammary gland undergoes massive cell death and tissue remodeling with regression of the epithelial structures in order to return to a virgin-like state. Involution is characterized by three major events: Programmed cell death of epithelial cells, degradation of the basement membrane and ECM remodeling, and, finally, adipocyte repopulation with a concomitant loss of the lobular–alveolar structure (Figure 2) [68–70]. Several signaling pathways are known to modulate mammary gland involution. Milk stasis within the gland activates programmed cell death of epithelial secretory cells that are no longer needed; this process is ruled by STAT3 and NF-κB transcription factors, which are rapidly activated upon cessation of suckling stimuli [68,72,73].

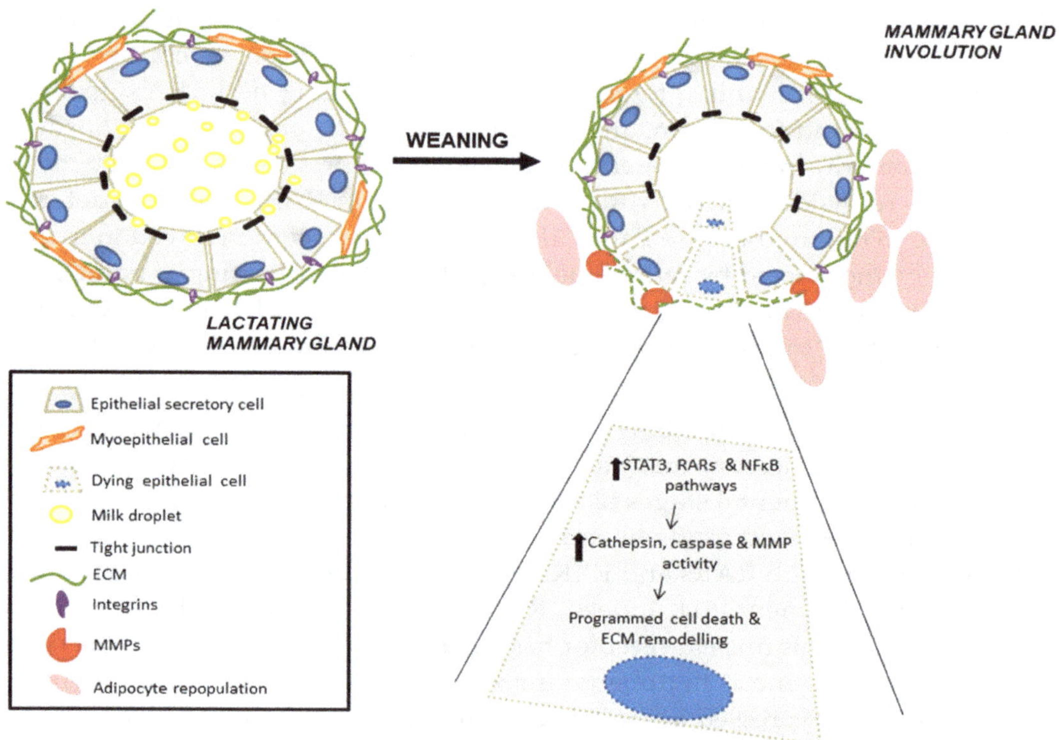

Figure 2. Schematic model of mammary gland involution. Lactation is characterized by an alveolar architecture lined by secretory mammary epithelial cells and contractile myoepithelial cells underneath. After weaning, milk stasis within the lumen and other local factors initiate involution of the mammary gland. At this point, cell shedding and cell death (cells with dotted lines) begins by 12 h after milk stasis, but lactation is still reversible until 48 h of weaning. Beyond this time point, epithelial tight junctions are disrupted, followed by extracellular matrix (ECM) remodeling and adipocyte re-differentiation [68,70,72,73]. MMP, metalloprotease; RAR, retinoic acid receptor; STAT3, signal transducer and activator of transcription 3; NF-kB, nuclear factor kappa B.

One could hypothesize that since milk production has ceased during this stage and blood flow to the gland also decreases, vitamin A recruitment to the gland would also be reduced, thus inhibiting the whole signaling pathway. Surprisingly, vitamin A plays an important role during weaning, not as a micronutrient to be secreted within milk, but as a signaling molecule instead. The RA signaling pathway is fully activated during mammary gland involution. Cytoplasmic transporter CRABP II and CRBP-I carrier proteins, together with several isoforms of RAR and RXRα, are significantly increased during involution. Besides, as previously described, RARα exerts its effect by binding to gene promoters such as the metalloprotease 9 (MMP-9) promoter, which induces MMP-9 mRNA and protein levels and, finally, proteinase activity [67]. The role of retinoids in matrix remodeling is reinforced by the fact that administration of an acute dose of retinol palmitate to control lactating rats also induced MMP-9 expression. This emphasizes the importance of retinoids in vivo to regulate mammary gland involution [67,68].

5. Vitamin A and Carotenoid Uptake by the Mammary Gland during Lactation

Vitamin A is transferred to the offspring by limited placental transfer during gestation, and mostly through maternal milk during the neonatal period. Because of the limited transplacental transfer, mammal newborns have low stores of vitamin A, depending significantly on the lactation period to acquire enough reserves and maintain adequate growth and development [37,44,45,74–79].

Lactation is characterized by widespread changes in the metabolism of different tissues to ensure a sufficient supply of nutrients to the mammary gland for milk production [80]. Among these changes, LPL in adipose tissue is inhibited; meanwhile, this enzyme is activated in the mammary tissue, therefore triglycerides are redirected to the latter [53–55]. Regarding amino acid and glutathione metabolism, there is also redistribution from the liver to the mammary gland, together with a nitrogen-sparing mechanism [81–85]. In addition, several physiological changes are required to ensure proper milk production, such as hyperphagia, liver and mammary gland hypertrophy, increased cardiac output, and increased blood flow to the gland. In this sense, substrate uptake by the lactating mammary gland is determined by several factors: (1) Increased availability of the substrates, which is met by hyperphagia and increased blood flow and substantial redistribution from different tissues to the mammary gland [81,82]; (2) transport mechanisms with increased expression of several carriers [85]; and (3) increased metabolism of nutrients within the gland [83,84]. All of these factors are under tight regulation by local and general effectors and contribute to milk production (Figure 3).

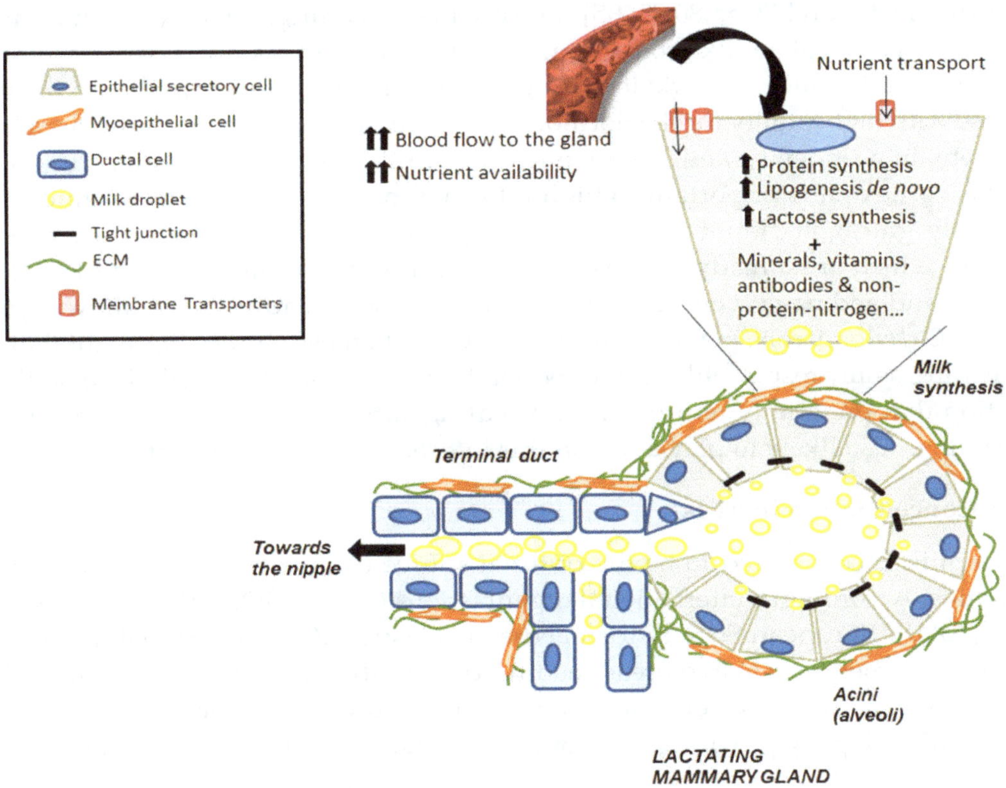

Figure 3. Metabolic events that lead to milk synthesis in alveolar cells from lactating mammary gland. During lactation, increased blood flow and intertissue redistribution of nutrients toward the mammary gland, together with increased membrane transporters, ensure bioavailability of precursors for milk synthesis within the epithelial cells. Both lipid and carbohydrate anabolism are increased, as is protein synthesis. Within the apex of the alveoli, milk-lipid droplets are formed and released toward the lumen with other milk components such as vitamins, minerals, and salts [81–85].

Vitamin A sources for the mammary gland comprise REs and carotenoids packed in the chylomicrons synthesized from dietary intake, and serum retinol (RBP4–retinol), which does not vary over a wide range of vitamin A ingestion and will be esterified within the mammary gland. During lactation, hyperphagia allows for higher vitamin A and carotenoid intake, which is associated with increased redistribution to the mammary tissue and thus to the secreted milk. REs associated with chylomicrons from the diet travel through the lymph and plasma, reaching extrahepatic tissues before getting to the liver. During breastfeeding, a great proportion of this vitamin A from the diet is redirected, preferably to lactating mammary tissue, as the activity of LPL in the mammary gland is a determinant for this highest uptake by the gland [53–55]. Indeed, the higher activity of LPL in thr mammary gland and the depressed activity in other tissues, such as adipose tissue, triggers the transfer of fatty acids, partial triglycerides, some unesterified cholesterol, and fat-soluble vitamins to the parenchymal cells of the gland during lactation (Figure 1). Once inside the mammary secretory epithelial cells, retinol is found to be bound to CRBPs, which will facilitate metabolism or excretion of this compound. In fact, it has been reported that CRBP-I and CRBP-III are both expressed in the mammary gland at different developmental stages. CRBP-III-null mice showed reduced RE levels in milk, suggesting that this isoform plays a role in retinol metabolism within lactating mammary tissue [86]. Human-milk vitamin A is present almost exclusively as REs, mainly retinyl palmitate, in the lipid fraction of the milk.

Hormonal changes are responsible for this nutrient redistribution and higher uptake within the mammary tissue. Preceding parturition, a number of hormones (insulin, steroids, and prolactin) play a role in preparing the gland for lactation [76]. Several studies using animal models have elucidated the role of these hormones in the intertissue flux of nutrients, together with the metabolic adaptations that occur during lactation [53–55,80,83–85]. During breastfeeding, the regulation of metabolism in lactating rats, and in particular milk production, appears to depend mainly on two hormones, prolactin and insulin. The insulin/glucagon ratio in lactation is decreased, but the number of insulin receptors, especially those with high affinity for the hormone, are increased in lactating mammary gland, contrary to what happens in adipocytes and hepatocytes, where the number of insulin receptors does not change. In this context, it is important to highlight that mammary tissue lacks glucagon receptors, and consequently, glucagon cannot affect mammary gland metabolism. On the other hand, prolactin levels in serum, which are already increased at the end of gestation, enhance LPL activity within the mammary gland and negatively regulate LPL activity within adipocytes, allowing for increased metabolism of RE-chylomicrons in mammary tissue. Overall, these studies highlight that high plasma prolactin levels are mainly responsible for the cooperative changes in the metabolism of different tissues during lactation that preferably redirect the circulating substrates to the mammary gland for milk synthesis; insulin is also likely to play a role in this intertissue flux of nutrients [25,53–55,76,80,83,85].

6. Vitamin A Concentration in Milk

Maternal milk is considered to be the optimal source of nutrition for infants and contains all essential vitamins. Accordingly, international organizations (e.g., WHO, UNICEF, American Academy of Pediatrics (AAP), European Society for Paediatric Gastroenterology Hepatology and Nutrition (ESPGHAN)) recommend exclusive breastfeeding during the first 6 months of life [17,41,44]. It is species-specific and a complete food adapted to the requirements for the survival and healthy development of offspring, by providing macronutrients (fats, carbohydrates, proteins, and free amino acids), micronutrients (vitamins and minerals), protective factors, and other important components for growth, such as cytokines, oligosaccharides, growth factors, and hormones [17,42,75–77]. A recent meta-analysis concluded that breast milk is not only a perfect nutritional supply for the infant, but is also probably the most specific personalized medication, at a time in life when genetic expression is being achieved. Breastfeeding provides protection against childhood infections and malocclusion, and is probably related to reductions in instances of overweight and diabetes, and globally could prevent 823,000 deaths of children younger than 5 years annually [87]. However, even in low- and middle-income countries, where breastfeeding duration is longer than in high-income countries, only 37% of children under 6 months of age are exclusively breastfed [87].

The milk produced in the first days after birth (colostrum) is higher in proteins, vitamins A, B12, and K, and immunoglobulins and lower in fat content than mature milk [42,76,88]. Rapid changes occur in breast milk composition during the first week postpartum, and it can be considered mature approximately 15 days after birth [76]. The volume and composition of breast milk are not homogeneous; the milk differs over time and between species, and it also depends on the demands made by the infant and the nutritional status of the mother in the same species. Maternal intake influences the macro- and micronutrient content of breast milk, as well as its immunological properties [44,47,89]. Indeed, the amount of retinol concentration in milk seems to be independent of serum retinol levels. On the contrary, several reports have revealed a strong correlation between vitamin A and carotenoid content in the diet during pregnancy and lactation and the amount of these micronutrients secreted in breast milk [17,43,90,91]. Due to the positive relationship between dietary intake of carotenoids and breastmilk concentration, breastfeeding mothers should have a diet abundant in this micronutrient. Therefore, the recommended dietary allowance (RDA) is higher for pregnant and lactating women than for non-pregnant women [17,19,31,41–43,48,75,90,92].

The concentration of vitamin A in human milk decreases over the course of lactation; it is maximal in the colostrum and reaches a plateau in mature milk. In healthy mothers, the vitamin A concentration varies from 5 to 7 μM in colostrum, 3 to 5 μM in transitional milk, and 1.4 to 2.6 μM in mature milk. The higher concentrations of retinol in colostrum allow tissue stores in the newborn to be rapidly replenished after limited placental transfer during gestation [25,76,88,90,92]. The newborn has a small amount of retinol pools in the liver (range 0–0.34 μmol/g in normal birth weight babies), achieved through the placental route, with maternal milk as the most important source of vitamin A [37,44,45,74–79]. Preterm birth aggravates the situation, since vitamin A liver stores are even lower, as the placental route has been cut off. These babies show lower plasma levels of retinol and retinol binding protein (RBP) at birth compared with full-term newborns. To compensate this deficit in retinol liver pools, it was observed that transitional milk in prematurity had a significant increase in micronutrient levels [91]. Milk retinol concentration in colostrum is lower in mothers of preterm babies (~3 μM) than in mothers of full-term babies [25,91]; however, it increases in transitional milk to values similar to those observed in milk from mothers of full-term babies (3.5 μM). There are no differences in mature milk between preterm and full-term, with milk retinol concentration of ~2 μM in mothers of preterm babies [91]. In this context, it is noteworthy that retinol level in preterm milk seems to be independent of the degree of prematurity [91].

During the first 6 months of life, infants from well-nourished mothers who are exclusively breastfed will accumulate around 310 μmol of vitamin A in the liver, approximately 60-fold higher than vitamin A accumulated throughout gestation by the transplacental pathway [25,88,90]. In fact, it has been reported that partial breastfeeding continues to provide a significant proportion of the recommended intake in infants after 6 months: 42% from 6 to 12 months and 61% during the second year in cases where vitamin A levels are low in the diet after weaning [78].

7. Deficiency of Vitamin A and Carotenoids during Pregnancy and Lactation

Vitamin A is necessary to maintain epithelial tissues, vision, and immune function. Breastfeeding from vitamin A-depleted mothers predisposes infants to the consequences of deficiency. Furthermore, VAD cannot be compensated by postnatal supplementation. As previously mentioned, pregnant and breastfeeding women are considered to be at risk of VAD in developing countries, where vitamin A in the diet is provided mainly as precursor carotenoids with lower bioavailability and efficiency to be converted into retinol. In this sense, several recent studies have shown that low dietary intake correlates with lower concentrations of vitamin A in milk of nursing mothers in Brazil [93,94], African countries [95–99], and Southeast Asia [26]. Thus, vitamin A supplementation for lactating mothers in these areas is regarded as a practical public health strategy to support maternal breastfeeding of newborns, more so of premature babies [25,40,90,92,100,101].

Serum retinol concentration is used to assess vitamin A status, with values below a cutoff of 0.70 μmol/L representing VAD, and below 0.35 μmol/L representing severe VAD. For pregnancy or lactation, the cutoff value is higher, and serum retinol concentration below 1.05 μmol/L reflects low vitamin A status among pregnant and lactating women [16]. The WHO Global Database estimated that clinical VAD (with night blindness and Bitot's spots) and biochemical VAD (with serum retinol concentration <0.70 μmol/L) affected 7 and 219 million preschool-aged children, respectively [16]. Regarding estimations in pregnant women, 19.8 million had low vitamin A status (serum retinol or breast milk concentration < 1.05 μmol/L), of whom 7.2 million were deficient in vitamin A (<0.70 μmol/L) and 6.2 million experienced gestational night blindness. These estimates found that nearly two-thirds of the women with night blindness lived in South and Southeast Asia [16,77,102].

However, it is important to point out that even in Western countries, where vitamin A- and β-carotene-rich foods are normally available, there are groups at risk for low vitamin A levels [16,45, 77,103,104]. One-fifth of the population in developed countries does not get the full recommended intake, with plasma and liver concentrations of vitamin A lower than those accepted as normal [104]. This situation can be aggravated by the increasingly common tendency to reduce fat intake in the diet and to engage in uncontrolled weight loss diets. Therefore, in these countries, it has been considered as subclinical vitamin A deficiency, which has increased markedly worldwide in the last decades [16,32,33,40]. Although calorie and protein content are largely unaffected by a woman's diet, there are some micronutrients in breast milk that will only be at adequate levels if there is sufficient dietary intake. Nutritional supplements should be given to these mothers to fulfill the requirements of micronutrients such as vitamin A in newborns [19,48,103]. It is well established that maternal VAD in pregnancy leads to placental dysfunction, fetal loss, congenital malformations, and preterm birth. Vitamin A-deficient mothers will produce breast milk that is low in the vitamin, consequently triggering VAD in the offspring. During lactation, if breast milk does not provide the neonate with appropriate vitamin A levels, the immune system might be affected, raising the risk for infectious diseases. Indeed, respiratory tract infections and complications during viral infections (e.g., measles) are increased in children with VAD [45]. Also, lung development could be compromised, increasing the risk for bronchopulmonary disease [45]. Indeed, recommended vitamin A during pregnancy, and especially during lactation, increases considerably, an almost 2-fold increase compared to non-pregnancy in terms of RDA [18,31,37,45,74,77,92,102]. A low neonatal store not only increases the risk of infectious diseases in the perinatal period, but also could have a negative effect on health later on in life [45–47]. The most specific clinical effect and one of the first manifestations of VAD is xerophthalmia with nyctalopia. If untreated, this can progress to night blindness; depressed immunity; squamous metaplasia of mucous epithelium in several organs; hyperkeratosis; disturbances in cell differentiation, organ development, growth, and reproduction; increased risk of infection; and mortality [16,32,33,38,43,46,74,102]. Similarly, VAD during pregnancy in experimental animals led to the formation of hypoplastic organs or alterations in fetal organs, such as eyes, brain, kidneys, and lungs, and even to the death and resorption of fetuses, depending on the severity of the deficiency [105–107].

8. Conclusions

Vitamin A plays a role in mammary gland metabolism during lactation. On the one hand, RA is essential for mammary gland development and, later on, in secretory epithelia to achieve adequate milk production. On the other hand, retinoids, through the RARα-dependent signaling pathway, have also been shown to regulate, at least in part, the weaning process, where epithelial cell death is coupled with tissue remodeling. Nevertheless, RA should not be considered exclusively as a signaling molecule controlling the development of mammary tissue, but also as a micronutrient essential for fetal and neonatal development. In this sense, the fetal liver stores only a small amount of vitamin A during gestation; therefore, the neonate depends on the external supply from the mother's milk.

An appropriate dietary intake of retinol and β-carotene during pregnancy and lactation together with the intertissue flux of different nutrients in the gland during lactation influence vitamin A concentration in breast milk. This is important in the long term, not only for maternal health, but also for the offspring, because vitamin A is involved in postnatal physiological functions.

Author Contributions: J.R.V. and T.B. were responsible for the general structure of the paper. J.R.V., T.B., M.T.C., and R.Z. performed the literature search, compiled and analyzed the data, drafted the manuscript, and designed the drawings. The final version was discussed by all authors, who gave their approval before submission. All authors have read and agreed to the published version of the manuscript.

References

1. McLaren, D.S.; Kraemer, K. Vitamin A in nature. *World Rev. Nutr. Diet* **2012**, *103*, 7–17. [CrossRef] [PubMed]
2. De Luca, L.M. Retinoids and their receptors in differentiation, embryogenesis and neoplasia. *FASEB J.* **1991**, *5*, 2924–2933. [CrossRef] [PubMed]
3. Livrea, M.A.; Tesoriere, L. Antioxidant activity of vitamin A within lipid environments. In *Fat-Soluble Vitamins*; Subcellular Biochemistry; Springer: Boston, MA, USA, 1998; Volume 30, pp. 113–143. [CrossRef]
4. Barber, T.; Borrás, E.; Torres, L.; García, C.; Cabezuelo, F.; Lloret, A.; Pallardó, F.V.; Viña, J.R. Vitamin A deficiency causes oxidative damage to liver mitochondria in rats. *Free Radic. Biol. Med.* **2000**, *29*, 1–7. [CrossRef]
5. Clagett-Dame, M.; Knutson, D. Vitamin A in reproduction and development. *Nutrients* **2011**, *3*, 385–428. [CrossRef] [PubMed]
6. Gimeno, A.; Zaragozá, R.; Vivó-Sesé, I.; Viña, J.R.; Miralles, V.J. Retinol, at concentration greater than the physiological limit, induces oxidative stress and apoptosis in human dermal fibroblasts. *Exp. Dermatol.* **2004**, *13*, 45–54. [CrossRef]
7. Rhinn, M.; Dollé, P. Retinoic acid signaling during development. *Development* **2012**, *139*, 843–858. [CrossRef]
8. Ross, A.C. Vitamin A and retinoic acid in T cell-related immunity. *Am. J. Clin. Nutr.* **2012**, *96*, 1166S–1172S. [CrossRef]
9. Sommer, A.; Vyas, K.S. A global clinical view on vitamin A and carotenoids. *Am. J. Clin. Nutr.* **2012**, *96*, 1204S–1206S. [CrossRef]
10. Esteban-Pretel, G.; Marín, M.P.; Renau-Piqueras, J.; Barber, T.; Timoneda, J. Vitamin A deficiency alters rat lung alveolar basement membrane: Reversibility by retinoic acid. *J. Nutr. Biochem.* **2010**, *21*, 227–236. [CrossRef]
11. Zielinska, M.A.; Wesołowska, A.; Pawlus, B.; Hamułka, J. Health Effects of Carotenoids during Pregnancy and Lactation. *Nutrients* **2017**, *9*, 838. [CrossRef]
12. Chambon, P. A decade of molecular biology of retinoic acid receptors. *FASEB J.* **1996**, *10*, 940–954. [CrossRef] [PubMed]
13. Ziouzenkova, O.; Orasanu, G.; Sharlach, M.; Akiyama, T.E.; Berger, J.P.; Viereck, J.; Hamilton, J.A.; Tang, G.; Dolnokowski, G.G.; Vogel, S.; et al. Retinaldehyde represses adipogenesis and diet-induced obesity. *Nat. Med.* **2007**, *13*, 695–702. [CrossRef] [PubMed]
14. Berry, D.C.; Noy, N. Signaling by Vitamin A and Retinol-Binding Protein in Regulation of Insulin Responses and Lipid Homeostasis. *Biochim. Biophys. Acta* **2012**, *1821*, 168–176. [CrossRef] [PubMed]
15. Al Tanoury, Z.; Piskunov, A.; Rochette-Egly, C. Vitamin A and Retinoid Signaling: Genomic and Nongenomic Effects. *J. Lipid Res.* **2013**, *54*, 1761–1775. [CrossRef] [PubMed]
16. WHO, World Health Organization. Global prevalence of vitamin A deficiency in populations at risk 1995–2005. In *WHO Global Database on Vitamin A Deficiency*; World Health Organization: Geneva, Switzerland, 2009; ISBN 978-92-4-159801-9.
17. Emmett, P.M.; Rogers, I.S. Properties of human milk and their relationship with maternal nutrition. *Early Hum. Dev.* **1997**, *9*, S7–S28. [CrossRef]
18. Strobel, M.; Tinz, J.; Biesalski, H.K. The importance of β-carotene as a source of vitamin A with special regard to pregnant and breastfeeding women. *Eur. J. Nutr.* **2007**, *46*, 1–20. [CrossRef]
19. Cruz, S.; Pereira da Cruz, S.; Ramalho, A. Impact of Vitamin A Supplementation on Pregnant Women and on Women Who Have Just Given Birth: A Systematic Review. *J. Am. Coll. Nutr.* **2018**, *37*, 243–250. [CrossRef]

20. Borel, P.; Desmarchelier, C. Genetic Variations Associated with Vitamin A Status and Vitamin A Bioavailability. *Nutrients* **2017**, *9*, 246. [CrossRef]
21. Das, B.C.; Thapa, P.; Karki, R.; Das, S.; Mahapatra, S.; Liu, T.C.; Torregroza, I.; Wallace, D.P.; Kambhampati, S.; Van Veldhuizen, P.; et al. Retinoic Acid Signaling Pathways in Development and Diseases. *Bioorg. Med. Chem.* **2014**, *22*, 673–683. [CrossRef]
22. Harrison, E.H.; Curley, R.W., Jr. Carotenoids and Retinoids: Nomenclature, Chemistry, and Analysis. In *The Biochemistry of Retinoid Signaling II*; Subcellular Biochemistry; Springer: Dordrecht, The Netherlands, 2016; Volume 81, pp. 1–19. [CrossRef]
23. Eroglu, A.; Harrison, E.H. Carotenoid metabolism in mammals, including man: Formation, occurrence, and function of apocarotenoids. *J. Lipid Res.* **2013**, *54*, 1719–1730. [CrossRef]
24. Kim, Y.K.; Wassef, L.; Chung, S.; Jiang, H.; Wyss, A.; Blaner, W.S.; Quadro, L. β-Carotene and its Cleavage Enzyme β-Carotene-15,15′-oxygenase (CMOI) Affect Retinoid Metabolism in Developing Tissues. *FASEB J.* **2011**, *25*, 1641–1652. [CrossRef] [PubMed]
25. Combs, G.F., Jr.; McClung, J.P. *The Vitamins: Fundamental Aspects in Nutrition and Health*; Academic Press, Elsevier: New York, NY, USA, 2017. [CrossRef]
26. Wieringa, F.T.; Dijkhuizen, M.A.; Berger, J. Micronutrient deficiencies and their public health implications for South-East Asia. *Curr. Opin. Clin. Nutr. Metab. Care* **2019**, *22*, 479–482. [CrossRef] [PubMed]
27. Tang, G.; Qin, J.; Dolnikowski, G.G.; Russell, R.M.; Grusak, M.A. Golden rice is an effective source of vitamin A. *Am. J. Clin. Nutr.* **2009**, *89*, 1776–1783. [CrossRef] [PubMed]
28. Diretto, G.; Al-Babili, S.; Tavazza, R.; Scossa, F.; Papacchioli, V.; Migliore, M.; Beyer, P.; Giuliano, G. Transcriptional-metabolic networks in beta-carotene-enriched potato tubers: The long and winding road to the golden phenotype. *Plant Physiol.* **2010**, *154*, 899–912. [CrossRef]
29. Moghissi, A.A.; Pei, S.; Liu, Y. Golden Rice: Scientific, Regulatory and Public Information Processes of a Genetically Modified Organism. *Crit. Rev. Biotechnol.* **2016**, *36*, 535–541. [CrossRef]
30. Govender, L.; Pillay, K.; Siwela, M.; Modi, A.T.; Mabhaudhi, T. Improving the Dietary Vitamin A Content of Rural Communities in South Africa by Replacing Non-Biofortified white Maize and Sweet Potato with Biofortified Maize and Sweet Potato in Traditional Dishes. *Nutrients* **2019**, *11*, 1198. [CrossRef]
31. NAS, National Academy of Sciences. Dietary References Intakes: The Essential Guide to Nutrient Requirements. In *Food and Nutrition Board*; National Academic Press: Washington, DC, USA, 2006; Available online: http://www.nap.edu/catalog.php?record_id511537#toc (accessed on 25 June 2019).
32. Underwood, B.A. Vitamin A Deficiency Disorders: International Efforts to Control a Preventable "Pox". *J. Nutr.* **2004**, *134*, 231S–236S. [CrossRef]
33. Sommer, A. Vitamin A deficiency and clinical disease: An historical overview. *J. Nutr.* **2008**, *138*, 1835–1839. [CrossRef]
34. Weber, D.; Grune, T. The contribution of β-carotene to vitamin A supply of humans. *Mol. Nutr. Food Res.* **2012**, *56*, 251–258. [CrossRef]
35. Priyadarshani, A.M. A Review on Factors Influencing Bioaccessibility and Bioefficacy of Carotenoids. *Crit. Rev. Food Sci. Nutr.* **2015**, *13*. [CrossRef]
36. Barber, T.; Esteban-Pretel, G.; Marín, M.P.; Timoneda, J. Vitamin A: An Overview. In *Vitamin A and Carotenoids: Chemistry, Analysis, Function and Effects*; Preedy, V.R., Ed.; The Royal Society of Chemistry: London, UK, 2012; pp. 396–416. ISBN 978-1-84973-368-7. [CrossRef]
37. McCauley, M.E.; van den Broek, N.; Dou, L.; Othman, M. Vitamin A supplementation during pregnancy for maternal and newborn outcomes. *Cochrane Database Syst. Rev.* **2015**, *10*. [CrossRef] [PubMed]
38. McLaren, D.S.; Kraemer, K. *Manual on Vitamin Deficiency Disorders (VADD)*, 3rd ed.; Sight and Life Press: Basel, Switzerland, 2012; ISBN 978-3-906412-58-0.
39. Lieber, C.S. Alcohol: Its metabolism and interaction with nutrients. *Annu. Rev. Nutr.* **2000**, *20*, 395–430. [CrossRef] [PubMed]
40. Timoneda, J.; Rodríguez-Fernández, L.; Zaragozá, R.; Marín, M.P.; Cabezuelo, M.T.; Torres, L.; Viña, J.R.; Barber, T. Vitamin A Deficiency and the Lung. *Nutrients* **2018**, *10*, 1132. [CrossRef] [PubMed]
41. Zielinska, M.A.; Hamulka, J.; Wesolowska, A. Month of Lactation and Its Associations with Maternal Dietary Intake and Anthropometric Characteristics. *Nutrients* **2019**, *11*, 193. [CrossRef]
42. Allen, L.H. Multiple micronutrients in pregnancy and lactation: An overview. *Am. J. Clin. Nutr.* **2005**, *81*, 1206S–1212S. [CrossRef]

43. Bravi, F.; Wiens, F.; Decarli, A.; Dal Pont, A.; Agostoni, C.; Ferraroni, M. Impact of maternal nutrition on breast-milk composition: A systematic review. *Am. J. Clin. Nutr.* **2016**, *104*, 646–662. [CrossRef]
44. Erick, M. Breast milk is conditionally perfect. *Med. Hypotheses* **2018**, *111*, 82–89. [CrossRef]
45. Biesalski, H.K.; Nohr, D. The importance of vitamin A during pregnancy and childhood: Impact on lung function. In *Vitamin A and Carotenoids: Chemistry, Analysis, Function and Effects*; Preedy, V.R., Ed.; The Royal Society of Chemistry: London, UK, 2012; pp. 532–554. ISBN 978-1-84973-368-7. [CrossRef]
46. Biesalski, H.K.; Black, R.E. Hidden Hunger. Malnutrition and the First 1000 Days of Life: Causes, Consequences and Solutions. *World Rev. Nutr. Diet* **2016**, *115*, 134–141. [CrossRef]
47. Davisse-Paturet, C.; Adel-Patient, K.; Divaret-Chauveau, A.; Pierson, J.; Lioret, S.; Cheminat, M.; Dufourg, M.-N.; Charles, M.-A.; de Lauzon-Guillain, B. Breastfeeding Status and Duration and Infections, Hospitalizations for Infections, and Antibiotic Use in the First Two Years of Life in the ELFE Cohort. *Nutrients* **2019**, *11*, 1607. [CrossRef]
48. Soares, M.M.; Silva, M.A.; Garcia, P.P.C.; Silva, L.S.D.; Costa, G.D.D.; Araújo, R.M.A.; Cotta, R.M.M. Effect of vitamin A suplementation: A systematic review. *Cien. Saude Colet.* **2019**, *24*, 827–838. [CrossRef]
49. Blomhoff, R.; Blomhoff, H.K. Overview of retinoid metabolism and function. *J. Neurobiol.* **2006**, *66*, 606–630. [CrossRef] [PubMed]
50. D'Ambrosio, D.N.; Clugston, R.D.; Blaner, W.S. Vitamin A Metabolism: An Update. *Nutrients* **2011**, *3*, 63–103. [CrossRef] [PubMed]
51. Blaner, W.S.; Li, Y.; Brun, P.J.; Yueng, J.J.; Lee, S.A.; Clugston, R.D. Vitamin A Absorption, Storage and Mobilization. In *The Biochemistry of Retinoid Signaling II*; Subcellular Biochemistry; Springer: Dordrecht, The Netherlands, 2016; Volume 81, pp. 95–126. [CrossRef]
52. Saeed, A.; Dullaart, R.P.F.; Schreuder, T.C.M.A.; Blokzijl, H.; Faber, K.N. Disturbed Vitamin A Metabolism in Non-Alcoholic Fatty Liver Disease (NAFLD). *Nutrients* **2018**, *10*, 29. [CrossRef] [PubMed]
53. Hang, J.; Rillema, J.A. Prolactin's effects on lipoprotein lipase (LPL) activity and on LPL mRNA levels in cultured mouse mammary gland explants. *Proc. Soc. Exp. Biol. Med.* **1997**, *214*, 161–166. [CrossRef]
54. Zhao, W.S.; Hu, S.L.; Yu, K.; Wang, H.; Wang, W.; Loor, J.; Luo, J. Lipoprotein Lipase, Tissue Expression and Effects on Genes Related to Fatty Acid Synthesis in Goat Mammary Epithelial Cells. *Int. J. Mol. Sci.* **2014**, *15*, 22757–22771. [CrossRef]
55. Jensen, D.R.; Gavigan, S.; Sawicki, V.; Witsell, D.L.; Eckel, R.H.; Neville, M.C. Regulation of Lipoprotein lipase activity and mRNA in the mammary gland of the lactating mouse. *Biochem. J.* **1994**, *298*, 321–327. [CrossRef]
56. Noy, N. Vitamin A transport and cell signaling by the retinol-binding protein receptor STRA6. In *The Biochemistry of Retinoid Signaling II*; Subcellular Biochemistry; Springer: Dordrecht, The Netherlands, 2016; Volume 81, pp. 77–94. [CrossRef]
57. Inman, J.L.; Robertson, C.; Mott, J.D.; Bissell, M.J. Mammary gland development: Cell fate specification, stem cells and the microenvironment. *Development* **2015**, *142*, 1028–1042. [CrossRef]
58. Fata, J.E.; Chaudhary, V.; Khokha, R. Cellular turnover in the mammary gland is correlated with systemic levels of progesterone and not 17beta-estradiol during the estrous cycle. *Biol. Reprod.* **2001**, *65*, 680–688. [CrossRef]
59. Stingl, J.; Raouf, A.; Emerman, J.T.; Eaves, C.J. Epithelial progenitors in the normal human mammary gland. *J. Mammary Gland Biol. Neoplasia* **2005**, *10*, 49–59. [CrossRef]
60. Cho, K.W.; Kwon, H.J.; Shin, J.O.; Lee, J.M.; Cho, S.W.; Tickle, C.; Jung, H.S. Retinoic acid signaling and the initiation of mammary gland development. *Dev. Biol.* **2012**, *365*, 259–266. [CrossRef]
61. Wang, Y.A.; Shen, K.; Wang, Y.; Brooks, S.C. Retinoic acid signaling is required for proper morphogenesis of mammary gland. *Dev. Dyn.* **2005**, *234*, 892–899. [CrossRef] [PubMed]
62. Cohn, E.; Ossowski, L.; Bertran, S.; Marzan, C.; Farias, E.F. RARα1 control of mammary gland ductal morphogenesis and wnt1-tumorigenesis. *Breast Cancer Res.* **2010**, *12*, R79. [CrossRef] [PubMed]
63. Honeth, G.; Lombardi, S.; Ginestier, C.; Hur, M.; Marlow, R.; Buchupalli, B.; Shinomiya, I.; Gazinska, P.; Bombelli, S.; Ramalingam, V.; et al. Aldehyde dehydrogenase and estrogen receptor define a hierarchy of cellular differentiation in the normal human mammary epithelium. *Breast Cancer Res.* **2014**, *16*, R52. [CrossRef] [PubMed]
64. Pierzchalski, K.; Yu, J.; Norman, V.; Kane, M.A. CrbpI regulates mammary retinoic acid homeostasis and the mammary microenvironment. *FASEB J.* **2013**, *27*, 1904–1916. [CrossRef]

65. Montesano, R.; Soulié, P. Retinoids induce lumen morphogenesis in mammary epithelial cells. *J. Cell Sci.* **2002**, *115*, 4419–4431. [CrossRef]
66. Arisi, M.F.; Starker, R.A.; Addya, S.; Huang, Y.; Fernandez, S.V. All trans-retinoic acid (ATRA) induces re-differentiation of early transformed breast epithelial cells. *Int. J. Oncol.* **2014**, *44*, 1831–1842. [CrossRef]
67. Zaragozá, R.; Gimeno, A.; Miralles, V.J.; García-Trevijano, E.R.; Carmena, R.; García, C.; Mata, M.; Puertes, I.R.; Torres, L.; Viña, J.R. Retinoids induce MMP-9 expression through RAR alpha during mammary gland remodeling. *Am. J. Physiol. Endocrinol. Metab.* **2007**, *292*, E1140–E1148. [CrossRef]
68. Zaragozá, R.; García-Trevijano, E.R.; Lluch, A.; Ribas, G.; Viña, J.R. Involvement of Different networks in mammary gland involution after the pregnancy/lactation cycle: Implications in breast cancer. *IUBMB Life* **2015**, *67*, 227–238. [CrossRef]
69. McNally, S.; Stein, T. Overview of Mammary Gland Development: A Comparison of Mouse and Human. *Methods Mol. Biol.* **2017**, *1501*, 1–17. [CrossRef]
70. Jena, M.K.; Jaswal, S.; Kumar, S.; Mohanty, A.K. Molecular mechanism of mammary gland involution: An update. *Dev. Biol.* **2019**, *445*, 145–155. [CrossRef]
71. Zile, M.H. Function of vitamin A in vertebrate embryonic development. *J. Nutr.* **2001**, *131*, 705–708. [CrossRef] [PubMed]
72. Torres, L.; Serna, E.; Bosch, A.; Zaragozá, R.; García, C.; Miralles, V.J.; Sandoval, J.; Viña, J.R.; García-Trevijano, E.R. NF-KB as a node for signal amplification during weaning. *Cell Physiol. Biochem.* **2011**, *28*, 833–846. [CrossRef] [PubMed]
73. Hughes, K.; Watson, C.J. The Multifaceted Role of STAT3 in Mammary Gland Involution and Breast Cancer. *Int. J. Mol. Sci.* **2018**, *19*, 1695. [CrossRef] [PubMed]
74. Underwood, B.A. The Role of Vitamin A in Child Growth, Development and Survival. In *Nutrient Regulation during Pregnancy, Lactation, and Infant Growth*; Advances in Experimental Medicine and Biology; Allen, L., King, J., Lönnerdal, B., Eds.; Springer: Boston, MA, USA, 1994; Volume 352, pp. 201–208. [CrossRef]
75. Report on Health and Social Subjects. 32. Present day practice in infant feeding: Third report. Report of a working party of the Panel on Child Nutrition Committee on Medical Aspects of Food Policy. *Rep. Health Soc. Subj.* **1988**, *32*, 1–66.
76. De Vries, J.Y.; Pundir, S.; Mckenzie, E.; Keijer, J.; Kussmann, M. Maternal Circulating Vitamin Status and Colostrum Vitamin Composition in Healthy Lactating Women—A Systematic Approach. *Nutrients* **2018**, *10*, 687. [CrossRef] [PubMed]
77. WHO, World Health Organization. *Essential Nutrition. Actions: Improving Maternal, Newborn, Infant and Young Child Health and Nutrition*; World Health Organization: Geneva, Switzerland, 2013. Available online: https://www.who.int/nutrition/publications/infantfeeding/essential_nutrition_actions/en/ (accessed on 20 May 2019).
78. Ross, J.S.; Harvey, P.W. Contribution of breastfeeding to vitamin A nutrition of infants: A simulation model. *Bull. World Health Organ.* **2003**, *81*, 80–86.
79. Da Silva, A.G.C.L.; de Sousa Rebouças, A.; Mendonça, B.M.A.; Silva, D.C.N.E.; Dimenstein, R.; Ribeiro, K.D.D.S. Relationship between the dietary intake, serum, and breast milk concentrations of vitamin A and vitamin E in a cohort of women over the course of lactation. *Matern. Child Nutr.* **2019**, *15*, e12772. [CrossRef]
80. Williamson, D.H. Regulation of metabolism during lactation in the rat. *Reprod. Nutr. Dev.* **1986**, *26*, 597–603. [CrossRef]
81. Barber, T.; García de la Asunción, J.; Puertes, I.R.; Viña, J.R. Amino acid metabolism and protein synthesis in lactating rats fed on a liquid diet. *Biochem. J.* **1990**, *270*, 77–82. [CrossRef]
82. Barber, T.; Triguero, A.; Martínez-López, I.; Torres, L.; García, C.; Miralles, V.J.; Viña, J.R. Elevated expression of liver gamma-cystathionase is required for the maintenance of lactation in rats. *J. Nutr.* **1999**, *129*, 928–933. [CrossRef]
83. Canul-Medina, G.; Fernandez-Mejia, C. Morphological, hormonal, and molecular changes in different maternal tissues during lactation and post-lactation. *J. Physiol. Sci.* **2019**. [CrossRef] [PubMed]
84. Zaragozá, R.; García, C.; Rus, A.D.; Pallardó, F.V.; Barber, T.; Torres, L.; Miralles, V.J.; Viña, J.R. Inhibition of liver trans-sulphuration pathway by propargylglycine mimics gene expression changes found in the mammary gland of weaned lactating rats: Role of glutathione. *Biochem. J.* **2003**, *373*, 825–834. [CrossRef] [PubMed]

85. De la Asunción, J.G.; Devesa, A.; Viña, J.R.; Barber, T. Hepatic amino acid uptake is decreased in lactating rats. In vivo and in vitro studies. *J. Nutr.* **1994**, *124*, 2163–2171. [CrossRef] [PubMed]
86. Piantedosi, R.; Ghyselinck, N.; Blaner, W.S.; Vogel, S. Cellular retinol-binding protein type III is needed for retinoid incorporation into milk. *J. Biol. Chem.* **2005**, *280*, 24286–24292. [CrossRef] [PubMed]
87. Victora, C.G.; Bahl, R.; Barros, A.J.; França, G.V.; Horton, S.; Krasevec, J.; Murch, S.; Sankar, M.J.; Walker, N.; Rollins, N.C.; et al. Breastfeeding in the 21st century: Epidemiology, mechanisms, and lifelong effect. *Lancet* **2016**, *387*, 475–490. [CrossRef]
88. Dror, D.K.; Allen, L.H. Retinol-to-Fat Ratio and Retinol Concentration in Human Milk Show Similar Time Trends and Associations with Maternal Factors at the Population Level: A Systematic Review and Meta-Analysis. *Adv. Nutr.* **2018**, *9* (Suppl. 1), 332S–346S. [CrossRef]
89. Van de Pavert, S.A.; Ferreira, M.; Domingues, R.G.; Ribeiro, H.; Molenaar, R.; Moreira-Santos, L.; Almeida, F.F.; Ibiza, S.; Barbosa, I.; Goverse, G.; et al. Maternal Retinoids Control Type 3 Innate Lymphoid Cells and Set the Offspring Immunity. *Nature* **2014**, *508*, 123–127. [CrossRef]
90. Debier, C.; Larondelle, Y. Vitamins A and E: Metabolism, roles and transfer to offspring. *Br. J. Nutr.* **2005**, *93*, 153–174. [CrossRef]
91. Lima, M.S.; da Silva Ribeiro, K.D.; Pires, J.F.; Bezerra, D.F.; Bellot, P.E.; de Oliveira Weigert, L.P.; Dimenstein, R. Breast milk retinol concentration in mothers of preterm newborns. *Early Hum. Dev.* **2017**, *106–107*, 41–45. [CrossRef]
92. Bastos Maia, S.; Rolland Souza, A.S.; Costa Caminha, M.F.; Lins da Silva, S.; Callou Cruz, R.S.B.L.; Carvalho Dos Santos, C.; Batista Filho, M. Vitamin A and Pregnancy: A Narrative Review. *Nutrients* **2019**, *11*, 681. [CrossRef]
93. Machado, M.R.; Kamp, F.; Nunes, J.C.; El-Bacha, T.; Torres, A.G. Breast Milk Content of Vitamin A and E from Early- to Mid-Lactation is Affected by Inadequate Dietary Intake in Brazilian Adult Women. *Nutrients* **2019**, *11*, 2025. [CrossRef] [PubMed]
94. Bezerra, D.S.; Ribeiro, K.D.S.; Lima, M.S.R.; Pires Medeiros, J.F.; da Silva, A.G.C.L.; Dimenstein, R.; Osório, M.M. Retinol status and associated factors in mother-newborn pairs. *J. Hum. Nutr. Diet.* **2019**. [CrossRef] [PubMed]
95. Hanson, C.; Lyden, E.; Anderson-Berry, A.; Kocmich, N.; Rezac, A.; Delair, S.; Furtado, J.; Van Ormer, M.; Izevbigie, N.; Olateju, E.K.; et al. Status of Retinoids and Carotenoids and Associations with Clinical Outcomes in Maternal-Infant Pairs in Nigeria. *Nutrients* **2018**, *10*, 1286. [CrossRef] [PubMed]
96. Abebe, Z.; Haki, G.D.; Schweigert, F.J.; Henkel, I.M.; Baye, K. Low breastmilk vitamin A concentration is prevalent in rural Ethiopia. *Eur. J. Clin. Nutr.* **2019**, *73*, 1110–1116. [CrossRef] [PubMed]
97. Wessells, K.R.; Young, R.R.; Ferguson, E.L.; Ouédraogo, C.T.; Faye, M.T.; Hess, S.Y. Assessment of dietary intake and nutrient gaps, and development of food-based recommendations, among pregnant and lactating women in Zinder, Niger: An optifood linear programming analysis. *Nutrients* **2019**, *11*, 72. [CrossRef] [PubMed]
98. Kaliwile, C.; Michelo, C.; Titcomb, T.J.; Moursi, M.; Donahue Angel, M.; Reinberg, C.; Bwembya, P.; Alders, R.; Tanumihardjo, S.A. Dietary intake patterns among lactating and non-lactating women of reproductive age in rural Zambia. *Nutrients* **2019**, *11*, 288. [CrossRef] [PubMed]
99. Petry, N.; Jallow, B.; Sawo, Y.; Darboe, M.K.; Barrow, S.; Sarr, A.; Ceesay, P.O.; Fofana, M.N.; Prentice, A.M.; Wegmüller, R.; et al. Micronutrient Deficiencies, Nutritional Status and the Determinants of Anemia in Children 0–59 Months of Age and Non-Pregnant Women of Reproductive Age in The Gambia. *Nutrients* **2019**, *11*, 2275. [CrossRef]
100. Meyer, S.; Gortner, L.; NeoVitaA Trial investigators. Up-date on the NeoVitaA Trial: Obstacles, challenges, perspectives, and local experiences. *Wien. Med. Wochenschr.* **2017**, *167*, 264–270. [CrossRef]
101. Atalhi, N.; El Hamdouchi, A.; Barkat, A.; Elkari, K.; Hamrani, A.; El Mzibri, M.; Haskell, M.J.; Mokhtar, N.; Aguenaou, H. Combined consumption of a single high-dose vitamin A supplement with provision of vitamin A fortified oil to households maintains adequate milk retinol concentrations for 6 months in lactating Moroccan women. *Appl. Physiol. Nutr. Metab.* **2019**. [CrossRef]
102. WHO, World Health Organization. *Micronutrients Deficiencies*; World Health Organization: Geneva, Switzerland, 2018; Available online: http://www.who.int/nutrition/topics/vad/en/ (accessed on 5 May 2019).

103. Copp, K.; DeFranco, E.A.; Kleiman, J.; Rogers, L.K.; Morrow, A.L.; Valentine, C.J. Nutrition Support Team Guide to Maternal Diet for the Human-Milk-Fed Infant. *Nutr. Clin. Pract.* **2018**, *33*, 687–693. [CrossRef]
104. Hanson, C.; Schumacher, M.; Lyden, E.; Furtado, J.; Van Ormer, M.; McGinn, E.; Rilett, K.; Cave, C.; Johnson, R.; Weishaar, K.; et al. Status of vitamin A and related compounds and clinical outcomes in maternal-infant pairs in the midwestern United States. *Ann. Nutr. Metab.* **2017**, *71*, 175–182. [CrossRef] [PubMed]
105. Wolbach, S.B.; Howe, P.R. Tissue changes following deprivation of fat-soluble A vitamin. *J. Exp. Med.* **1925**, *42*, 753–777. [CrossRef] [PubMed]
106. Wilson, J.G.; Roth, C.B.; Warkany, J. An analysis of the syndrome of malformations induced by maternal vitamin A deficiency. Effects of restoration of vitamin A at various times during gestation. *Am. J. Anat.* **1953**, *92*, 189–217. [CrossRef] [PubMed]
107. Takahashi, Y.I.; Smith, J.E.; Winick, M.; Goodman, D.S. Vitamin A deficiency and fetal growth and development in the rat. *J. Nutr.* **1975**, *105*, 1299–1305. [CrossRef] [PubMed]

9

Milk Therapy: Unexpected Uses for Human Breast Milk

Malgorzata Witkowska-Zimny *, Ewa Kamińska-El-Hassan and Edyta Wróbel

Department of Biophysics and Human Physiology, Medical University of Warsaw, Chalubinskiego 5, 02-004 Warsaw, Poland; malirob@poczta.onet.pl (E.K.-E.-H.); mwzgenetyka@onet.pl (E.W.)
* Correspondence: mwitkowska@wum.edu.pl

Abstract: Background: Human breast milk provides a child with complete nutrition but is also a popular therapeutic remedy that has been used in traditional, natural pharmacopeia, and ethnomedicine for many years. The aim of this current review is to summarize studies of non-nutritional uses of mothers' milk. Methods: Two databases (PubMed and Google Scholar) were searched with a combination of twelve search terms. We selected articles that were published between 1 January 2010, and 1 January 2019. The language of publication was limited to English. Results: Fifteen studies were included in the systematic review. Ten of these were randomized controlled trials, one was a quasi-experimental study, two were in vitro studies, and four employed an animal research model. Conclusions: Many human milk components have shown promise in preclinical studies and are undergoing active clinical evaluation. The protective and treatment role of fresh breast milk is particularly important in areas where mothers and infants do not have ready access to medicine.

Keywords: human milk benefits; colostrum; milk therapy; bioactive factors

---

1. Introduction

Human breast milk (HBM) is perhaps the most important functional food known. It is a dynamic food with both nutritional and health benefits for neonates and infants. Human milk has powerful immunological properties, protecting infants from respiratory diseases, middle ear infections, and gastro-intestinal diseases. It is now appreciated that human breast milk has health impacts that are lifelong, with breastfeeding showing protective effects against diabetes mellitus, obesity, hyperlipidemia, hypertension, cardiovascular diseases, autoimmunity, and asthma [1]. However, human milk is also a popular therapeutic remedy that has been applied as a part of traditional, natural pharmacopeia, and ethnomedicine for many years. Public health nurses have reported on the effects of fresh colostrum and human milk as a treatment for conjunctivitis, chapped nipples, rhinitis, infections of the skin and soft tissues. The discovery of growth factors, cytokines, and a heterogeneous population of cells—including stem cells, probiotic bacteria, and the HAMLET complex (human alpha-lactalbumin made lethal to tumor cells)—in human milk has led to researchers' increased interest in human breast milk as a natural medicine. In recent years, human milk has been the focus of many types of evidence-based research. There have been a number of reports on the topical application of human milk as an effective treatment for diaper rash, atopic eczema, diaper dermatitis, and umbilical cord separation [2–4]. The protective and treatment role of human milk is particularly important in areas where mothers and infants do not have ready access to medicine, such as in developing countries. In these situations, milk therapy is often a determining factor of infant recovery and survival. For this reason, more clinical trials and research into mothers' milk come from low and middle-income countries in Africa and Asia. Many human milk components have shown promise in preclinical studies and are undergoing active clinical evaluation. A few milk-derived therapeutic preparations are available to clinicians. The study of human milk has resulted in abundant opportunities for translational medicine. However, complementary and alternative medicine (CAM) therapies often fare unfavorably under the scrutiny of evidence-based practice (EBP), due to the lack of or shortage of research and the inherent differences in healing ideology. Yet excess medicalization and pharmaceuticalization can lead to the extension of the medical gaze to human conditions. Physically maladaptive outliers have been treated as diseases and pulled into the realm of medicine. Many "non-disease" states can creep up into medicine, and with time become medicalized due to the redefining of many conditions that were long considered social or psychological phenomena as disease states. Processes regarded as natural are now looked at medical problems or diseases. Unnecessary medicalization leads to great social and financial cost, as well as increased anxiety and the risk for complication from further workups for incidental or clinically unimportant findings. The growth of research and reflections on medicalization has led to the proposal of other parallel concepts, such as biomedicalization. These tools could be useful in the analysis of human enhancement and can be defined as contributing to a "bionic society". Medicalization risks neglecting the role of social determinants, natural therapies, and ethnomedicine in shaping human health. On the other hand, where individuals do not have ready access to medicine—particularly in developing countries—knowledge, skills, and practices based on the theories and experiences indigenous to different cultures, whether explicable or not, are used in the maintenance of health as well as in the prevention, improvement, and treatment of illness.

There is no doubt that incorporating traditional and modern evidence-based medicine (EBM) as integral parts of the formal health-care system is important and likely to be achieved in many countries. The aim of the current review is to summarize studies of non-nutritional usage of mothers' milk. Due to its low cost, wide availability, and lack of undesirable effects, mothers' milk has the potential to play a role in human health and in evidence-based therapy.

2. Methods

The literature review was performed by conducting an electronic search of PubMed and Google Scholar. No filter or limitation was used during the search. Reference lists from selected studies were manually scanned to identify any other relevant studies. The electronic search used the following keywords and medical subject headings (MeSH) terms: Human milk; breast milk, mother milk, colostrum, atopic eczema, diaper dermatitis, nipple pain, breast inflammation, umbilical cord separation, neonatal conjunctivitis, HAMLET, topical treatment. The two authors independently searched databases and reviewed articles. Bibliographic references to retrieved reviews and studies were searched for additional articles. We included articles that were published between 1 January 2010, and 1 January 2019. The language of publication was limited to English.

From total of 1503 initially screened articles, only 15 fulfilled all the inclusion criteria. The following criteria needed to be fulfilled for a study to be included in this review: (1) Topical application of human milk or human milk active factors versus control; (2) in the case of human studies, participants had to be newborns; (3) in the case of animal models, HBM in vitro assessment had to be included. Articles that did not provide sufficient information from the title and abstract were included for further evaluation, and reading was done in full. Records were first selected after which 1469 were excluded based on excluded criteria: Did not report the data of interest, the language of publication, no access to the full text, conference proceeding, reviews. There was no restriction of study designs included. In order to limit bias in the inclusion–exclusion process, the selection was made on the basis of the consensus of two authors. The Cohen's kappa index was calculated to assess the agreement between the two reviewers and any discrepancy was resolved by consensus or by a third reviewer. The reviewers were not blind to author, institutions, or manuscript journals. Data extraction and analysis were performed by the same two reviewers. Figure 1 presents a flow diagram of the review process while Table 1 summarizes the studies that were included.

Table 1. Articles included in this review, with study details.

References	Intervention/Study Type	Sample Size	The Dropout Rate	Study Design	Outcomes	Main Findings
Berents et al. (2015) [5]	Atopic eczema/Randomized clinical trial	18 participants	33%	HBM or emollient was applied on the spot, three times a day for four weeks. The severity and area of the eczema spots was calculated weekly by SCORAD.	Both control and intervention areas of the eczema spots were increased during the intervention. At inclusion mean SCORAD (SCORing Atopic Dermatitis) was 35 and at the end of study 34.	No effect with topical application of HBM was found.
Kasrae et al. (2015) [6]	Atopic eczema/Randomized clinical trial	116 participants	10%	HBM or hydrocortisone 1% was applied twice a day for 21 days on the affected area. Efficiency of the treatment was defined by SCORAD index.	The frequency of healed infants was 81.5% and 76% in HBM and 1% hydrocortisone groups on day 21, respectively ($p < 0.24$).	HBM was as effective as 1% hydrocortisone.
Farahani et al. (2013) [7]	Diaper dermatitis/Randomized clinical trial	152 participants	4.6%	HBM or hydrocortisone 1% was applied for 7 days on the affected area. The efficiency of the treatment was evaluated at 3 and 7 days by a 6-point scale.	The severity score was not different between the topical HBM and hydrocortisone 1% groups at 3 and 7 days ($p < 0.95$).	HBM was as effective as 1% hydrocortisone.
Gozen et al. (2014) [8]	Diaper dermatitis/Randomized clinical trial	70 participants	10%	HBM and barrier cream containing 40% zinc oxide and cod liver oil was applied on diaper dermatitis change for 5 days and the postlesion score was establish by a 4-point scale.	The condition of dermatitis was improved in 60% of infant from HBM group and 93.6% treated with barrier cream. The postlesion score of barrier cream group was lower than HBM group ($p = 0.002$).	Barrier cream was more effective than HBM.
Seifi et al. (2017) [9]	Diaper dermatitis/Randomized clinical trial	30 participants	0	Infants suffering from diaper dermatitis assigned to HBM group and the control group were followed up for 5 days and the efficiency of the treatment was evaluated by a 5-point scale rash severity.	In the control group 26.1% infants showed improvement, in HBM group—80%. HBM has decreased the incidence of anal dermatitis rash ($p = 0.009$).	A positive effect with topical application of HBM was found.
Abou-Dakn et al. (2011) [10]	Painful and damaged nipples/No full randomized clinical trial	84 participants	14%	The efficacy of HBM and lanolin on pain and damage nipples was assessed on the 10-range Visual Analog Scale (VAS) and the Nipple Trauma Score (NTS) over 14 days after delivery.	Lanolin was more effective than HBM, including faster healing of nipple trauma and reducing nipple pain ($p = 0.043$).	No positive effect with topical application of HBM was found.
Golshan and Hossein (2013) [11]	Umbilical cord care/Randomized clinical trial	316 participants	5%	The neonates were divided into three groups: Topical ethanol or HBM application twice a day, the control group kept the stump dry. Umbilical separation time and local infection frequency were considered.	Umbilical separation time in human milk group was significantly shorter (6.5 days) than in ethanol (8.94 days) ($p < 0.0001$) and drying groups (7.54 days) ($p < 0.003$).	A positive effect with topical application of HBM was found.
Aghamohammadi et al. (2012) [12]	Umbilical cord care/Randomized clinical trial	152 participants	14.5%	The umbilical separation time was compared in the group of topical HBM application (three times a day) and dry cord care for 10 days.	Median time of cord separation in human milk application group (150.95 ± 28.68 h) was significantly shorter than dry cord care group (180.93 ± 37.42 h) ($p < 0.001$).	A positive effect with topical application of HBM was found.
Abbaszadeh et al. (2016) [13]	Umbilical cord care/Randomized clinical trial	174 participants	6.9%	The infant from HBM group received topical application of milk and group 2 chlorhexidine solution 4% to the umbilical stump 2 times a day. Follow-up and visit at home were done.	The mean cordseparation time in the human milk group (7.14 ± 2.15 days) was shorter than the chlorhexidine group (13.28 ± 6.79 days) ($p < 0.001$).	A positive effect with topical application of HBM was found.

Table 1. *Cont.*

References	Intervention/Study Type	Sample Size	The Dropout Rate	Study Design	Outcomes	Main Findings
Ghaemi et al. (2014) [14]	Neonatal conjunctivitis/Randomized clinical trial	300 preterm neonates	10.6%	The intervention group with culture-negative eye swab received two drops of HBM in each eye or erythromycin ointment (0.5%), control group—no treatment. All neonates were followed for the occurrence of clinical conjunctivitis for 28 days.	The beneficial preventive effects of colostrum against neonatal conjunctivitis ($p = 0.036$).	A positive effect with application of HBM was found.
Asena et al. (2017) [15]	Corneal epithelial wound/Randomized trial on mice model	24 female experimental corneal epithelial defect mice model	0	A central corneal epithelial defect was created in mice and HBM, autologous serum, artificial tears four times a day was applied for 3 days. Histopathological and electron microscopy examination was performed.	Topical human breast milk drops causedfaster and better healing of central corneal epithelial defect than serum drops, artificial tears and in the control group ($p < 0.001$).	A positive effect with application of HBM was found.
Beynham et al. (2013) [16]	Antimicrobial effect on pediatric conjunctivitis/in vitro study	milk from 23 women/9 bacterial species tested	not applicable	The inhibitory effects of HBM against three common ocular pathogens were assessed. Zones of inhibition by milk samples, sterile saline, and trimethoprim ophthalmic solution were measured	Growth of *N gonorrhoeae*, *M catarrhalis*, *M viridans* was significantly inhibited ($p \leq 0.01$) by human milk samples.	A positive effect with application of HBM was found.
Diego et al. (2016) [17]	Dry eye syndrome/Animal in vivo study	91 BALB/c mice	0	The animals with dry eye syndrome were treated with HBM, nopal, nopal extract derivatives, or cyclosporine four times daily for 7 days. Punctate staining and preservation of corneal epithelial thickness were used as indices of therapeutic efficacy.	Reduction in corneal epithelial thickness was largely prevented by administration of HBM (33.2 ± 2.5 μm).	HBM decreased epithelial damage.
Mossberg et al. (2010) [18]	Bladder cancer treatment/animal model and in vitro studies	6 C57BL mice bladder cancer model	0	Bladder tumors cells and bladder mice cancel models were instilled by HAMLET. Effects of HAMLET on tumor size and apoptosis were analyzed.	HAMLET caused a dose dependent decrease in MB49 cell viability in vitro. Five intravesical HAMLET instillations significantly decreased tumor size anddelayed development in vivo compared to controls.	HAMLET from HBM delays bladder cancer development.
Puthia et al. (2014) [19]	Colon cancer prevention and treatment/animal model and in vitro studies	$Apc^{Min/+}$ mice colorectal tumors model	0	HAMLET was given in therapeutic and prophylactic regimens. Tumor burden and animal survival were compared, and biochemistry and molecular methods were used to determine effects on colon cancer cells.	Peroral HAMLET administration reduced tumor progression and mortality in $Apc^{Min/+}$ mice.	HAMLET from HBM delays colon cancer development.

HBM: Human breast milk; HAMLET: human alpha-lactalbumin made lethal to tumor cells.

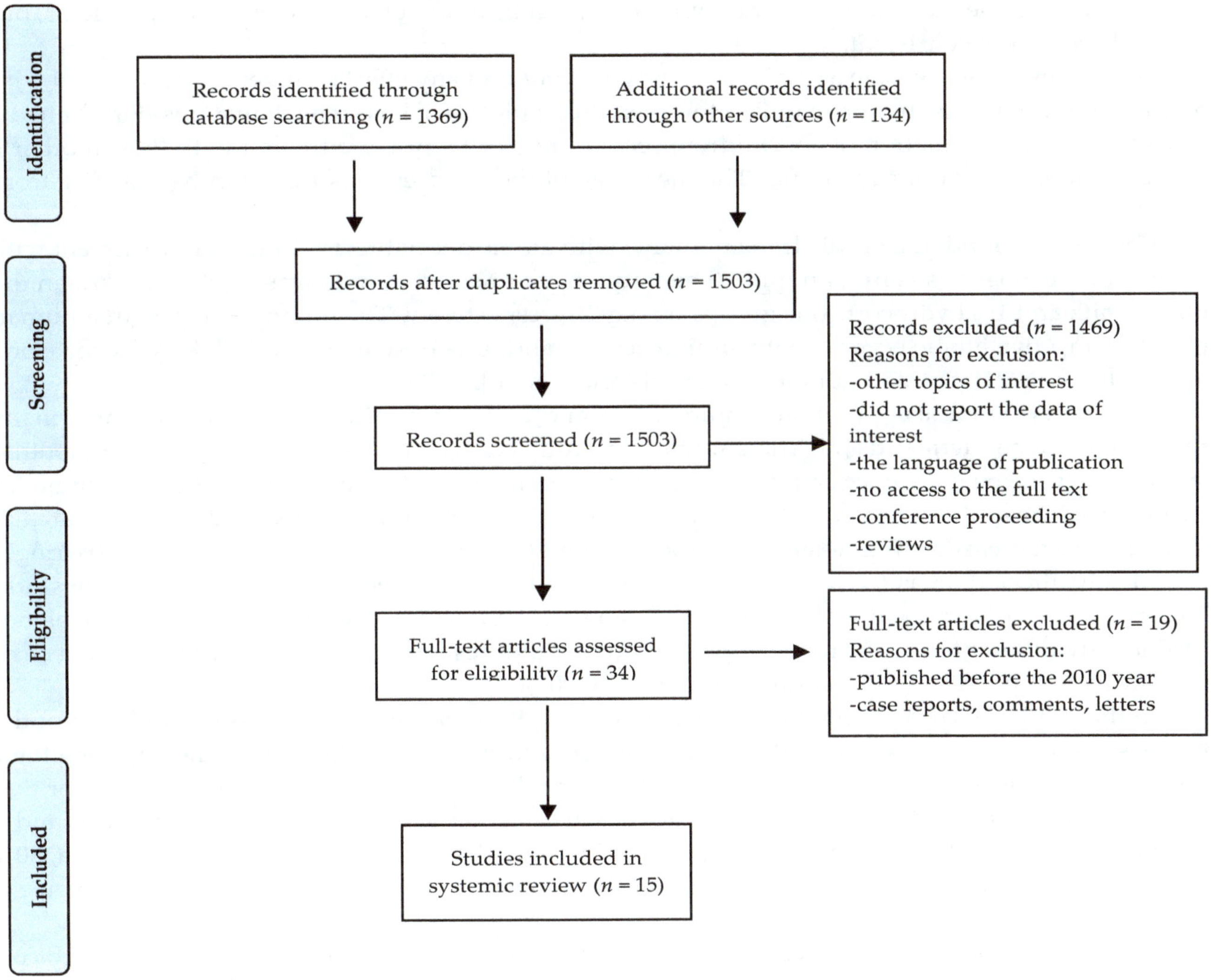

Figure 1. Flow diagram.

We present a narrative summary of studies, rather than a meta-analysis, because of the heterogeneity in measurement tools, populations, interventions, and design (whether qualitative or observational). The reporting in this review follows the Preferred Reporting Items for Systematic Reviews and MetaAnalysis (PRISMA) guidelines, where warranted.

3. Results

Fifteen studies were of sufficient quality to be included in the systematic review. All of these had been published in peer-reviewed journals. The agreement between the reviewers was substantial: $\kappa = 0.625$ ($p = 0.02$). Seven studies were conducted in Iran, two in the USA, two in each of Turkey and Sweden, and one in each of Norway and Germany (Table 1).

Ten of these fifteen studies were randomized controlled trials (two on experimental mice models), and one was a quasi-experimental study. We also considered two in vitro studies and four with animal research models. We decided to include these because they have practical implication for clinical trials and, in our opinion, are examples of translational science.

Below we briefly describe the studies by medical problem.

3.1. Skin Problems: Atopic Eczema and Diaper Dermatitis

Recently, a few studies have been published on the topical anti-inflammatory effects of human breast milk in the treatment of skin problems, such as atopic eczema and diaper dermatitis [6,20,21].

Our systematic review included five randomized clinical trials devoted to infants' skin problems, but the results were not consistent.

Berents and colleagues, in a small pilot study, did not find any effect on eczema spots treated with topical application of fresh human milk. However, this clinical trial has some limitations. First, it had a very small study population of six children; second, two of them were treated with their mother's milk produced for a younger sibling. The mean age of the children was 18.5 months (ranging from 4 to 32) [5].

Kasrae et al. randomized 104 Iranian infants with atopic dermatitis for 21 days of treatment with 1% hydrocortisone versus human milk. The frequency of healed infants was 81.5% and 76% in the human milk and 1% hydrocortisone groups on day 21, respectively. The findings suggest that human milk can improve atopic eczema with similar results and is as easy to apply as 1% hydrocortisone ointment ($p < 0.001$), but without the side-effects and cost [6].

The effects of topical application of human milk and 1% hydrocortisone were also compared in the treatment of diaper dermatitis [7]. The randomized group consisted of 141 infants (aged 0–24 months). Parents received general advice about diaper rash care and were instructed to apply the medication for seven days. The mothers assigned to use milk were asked to rub milk gently on the affected area at the end of each breastfeeding session. Hydrocortisone 1% in an ointment base was applied sparingly to clinically affected areas twice a day. The children were reassessed on days 3 and 7 of the study. The presence of diaper rash was noted daily using a six-point scale, and in both groups, was not significantly different after the topical application of either tested medication.HBM was as effective and safe as hydrocortisone 1% ointment alone ($p < 0.001$).

In the randomized controlled trials by Seifi et al., 30 Iranian infants (between 0 and 12 months of age) suffering from diaper dermatitis were divided into two matched groups: One applying their mother's milk three times a day to the affected area, and a control without any application for five days. The findings revealed positive effects of human milk on the healing of diaper dermatitis and a significant difference between both groups. Out of 15 infants with mild or moderate erythema, 80% improved during the five-day study, whereas in the control group 26.1% infants showed improvement ($p = 0.009$) [9].

Gozen et al. tested the effectiveness of human milk and barrier cream (40% zinc oxide with cod liver oil formulation) on the healing of diaper dermatitis. The population of the trial included 63 term and preterm newborns with developed diaper dermatitis in neonatal intensive care units, divided into two groups. There were no statistically significant differences between the groups in terms of the mean number of clinical improvement days, but the postlesion score in the barrier cream group was lower than in human milk group ($p = 0.002$) [8]. As the researchers stated, neonatal intensive care units typically host infants with disorders and who are on antibiotics. Hence, negative findings can be difficult to discuss and compare with other study data.

3.2. Nipple Problems

A common breastfeeding difficulty for mothers is painful nipples. One traditional non-pharmacological intervention to reduce nipple pain in breastfeeding women is topical treatment with expressed breast milk. Abou-Dakn et al. carried out clinical trials to evaluate the efficacy of lanolin versus breast milk on painful and damaged nipples during lactation [10]. They evaluated 84 lactating mothers from Berlin who developed nipple pain while breastfeeding within 72h after delivery. The first group was instructed after each feed to express a few drops of breast milk and massage them into the nipples and areola, allowing to air-dry. The second group patted the nipples dry after each feeding session and applied a pea-sized amount of lanolin to the nipple and areola, keeping this area covered. During a number of visits over two weeks, the nipple trauma score was used to evaluate healing rates and the visual analog scale (VAS) was employed to judge the pain intensity. Significantly lower pain levels were detected in the lanolin group, and these decreased with the continuation of treatment. Lanolin was more effective than HBM, including faster healing of nipple trauma ($p = 0.043$). According to many studies, the women who applied expressed breast milk had significantly lower perceptions of nipple pain following four to five days of treatment than the women who applied lanolin. However, this beneficial effect was not maintained after six to seven days of treatment. At no assessment were there any group differences in nipple pain perceptions between the women who applied expressed breast milk and the women who had applied lanolin, warm compresses, or nothing [22].

3.3. Eye Problems

Treatment of ocular surface disease with human milk is documented in ancient Egyptian, Roman, Greek, and Byzantine texts and was traditionally used by mothers to treat infectious conjunctivitis. Ghaemi et al. have shown the beneficial preventive effects of colostrum against neonatal conjunctivitis on 89 breastfeeding neonates. The 269 preterm neonates were randomly divided into three groups: The first ($n = 89$) received two drops of colostrum in each eye, the second ($n = 82$) was treated with topical erythromycin ointment (0.5%), and the control group (97) received no treatment. The frequency of conjunctivitis was higher in the control group, followed by the group receiving topical application of colostrum and antibiotic ($p = 0.003$) [14]. However, colostrum does not have potential hazards or side effects and is easily accessible without extra cost. Diego et al. observed that human milk was able to preserve corneal epithelial thickness in the dry-eye mouse model. Epithelial damage, reflected in the punctate scores, decreased over four days of treatment with milk. This was the first study to demonstrate that human milk can preserve corneal epithelial thickness in a dry-eye model, and that preservation of corneal epithelial thickness was comparable to topical cyclosporine [17]. According to the study of Asena et al., topical human breast milk drops caused faster and better healing of central corneal epithelial defects in a mouse model than in the case of treatment with serum drops or artificial tears or in the control group ($p < 0.001$) [15]. They concluded that the rich contents of human breast milk may be an alternative to epithelial healers and artificial tears.

3.4. Umbilical Cord Care

Breast milk is widely reported to be used for umbilical cord care in developing countries, as evidenced by numerous publications. Since 1998, the World Health Organization (WHO) has advocated the use of dry umbilical cord care in high-resource settings but has also recommended research into the use of breast milk and colostrum in umbilical cord care [23]. There are several reports of the effectiveness of applying mother's milk in assisting umbilical cord separation [12,24]. However, in the PubMed database between 2010 and 2018, only three studies were randomized controlled trials. All were published in peer-reviewed journals and were conducted in Iran (see Table 1).

Aghamohammadi et al. randomized 130 singletons, all mature and healthy newborns born in hospital, and compared the effect of topical application of human milk and dry cord care on umbilical cord separation time. Newborns were breastfed. Mothers were asked not to cover the cord with diapers and not to bath the child until the cord had separated. All mothers received instructions, a form for recording symptoms of infection and cord bleeding, and a form for observation on the progress of care. The human milk group dropped milk on the remaining part of the cord and the cut edge, letting it dry, three times a day for two days after separation of the cord. Two days after cord separation, a physician checked the cord. The median time of the cord separation was 150.95 ± 28.68 hours in the human milk topical application group and 180.93 ± 37.42 hours in the dry cord care group ($p = 0.001$). The median number of bleeding days after cord separation was 1.2 ± 2.33 and 3.1 ± 3.77, respectively [12].

In the study of Golshan et al., 300 healthy neonates, delivered normally or by Cesarean section, were divided into three random groups, in which ethanol, their mother's milk, or dry cord care was applied. In the milk group, mothers washed the umbilical cord stump with their milk two times a day. Umbilical separation time in neonates of the human milk group was 6.5 ± 1.93 days, whereas in the ethanol and dry care group this was 8.94 ± 2.39 and 7.54 ± 2.37 days, respectively. The frequency of omphalitis was not significantly different between the three groups. Umbilical separation time in the human milk group was significantly shorter than in the ethanol ($p < 0.0001$) and drying groups ($p < 0.003$) [11].

In a clinical trial by Abbaszadeh et al., 162 healthy, hospital-borne neonates were assigned to two groups, where cord care was performed using human milk or chlorhexidine. Human milk was applied to the umbilical cord every twelve hours for days after separation. The shortest cord separation time was 3 days in the topical human milk group (7.14 ± 2.15), while the longest was 53 days in chlorhexidine group (13.28 ± 6.79) ($p < 0.001$) [13].

All three studies recommend topical application of mother's milk for umbilical cord stump care, which leads to shorter cord separation time and can be used as an easy, cheap, natural, and noninvasive means of cord care.

3.5. The Antitumoricidal Effect of HAMLET

One example of translational medicine is the topical application of α-lactalbumin-oleic acid, a natural product from breast milk. The complex called human alpha-lactalbumin made lethal to tumor cells (HAMLET) was discovered by the Svanborg group when they were studying antiadhesive molecules in human milk [25].

HAMLET is formed during low-pH precipitation of the casein fraction, which allows for partial unfolding of the α-lactalbumin structure and binding with the fatty acid. HAMLET triggers rapid carcinoma cell detachment in vitro and in cancer patients after topical administration of the lyophilized complex. To form HAMLET, α-lactalbumin is obtained from human milk by chromatography. The partially unfold protein is subsequently bound to oleic acid on an ion-exchange matrix, and the complex is eluted with salt, purified, lyophilized, and frozen in aliquots for instillation [26].

The therapeutic efficacy of HAMLET has been demonstrated through in vitro research in animal models of glioblastoma, bladder cancer, and intestinal cancer; and in clinical studies targeting bladder cancers and skin papillomas [27,28]. Local HAMLET infusion was shown to delay the development of tumors and prolong survival in animal models of human cancer. In the study of Mossberg et al., groups of C57BL/6 mice with MB49-implanted murine bladder cancer cells were given instillations of HAMLET or phosphate buffered saline PBS for eight days. The HAMLET treated mice lacked detectable tumors more often than the controls (33% vs. 0%, $p < 0.02$) and the tumors were significantly reduced (mean score 1.9 vs. 2.5, respectively; $p < 0.02$) [18]. Puthia et al. tested whether HAMLET could be used for colon cancer therapy. Peroral HAMLET administration caused a significant reduction in the number of small intestinal tumors and in tumor size ($p < 0.0001$ for total tumor count), reduced polyps by about 58% ($p = 0.0001$), and improved survival ($p = 0.0103$) over the control group mice.

Through gene set enrichment analysis, the researchers concluded that the prophylactic and therapeutic effects of HAMLET are accompanied by well-defined series of stable changes in gene expression, affecting Wnt signaling and β-catenin, glycolysis, oxidative phosphorylation, and lipid metabolism in tumor tissue [19].

The same complex showed strong bactericidal activity against specific pathogens of the oral cavity and respiratory track, with the highest activity against the gram-positive organism *Streptococcus pneumoniae* by cell shrinkage, DNA condensation, and DNA degradation [29].

4. Discussion

The transfer of traditional medical knowledge is an ongoing process. It is important both for the preservation of traditional natural medicine, but also in the search for novel agents in treatment. Home remedies are generally believed to be natural ways to cure minor illnesses or conditions. They are usually cultural practices, traditions, customs, or folk remedies that have been passed down from generation to generation or from person to person. However, it should be kept in mind that there is not necessarily any medical proof that any of these treatments work, or whether they can cause more harm than good. Human milk is considered to be the gold standard in infant nutrition, providing optimal nutrients for normal growth and development. Apart from its nutritional benefits, human milk contains multiple bioactive and immunomodulatory components. The latter of these include growth and immunological factors, as well as micro-RNAs, cellular components such as leukocytes, epithelial cells, progenitor cells, and stem cells [30]. Furthermore, breast milk is also a continuous source of commensal and beneficial bacteria, including lactic acid bacteria and bifidobacteria [31,32]. The discovery of stem cells, the HAMLET complex, and probiotic bacteria in breast milk has resulted in increased interest in human breast milk as a natural medicine. The studies described here suggest safe and cost-effective non-nutritional uses of mothers' breast milk, though further evaluation of effectively is needed. Breast milk has natural antibacterial properties, so it can be used to treat a range of skin problems, including cuts and scrapes.

Common skin problems may appear during lactation and breastfeeding, particularly affecting the nipple, areola, and breast. Some medications used in the treatment of skin conditions are unsuitable during lactation. It has been shown that expressing a few drops of milk and rubbing them gently into the sore nipples, then allowing it to dry naturally, takes advantage of the healing properties of human milk. Many studies have indicated that bioactive components of human milk and microbiota have promise as adjuvants for wound healing [33,34]. From lesions of the corneal epithelium to lacerations of the skin, milk-treated groups healed faster than controls.

Breast milk is used in many cultures for skin irritations. Breast milk involves no risk of allergy, contains antibodies, epidermal growth factor (EGF), and erythropoietin, which may promote the growth and repair of skin cells. Human milk is a source of commensal bacteria that can play an anti-infectious, immunomodulatory role. Their possible function in the acceleration of conditions for skin biofilm formation can open new perspectives for the prevention and treatment of skin and wound healing diseases. Interestingly, the analysis of Simpson et al. showed that miRNAs are possible mediators of the observed preventative effects of atopic dermatitis [35].

The concentration, regulation, and individual variation between bioactive element, immune factors, various progenitor and mature cell types, and stage of lactation are not well established. Complexity and variability in human milk composition, and infants' responses to many human milk constituents may also explain some of the conflicting results of studies evaluating the effects of non-nutritional uses of human milk.

The studies considered here vary in methodology and in definition of outcomes, which leads to considerable heterogeneity. Human milk composition varies both within and between individuals, and this may partially explain the conflicting data.

However, the use of breast milk in the treatment of inflamed or injured eyes is not applicable in all cases. It should rather serve as complementary therapy, and not the only mode of treatment. At our present level of knowledge, non-nutritional uses of breast milk are certainly better suited to prevention than to a medicated process. However, in areas where mothers and infants do not have ready access to medicine, such as in developing countries, the application of breast milk is often a determining factor in infant recovery and survival.

4.1. Implications for Future Research

Fresh whole human milk and its components have potential as a novel therapeutic tool in the treatment of many diseases. In our opinion, the future implications of non-nutritional application are associated with particular components of breast milk, rather than with the whole milk.

In Hakansson's study of the antimicrobial activity of human milk, a complex of α-lactalbumin and oleic acid induced apoptosis in tumor cells without affecting healthy differentiated cells. HAMLET is a tumoricidal protein–lipid complex from human milk with broad effects against cancer cells of different origins. The mechanism of its action is unusual, as the complex interacts with a number of molecular targets and cellular components. Importantly, HAMLET does not have any toxic effects on healthy tissues in the treated patients and animals. HAMLET has been shown to be safe and effective in humans in two proof-of-concept human clinical trials: Convincing therapeutic efficacy was demonstrated in a topical skin papilloma study and in patients with bladder cancer (ClinicalTrials.gov

Identifier: NCT03560479) [33]. Publications on HAMLET are related to the establishment of a Swedish company, HAMLET Pharma, and the increased number of patents regarding this molecule. Based on these discoveries, HAMLET Pharma is developing natural tumor-killing drugs based on molecules with tumor selectivity. A HAMLET patent portfolio has been established with a number of patents issued worldwide. Intellectual property rights include patents covering the manufacturing and use of HAMLET and substances derived from HAMLET "second generation drug candidates".

Many studies highlight progenitor and breast milk stem cells. The presence of stem cells in human milk poses numerous questions and implications for breastfeeding, newborn, and maternal health, but also opens a new perspective of future potential applications of these cells in personal and regenerative medicine. The goals of future research should be to assess the function, potency, and therapeutic value of breast milk cells—including cell therapy for future applications—and should determine the direct or indirect effects of breast milk cell components on promoting immunological tolerance and newborn development, and also on providing effective and complementary treatment of diaper rash, atopic eczema, diaper dermatitis, umbilical cord separation, and eye problems. Without any doubt, future research on these topics will need to involve evidence-based medicine and clinical trials.

4.2. Limitations

Due to the limited and heterogeneous body of evidence that included animal studies, human intervention studies, and observational human studies, the risk of bias assessment for individual studies was not performed. The overall body of evidence was narratively discussed.

This article is limited by its emphasis on papers published in English in journal databases, so many useful local ethnomedical studies may have been missed. Evidence-based medicine focuses more on new approaches than on developing traditional folk and ethnobiological data, so many promising intervention studies are not published in papers indexed in PubMed with high impact factor. It is unclear whether a lack of institutional support and funding for clinical trials of natural products might be critical in the low number of studies.

4.3. Conclusions

The findings of this review provide information about possible non-nutritional uses of breast milk in postnatal care. Breast milk is a natural agent and is biologically suitable for the body, having no side effects; it is always available and can be used in all social and economic groups of society. The health implications of milk components—such as macronutrients, biologically active factors, and somatic cells—remain unknown or not well understood. The positive effects of HBM found by in vitro and animal studies must be substantiated by findings from clinical studies. The most reliable clinical studies for assessing the benefits of HBM are randomized, double-blinded, multicenter controlled trials but to date, they are very scarce.

Non-nutritional uses of human breast milk can be considered examples of personalized medicine. Further research including developed countries is recommended to find or confirm the results and to evaluate the effects of traditional therapies. This knowledge may also have the effect of convincing mothers to continue to breastfeed with their own milk, as a substance that possesses extraordinary properties, not only for nutrition.

Author Contributions: M.W.-Z. designed the model and analyzed and processed the data, drafted the manuscript; E.K.-E.-H. analyzed and processed the data, performed the analysis; E.W. designed the figures. All authors provided critical feedback and helped shape the research, analysis, and manuscript.

References

1. Kramer, M.S. "Breast is best": The evidence. *Early Hum. Dev.* **2010**, *86*, 729–732. [CrossRef] [PubMed]

2. Allam, N.; Megrin, W.; Talat, A. The effect of topical application of mother milk on separation of umbilical cord for newborn babies. *Am. J. Nurs. Sci.* **2015**, *4*, 288–296. [CrossRef]
3. Mahrous, E.S.; Darwish, M.M.; Dabash, S.A.; Marie, I.; Abdelwahab, S.F. Topical application of human milk reduces umbilical cord separation time and bacterial colonization compared to ethanol in newborns. *Transl. Biomed.* **2012**, *3*, 4.
4. Arroyo, R.; Martín, V.; Maldonado, A.; Jiménez, E.; Fernández, L.; Rodríguez, J.M. Treatment of infectious mastitis during lactation: Antibiotics versus oral administration of Lactobacilli isolated from breast milk. *Clin. Infect. Dis.* **2010**, *50*, 1551–1558. [CrossRef]
5. Berents, T.L.; Rønnevig, J.; Søyland, E.; Gaustad, P.; Nylander, G.; Løland, B.F. Topical treatment with fresh human milk versus emollient on atopic eczema spots in young children: A small, randomized, split body, controlled, blinded pilot study. *BMC Dermatol.* **2015**, *15*, 7. [CrossRef] [PubMed]
6. Kasrae, H.; AmiriFarahani, L.; Yousefi, P. Efficacy of topical application of human breast milk on atopic eczema healing among infants: A randomized clinical trial. *Int. J. Dermatol.* **2015**, *54*, 966–971. [CrossRef]
7. Farahani, L.A.; Ghobadzadeh, M.; Yousefi, P. Comparison of the effect of human milk and topical hydrocortisone 1% on diaper dermatitis. *Pediatr. Dermatol.* **2013**, *30*, 725–729. [CrossRef]
8. Gozen, D.; Caglar, S.; Bayraktar, S.; Atici, F. Diaper dermatitis care of newborns human breast milk or barrier cream. *J. Clin. Nurs.* **2014**, *23*, 515–523. [CrossRef]
9. Seifi, B.; Jalali, S.; Heidari, M. Assessment Effect of Breast Milk on Diaper Dermatitis. *Dermatol. Rep.* **2017**, *9*, 7044. [CrossRef]
10. Abou-Dakn, M.; Fluhr, J.W.; Gensch, M.; Wöckel, A. Positive effect of HPA lanolin versus expressed breastmilk on painful and damaged nipples during lactation. *Skin Pharmacol. Physiol.* **2011**, *24*, 27–35. [CrossRef]
11. Golshan, M.; Hossein, N. Impact of ethanol, dry care and human milk on the time for umbilical cord separation. *J. Pak. Med. Assoc.* **2013**, *63*, 1117–1119. [PubMed]
12. Aghamohammadi, A.; Zafari, M.; Moslemi, L. Comparing the effect of topical application of human milk and dry cord care on umbilical cord separation time in healthy newborn infants. *Iran J. Pediatr.* **2012**, *22*, 158–162. [PubMed]
13. Abbaszadeh, F.; Hajizadeh, Z.; Jahangiri, M. Comparing the Impact of Topical Application of Human Milk and Chlorhexidine on Cord Separation Time in Newborns. *Pak. J. Med. Sci.* **2016**, *32*, 239–243. [CrossRef] [PubMed]
14. Ghaemi, S.; Navaei, P.; Rahimirad, S.; Behjati, M.; Kelishadi, R. Evaluation of preventive effects of colostrum against neonatal conjunctivitis: A randomized clinical trial. *J. Educ. Health Promot.* **2014**, *3*, 63. [CrossRef]
15. Asena, L.; Suveren, E.H.; Karabay, G.; Dursun-Altinors, D. Human Breast Milk Drops Promote Corneal Epithelial Wound Healing. *Curr. Eye Res.* **2017**, *42*, 506–512. [CrossRef] [PubMed]
16. Baynham, J.T.; Moorman, M.A.; Donnellan, C.; Cevallos, V.; Keenan, J.D. Antibacterial effect of human milk for common causes of paediatric conjunctivitis. *Br. J. Ophthalmol.* **2013**, *97*, 377–379. [CrossRef] [PubMed]
17. Diego, J.L.; Bidikov, L.; Pedler, M.G.; Kennedy, J.B.; Quiroz-Mercado, H.; Gregory, D.G.; Petrash, J.M.; McCourt, E.A. Effect of human milk as a treatment for dry eye syndrome in a mouse model. *Mol. Vis.* **2016**, *22*, 1095–1102. [PubMed]
18. Mossberg, A.K.; Hou, Y.; Svensson, M.; Holmqvist, B.; Svanborg, C. HAMLET treatment delays bladder cancer development. *J. Urol.* **2010**, *183*, 1590–1597. [CrossRef] [PubMed]
19. Puthia, M.; Storm, P.; Nadeem, A.; Hsiung, S.; Svanborg, C. Prevention and treatment of colon cancer by peroral administration of HAMLET (human α-lactalbumin made lethal to tumour cells). *Gut* **2014**, *63*, 131–142. [CrossRef] [PubMed]
20. Chaumeil, C.; Liotet, S.; Kogbe, O. Treatment of severe eye dryness and problematic eye lesions with enriched bovine colostrum lactoserum. *Adv. Exp. Med. Biol.* **1994**, *350*, 595–599.
21. Mohammadzadeh, A.; Farhat, A.; Esmaeily, H. The effect of breast milk and lanolin on sore nipples. *Saudi Med. J.* **2005**, *26*, 1231–1234. [PubMed]
22. Pugh, L.C.; Buchko, B.L.; Bishop, B.A.; Cochran, J.F.; Smith, L.R.; Lerew, D.J. A comparison of topical agents to relieve nipple pain and enhance breastfeeding. *Birth* **1996**, *23*, 88–93. [CrossRef] [PubMed]
23. World Health Organization. *Care of the Umbilical Cord: A Review of the Evidence*; WHO: Geneva, Switzerland, 1998; p. 19.
24. Karumbi, J.; Mulaku, M.; Aluvaala, J.; English, M.; Opiyo, N. Topical umbilical cord care for prevention of infection and neonatal mortality. *Pediatr. Infect. Dis. J.* **2013**, *32*, 78–83. [CrossRef]

25. Håkansson, A.; Zhivotovsky, B.; Orrenius, S.; Sabharwal, H.; Svanborg, C. Apoptosisinduced by a human milkprotein. *Proc. Natl. Acad. Sci. USA.* **1995**, *92*, 8064–8068. [CrossRef] [PubMed]
26. Trulsson, M.; Yu, H.; Gisselsson, L.; Chao, Y.; Urbano, A.; Aits, S.; Mossberg, A.K.; Svanborg, C. HAMLET Binding to α-Actinin Facilitates Tumor Cell Detachment. *PLoS ONE* **2011**, *6*, e17179. [CrossRef] [PubMed]
27. Ho, J.C.S.; Nadeem, A.; Svanborg, C. HAMLET—A protein-lipid complex with broad tumoricidal activity. *Biochem. Biophys. Res. Commun.* **2017**, *482*, 454–458. [CrossRef]
28. Rath, A.E.; Duff, A.P.; Håkansson, A.P.; Vacher, C.S.; Li, G.J.; Knott, R.B.; Church, W.B. Structure and potential cellular targets of HAMLET-like anti-cancer compounds made from milk components. *J. Pharm. Pharm. Sci.* **2015**, *18*, 773–824. [CrossRef]
29. Hakansson, A.P.; Roche-Hakansson, H.; Mossberg, A.K.; Svanborg, C. Apoptosis-like death in bacteria induced by HAMLET, a human milk lipid-protein complex. *PLoS ONE* **2011**, *6*, e17717. [CrossRef]
30. Hassiotou, F.; Geddes, D.T. Immune cell-mediated protection of the mammary gland and the infant during breastfeeding. *Adv. Nutr.* **2015**, *6*, 267–275. [CrossRef]
31. McGuire, M.K.; McGuire, M.A. Human milk: Mother nature's prototypical probiotic food. *Adv. Nutr.* **2015**, *6*, 112–123. [CrossRef]
32. Witkowska-Zimny, M.; Kaminska-El-Hassan, E. Cells of human breast milk. *Cell Mol. Biol. Lett.* **2017**, *22*, 11. [CrossRef] [PubMed]
33. Gustafsson, L.; Leijonhufvud, I.; Aronsson, A.; Mossberg, A.K.; Svanborg, C. Treatment of skin papillomas with topical alpha-lactalbumin-oleic acid. *N. Engl. J. Med.* **2004**, *350*, 2663–2672. [CrossRef] [PubMed]
34. Heikkila, M.P.; Saris, P.E. Inhibition of Staphylococcus aureus by the commensal bacteria of human milk. *J. Appl. Microbiol.* **2003**, *95*, 471–478. [CrossRef]
35. Simpson, M.R.; Brede, G.; Johansen, J.; Johnsen, R.; Storrø, O.; Sætrom, P.; Øien, T. Human Breast MilkmiRNA, Maternal Probiotic Supplementation and Atopic Dermatitis in Offspring. *PLoS ONE* **2015**, *10*, e0143496. [CrossRef] [PubMed]

10

Predictors of Continued Breastfeeding at One Year among Women Attending Primary Healthcare Centers in Qatar

Amal Nasser, Fadumo Omer, Fatima Al-Lenqawi, Rehab Al-awwa, Tamam Khan, Asmaa El-Heneidy, Rana kurdi and Ghadir Al-Jayyousi *

Department of Public Health, College of Health Sciences, Qatar University, 2713 Doha, Qatar; an1205803@student.qu.edu.qa (A.N.); fo1203580@student.qu.edu.qa (F.O.); fa1203503@student.qu.edu.qa (F.A.-L.); ra1208955@student.qu.edu.qa (R.A.-a.); tk1202457@student.qu.edu.qa (T.K.); mph.asmaa@gmail.com (A.E.-H.); rana.kurdi@qu.edu.qa (R.k.)

* Correspondence: g.aljayyousi@qu.edu.qa

Abstract: The number of babies in Qatar being exclusively breastfed is significantly lower than the global target set by the World Health Organization. The purpose of this study was to assess knowledge, attitude, and practice (KAP), selected barriers, and professional support as well as their association with continued breastfeeding at one year of age. A sample of Qatari and non-Qatari mothers (N = 195) who attended a well-baby clinic held at primary health care centers in Qatar completed a self-administered questionnaire. Descriptive analysis, the Pearson Chi-squared test, and logistic regression were performed. Around 42% of the mothers stopped breastfeeding when their child was aged between 0 and 11 months old. Mothers who had only one or female child stopped breastfeeding between the ages of 0 and 6 months (p = 0.025, 0.059). The more optimal the breastfeeding practices followed by the mothers, the older the age of the infant when they stopped breastfeeding (p = 0.001). The following factors were inversely associated with breastfeeding duration: the mother's perceptions that she "did not know how to breastfeed," or "wasn't making enough milk," and the need "to return to work/school", with p = 0.022, 0.004, and 0.022, respectively. These findings present factors that should be considered when planning for health education and promotion programs to prolong breastfeeding duration in Qatar.

Keywords: breastfeeding; knowledge; practice; barriers; social support; professional support

---

1. Introduction

Exclusive breastfeeding contributes greatly to providing better health outcomes by preventing disease and promoting health in both the short and long term for mothers and their children [1]. It also reduces infant mortality from common childhood illnesses. Approximately 800,000 children's lives could be saved globally each year if every child was exclusively breastfed for the first six months of life [2].

Despite the established importance of breastfeeding, in the Middle East and North Africa (MENA), regional fact sheet-recommended levels are still not attained. The rate of exclusive breastfeeding continuation in Qatar is 12%, which is low when compared with the global rate of 37%. Qatar's rate is also significantly lower than the global target set by the World Health Organization, which calls for at least 50% of babies under six months of age to be exclusively breastfed by 2025 [3].

Mothers who do not breastfeed their infants and depend on formula milk may suffer from increased incidence of premenopausal breast cancer, ovarian cancer, retained gestational weight gain, type 2 diabetes, myocardial infarction, and metabolic syndrome. Additionally, infants who are not breastfed are more likely to suffer from infectious morbidity, childhood obesity, diabetes (types 1 and 2), leukemia, and sudden infant death syndrome [4].

Qatar ranks 10th in the world and third in the MENA region for diabetes. The nation has a comparative prevalence of diabetes of 22.9% and an estimated 283,000 diabetes patients between 20 and 75 years of age [5]. Therefore, understanding the factors affecting breastfeeding and how to enhance and prolong the duration of breastfeeding is vital for diabetes prevention in the region.

1.1. Continued Breastfeeding at One Year: A Core Indicator to Assess Breastfeeding Practices

Globally in 2015, the percentage of children with continued breastfeeding at one year of age was 74% [6]. Regionally, the proportion of children with continued breastfeeding up to one year in Oman was reported to be 95% in 2000. This is much higher than the rate of Qatar, where it was 4% among Qataris and 69.6% among non-Qataris (non-Qataris refer to any immigrant in Qatar—not only limited to Middle Eastern immigrants, but also Arabs from the Gulf Cooperation Council (GCC) region, other Arab regions, and non-Arab nationalities [7]). The World Health Organization uses core indicators to assess breastfeeding practices among women [8]. Since the majority of mothers in Qatar stop breastfeeding within one year, it is crucial to study the "continued breastfeeding at one year" indicator, which is defined as the proportion of children aged 12–15 months who are fed breast milk.

1.2. Factors Influencing Breastfeeding Continuation at One Year

Qatar is a rapidly developing country with massive reserves of oil and natural gas. Globally, it is considered to have the second-largest natural gas reserves. It is part of the GCC region and has a population of 2,700,000, which includes only 320,000 Qatari citizens. The remaining are residents from a large range of nationalities and comprise the main work force in the country.

Previous research has found that nationality, education, and financial status are among the factors that influence breastfeeding duration. Al-Darweesh and colleagues found that non-Kuwaiti women with postgraduate degrees practiced breastfeeding longer than other Kuwaiti women [9,10] and that rich families left traditional practices and used formula feeds [11].

Knowledge, attitude, and practice (KAP) of breastfeeding also contribute to continued breastfeeding at one year of age. In GCC countries, research found that breastfeeding knowledge among studied participants was highly adequate [12]. However, continued breastfeeding practices at one year were not sufficient, and was negatively influenced by mother's attitudes toward breastfeeding [13]. In addition, some breastfeeding practices have contributed to continued breastfeeding at one year of age, including mother–infant skin-to-skin contact (SSC) after birth, which was shown as an efficient method in supporting the continuation of breastfeeding [14]. However, pacifier usage and using only breast milk to feed infants six months and older without complementary foods were factors that were found to promote weaning [15,16].

Factors that are considered as barriers to continued breastfeeding include mothers' perception of pain, body image, body changes, embarrassment from breastfeeding in public, and breastfeeding at work. Barriers arising from social norms are also documented in the literature: some mothers subscribe to the norm "bigger is better," which means fat babies are healthier. This leads them to use bottled milk and introduce solid food earlier than recommended [9,11,17].

Social support provided by family members also shapes continued breastfeeding at one year of age. Women rely on support and advice from their mothers and grandmothers, who may provide practical support to continue breastfeeding for up to two years. Research has reported that support from a spouse was also positively associated with longer duration of breastfeeding [17,18]. With regards to professional support, healthcare professionals can also provide a vital role for breastfeeding mothers. Face-to-face pre-natal and postnatal classes proved to be effective in reducing early cessation of breastfeeding and promoted breastfeeding prevalence [19].

The unique context in Qatar causes more challenges to continued breastfeeding than in other GCC countries. A previous study reported that mothers in Saudi Arabia than Qatar are more open to breastfeeding in front of the family and in public [11]. Relatively little is known about breastfeeding continuation practices up to one year of age among mothers in Qatar. The purpose of this research is to study demographics, assess KAP regarding breastfeeding, explore barriers to breastfeeding, and study selected aspects of professional support and their association with continued breastfeeding at one year of age among mothers visiting primary healthcare centers in Qatar.

2. Materials and Methods

A cross-sectional study was conducted between February and June 2017. Participants were randomly selected mothers attending well-baby clinics at five primary healthcare centers in Doha, Qatar. The study locations were selected based on geographical distribution; they were also training sites for the first five authors.

A selection of Qatari and non-Qatari mothers who attended well-baby clinics was chosen. The target sample was 200 with 40 mothers per center. To be eligible for the study, mothers had to have given birth to their youngest baby in Qatar (participant baby), lived in Qatar for at least two-thirds of the pregnancy, and attended a well-baby clinic at one of the chosen centers. A total of 195 questionnaires were completed by participants.

The study was approved by the Qatar University Institutional Review Board (Research Ethics Approval No is QU-IRB 387-E/17) and was conducted in full agreement with the rules and regulations of the Primary Healthcare Care Cooperation (PHCC) Research Section. A consent form was read and signed by participants who agreed to participate prior to filling out the questionnaire.

2.1. Data Collection

Data were collected anonymously using a self-administered questionnaire, which was prepared in English and Arabic. Participants were randomly selected from the different five centers. We approached mothers in the well-baby clinic and briefly explained the purpose of the study. Mothers who agreed to participate were handed a consent form to sign prior to completing the questionnaire. A cover letter was attached to each questionnaire, addressing the purpose of the study and emphasizing confidentiality.

The estimated time for completion of the survey was 15–20 min. The opportunity to ask any question was given to the participants. Mothers completed the questionnaire and returned it to the data collectors. Participation was voluntary, and mothers were able to refuse any question they did not wish to respond to.

2.2. Overview of Survey

An extensive literature review of studies on breastfeeding was conducted to identify potential items of the study instrument. Based on the literature review, the questionnaire was adapted from validated surveys that have been used locally, regionally, and globally. It was translated into Arabic and subjected to a process of forward and backward translation by a research group at Qatar University. It was pretested on 20 mothers who attended well-baby clinics at primary health care institutions in Doha, and modifications were made as necessary so that it was clear and would provide accurate information.

The first section of the questionnaire related to socio-demographic characteristics of the participants, such as age, nationality, religion, education level for mothers and husbands, occupation, living with a husband, total monthly income, number of children, mode of delivery, last age of child, sex of child, and order. These questions were adapted from previous studies conducted in Saudi Arabia and Iran [9,10,17,19,20]. The second section covered breastfeeding knowledge, attitude, and practice. The breastfeeding knowledge part was used to assess the participants' knowledge of four aspects: benefits to the baby (it provides more protection from allergies compared to formula milk and reduces the risk of childhood obesity and chronic diseases such as diabetes), benefits to mothers (exclusive breastfeeding is beneficial in spacing births, achieving pre-pregnancy weight faster, and leads to a lower risk of developing breast and ovarian cancer), duration of breastfeeding, and effective feeding (breastfeeding should initiate immediately after delivery, infants should be exclusively breastfed for the first 6 months, breastfeeding is recommended up to one year of age, and the optimal age to stop breastfeeding is two years of age). These questions were adapted from previous research in Kuwait and Saudi Arabia [21,22]. For benefits to baby statements, a five-point Likert scale (1 = strongly agree and somewhat agree, 0 = somewhat disagree, strongly disagree, and neutral) was used to evaluate the participants' responses. For the benefits to mothers, duration of breastfeeding, and effectiveness of breastfeeding, items had several categories of responses (yes, no, or do not know).

The part on breastfeeding attitudes focused on reasons behind the adoption of breastfeeding, and items had response categories of yes, no, and do not know [21,22]. The breastfeeding practice questions asked about the number of children who were breastfed, the starting time of breastfeeding, the age of the child when mothers introduced formula or other milk, the practice of skin-to-skin contact, amount of water given to the baby after breastfeeding, and pacifier usage after delivery [7,9,14,21,23].

In the third section, participants were asked whether they had stopped breastfeeding, the age of the child when they completely stopped breastfeeding, and reasons that made women decide to stop breastfeeding. These questions were adapted from different studies [21,22]. Furthermore, there was a question reflecting social support ("Who had the most impact on you to continue breastfeeding?") and participants were able to select more than one answer. The choices included mother, partner, mother-in-law, and friends [21].

Section four was about professional support provided by healthcare providers for breastfeeding mothers. This section included questions about whether mothers received training about proper positioning during breastfeeding and support for feeding problems after delivery, if the importance of breast milk was explained by a physician, if they received breastfeeding health education, and if the hospital provided them with breastfeeding tools [16,19,22]. This section included five questions and items had two categories of responses (yes and no). At the end of the survey, an open-ended question was used to elicit the participants' opinion on how professionals can support mothers for prolonged breastfeeding.

2.3. Statistical Analysis

Data generated by the questionnaire were appropriately coded and analyzed using Software Package for Social Sciences (SPSS) version 23. Regarding the breastfeeding knowledge part, a correct response was scored as 1, while a wrong answer/"do not know" response was scored as 0. The knowledge score was calculated by adding the correct responses to 14 statements and categorized into three levels, which were poor (0–4), moderate (5–9), and good (10–14).

The first and second statements in the breastfeeding attitude part ("The community prefers breastfeeding over artificial feeding" and "Breastfeeding reduces family expenses") were scored as "yes" = 1, "no", "do not know" = 0. The third statement ("It is difficult for a breast feeder to take care of her family") was scored as "yes" = 1, "no", "do not know" = 0. To calculate the total attitude score, we classified those that answered two or three statements correctly as having a positive attitude, while others who answered zero or one statement correctly as having a negative attitude.

The breastfeeding practice part included nine questions. Out of these questions, five featured "yes" and "no", options—the correct answer was scored as 1 while a wrong answer was scored as 0. For the question "How many of your children did you breastfeed?", the response "all or some of them" was scored as 1, and the response "only the first child only or last child only" was scored as 0. For the question "When did you start breastfeeding?", the answer was scored as 1 if they answered that it had occurred within 1 or 6 h of delivery and was scored as 0 if they responded that it had occurred after 6 h of delivery, after 24 h of delivery, or that they did not breastfeed. The overall practice score was categorized into two levels, indicated as non-optimal (0–4) and optimal (5–9). Optimal practice means that mothers breastfed all or some of their children, practiced skin-to-skin contact, practiced breastfeeding within 1 or 6 h of delivery, did not introduce formula or other milk before 6 months of age, did not give water to the infant after every breastfeed, and did not use a pacifier after delivery.

In the third section, the answers to the question "Did you stop breastfeeding?" were scored as "yes" = 1 and "no" = 0. For the question "How old was your infant when you totally stopped breastfeeding?", the answers were scored as "Have not stopped" = 0, "0–6 months" = 1, "7–11 months" = 2, and "12 months or more" = 3. Questions about the reasons that made women decide to stop breastfeeding included nine statements. We scored the participants' responses as "not at all" = 0, and "a little", "somewhat", and "a lot" = 1. The last section, regarding professional support, included five questions for which the possible responses were "yes" and "no". A correct response was scored as 1 while a wrong response was scored as 0. Lastly, a thematic analysis was conducted for participants' responses to the open-ended question to understand the mothers' recommendations on how to prolong the duration of breastfeeding.

Descriptive analysis was performed for mothers' demographics, breastfeeding knowledge, attitude and practice, barriers, and professional support. The bivariate Chi-squared analysis was used to describe the categorical variables and study the association with outcome 1 "Did the mother stop breastfeeding?" and outcome 2 "Infant age when breastfeeding was stopped". A bar chart was used for breastfeeding adoption question, barriers, and professional support to show the comparison of each category in a frequency distribution. The significant variables from the Chi-squared test were used to fit a model about the possible predictors of outcomes one and two by performing multivariate logistic regression, p-values less than 0.05 were considered to be significant.

3. Results

The majority of the participants in this study were aged between 31 and 35 years (31.8%), were non-Qatari (around 60%), Muslim (87.7%), and had university education or higher (74.4%). In terms of the mother's occupation, 53.3% of the mothers were housewives and most of the participants (64.1%) had a monthly income between 0–20,000 QR ($5500) (Table 1). The majority of the participant babies were aged 12 months or older (57.7%), around 29.2% were aged 0–6 months, and 12.8% of the babies were aged 7–11 months.

Table 1. Socio-demographic characteristics of participants.

Characteristics	*N* (%)
Age	
21–25	36 (18.5%)
26–30	53 (27.2%)
31–35	62 (31.8%)
36–40	44 (22.6%)
Nationality	
Qatari	79 (40.50%)
Non-Qatari	115 (59.0%)
Religion	
Muslim	171 (87.7%)
Non-Muslim	24 (12.3%)
Mother's education	
High school or less	50 (26.6%)
University education or higher	145 (74.4%)
Mother's occupation	
Housewife	98 (53.3%)
Employee	86 (46.7%)

Table 1. *Cont.*

Characteristics	N (%)
Income	
0–20,000 ($5500)	123 (64.1%)
More than 20,000	69 (35.9%)
Smoking	
Yes	3 (1.5%)
Number of children	
One	58 (29.7%)
Two	52 (26.7%)
Three or more	85 (43.6%)
Delivery mode	
Normal delivery	122 (62.6%)
Caesarean section	73 (37.4)
Sex of last child	
Male	91 (46.7%)
Female	104 (53.3%)

3.1. Descriptive Analysis

Our study showed that overall breastfeeding knowledge based on four aspects (the benefits to the baby, the benefits to mothers, the duration of breastfeeding, and effective feeding) was possessed by 80% of the mothers.

The majority of the mothers (89%) reported a positive attitude towards breastfeeding. Most of the respondents agreed that "The community prefers breastfeeding over artificial feeding" (78.9%), and "Breastfeeding reduces family expenses" (82.5%). Around 76% of the mothers believed that breastfeeding did not affect taking care of the family when presented with the statement: "It is difficult for the breastfeeding mother to take care of her family." They also reported that the major reasons behind the adoption of breastfeeding were child health (44.3%), followed by cleanliness (20.9%), and religious reasons (19.3%). The latter is related to Islamic beliefs stated in the Holy Quran that "... mothers shall breastfeed their children for two whole years for those who desire to complete the appropriate duration of breastfeeding" (2:223) (Figure 1).

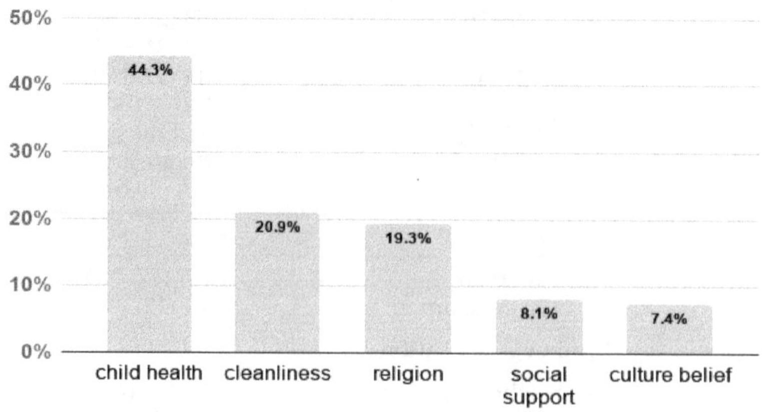

Figure 1. Reasons behind the adoption of breastfeeding among mothers attending the Primary Healthcare Care Cooperation (PHCC).

Regarding breastfeeding practices, around 94% of participants breastfed their children, and the majority (78.8%) initiated breastfeeding within the first 6 h of delivery (Table 2). Yet, around 78% of participants gave their children formula or other milk and most of them started this between the first and third month of the infant's life (40.6%). This may have influenced the exclusive breastfeeding rates among the participants at 1–3 months, 4–6 months, and after 6 months, which were 40%, 20%, and 10%, respectively.

Table 2. Breastfeeding practices by mothers attending primary healthcare centers

Statements (Variables)	N (%)
Had breastfed a child	182 (93.8%)
Number of children breastfed	
First child only or last child only	53 (28.2%)
All of them or some of them	135 (71.8%)
Practiced skin-to-skin contact	162 (85.7%)
Timepoint when breastfeeding started	
Within 1 or 6 h of delivery	152 (78.8%)
Did not breastfeed, or breastfed after 6 h but within 24 h of delivery	41 (21.2%)
Used formula or other milk	48 (77.5%)
Baby's age when the formula or other milk was introduced	
Less than 1 month	47 (29.4%)
1–3 months	65 (40.6%)
4–6 months	32 (20.0%)
More than 6 months	16 (10.0%)
Giving water to the baby is encouraged after every breastfeeding	72 (38.3%)
Use a pacifier after delivery	87 (46.3%)

Table 3 shows that, among mothers who had already stopped breastfeeding (76.8%), 42% had stopped before the age of 12 months. Participants explained that major factors prohibited them from continuing to breastfeed their infants. These reasons include being uncomfortable with breastfeeding in public (59.4%), not producing enough milk for their baby's needs (57%) and having to go back to work or school (43.6%) (Figure 2).

Table 3. Prevalence of outcomes 1 and 2.

Did you stop breastfeeding?	Yes			
	139 (76.8%)			
How old was your infant when you totally stopped breastfeeding?	Have not stopped	0–6 months	7–11 months	12 months or more
	42 (23.2%)	64 (35.4%)	12 (6.6%)	63 (34.8%)

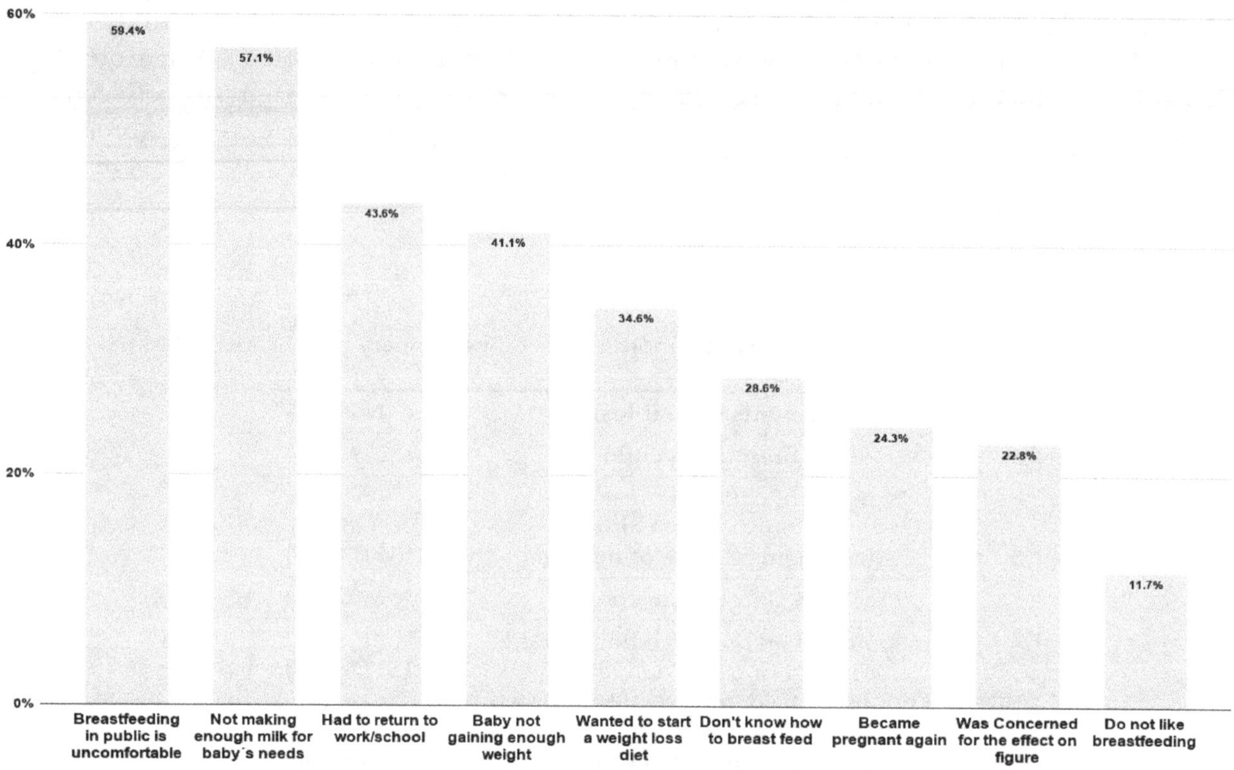

Figure 2. Barriers to continued breastfeeding as identified by mothers attending the PHCC.

However, participants reported that mothers had the most influence on their continuation of breastfeeding (52.90%), followed by partners and mothers-in-law (17.60%). Regarding professional support provided by healthcare providers at PHCCs, participants were mostly satisfied with the physicians' explanation regarding the importance of breastmilk, followed by breastfeeding health education messages provided during or after pregnancy. Only half of mothers received training about the proper position during breastfeeding and thought that there was enough support for feeding problems after delivery. Even though mothers received knowledge and information regarding the importance of breastfeeding, they were not provided the crucial skills needed to follow an effective feeding process and manage any feeding issue faced after delivery.

3.2. *Bivariate Analysis*

Table 4 presents the association of selected demographics of the participants, KAP, and barriers of continued breastfeeding with outcome 1 (if the mother stopped breastfeeding) and outcome 2 (infant age when stopped breastfeeding). The Chi-squared test showed that 81.3% of women who stopped breastfeeding were aged between 21 to 25 years old and, according to outcome 2 (infant age when stopped breastfeeding), 50% of these women stopped breastfeeding early (0–6 months of age). Qatari mothers who stopped breastfeeding when their infant was between 0 to 6 months of age represented 41.9% of the studied population. However, 36.8% of non-Qataris mothers continued breastfeeding to 12 months, which was longer compared to the Qataris mothers (31.1%).

Table 4. Association between sociodemographic and lifestyle variables and breastfeeding.

Variable		Did You Stop Breastfeeding? Yes	No	p-Value	Infant Age When Breastfeeding Was Stopped: Have not Stopped	0–6 Months	7–11 Months	≥12 Months	p-Value
		N (%)	N (%)		N (%)	N (%)	N (%)	N (%)	
Mother's age	21–25	26 (81.3%)	6 (18.8%)	0.644	6 (18.8%)	16 (50.0%)	1 (3.1%)	9 (28.1%)	0.370
	26–30	33 (70.2%)	14 (29.8%)		14 (29.8%)	14 (29.8%)	2 (4.3)	17 (36.2%)	
	31–35	46 (78%)	13 (22%)		13 (20.0%)	16 (27.1%)	7 (11.9%)	23 (39.0%)	
	36–40	34 (79.1%)	9 (20.9%)		9 (20.9%)	18 (41.9%)	2 (4.7%)	14 (32.6%)	
Nationality	Qatari	61 (82.4%)	13 (17.6%)	0.226	13 (17.6%)	31 (41.9%)	7 (9.5%)	23 (31.1%)	0.321
	Non-Qatari	77 (72.6%)	29 (27.4%)		29 (27.4)	33 (31.1%)	5 (4.7%)	39 (36.8%)	
Number of children	One	39 (79.6%)	10 (20.4%)	0.186	10 (20.4%)	24 (49.0%)	5 (10.2%)	10 (20.4%)	* 0.025
	Two	42 (84.0%)	8 (16.0%)		8 (16.0%)	17 (34.0%)	1 (2.0%)	24 (48.0%)	
	Three or more	58 (70.7%)	24 (29.3%)		24 (29.3%)	23 (28.0%)	6 (7.3%)	29 (35.4%)	
Sex of last child	Female	78 (80.4%)	19 (19.6%)	0.215	19 (19.6%)	43 (44.3%)	6 (6.2%)	29 (29.9%)	* 0.059
	Male	61 (72.6%)	23 (27.4%)		23 (27.4%)	21 (25.0%)	6 (7.1%)	34 (40.5%)	
Knowledge	Moderate	29 (80.6%)	7 (19.4%)	0.567	7 (19.4%)	15 (41.7%)	2 (5.6%)	12 (33.3%)	0.800
	Good	108 (76.1%)	34 (23.9%)		34 (23.9%)	47 (33.1%)	10 (7.0%)	51 (35.9%)	
Attitude	Negative	17 (89.5%)	2 (10.5%)	0.174	2 (10.5%)	8 (42.1%)	2 (10.5%)	7 (36.8%)	0.541
	Positive	121 (75.6%)	39 (24.4%)		39 (24.4%)	56 (35.0%)	10 (6.3%)	55 (34.4%)	
Practice	Bad	29 (87.9%)	4 (12.1%)	0.082	4 (12.1%)	21 (63.6%)	3 (9.1%)	5 (15.2%)	* 0.001
	Good	97 (73.5%)	35 (26.5%)		35 (26.5%)	37 (28.0%)	9 (6.8%)	51 (38.6%)	
Did not know how to breastfeed	Did not contribute to stopping	98 (75.4%)	32 (24.6%)	0.286	32 (24.6%)	37 (28.5)	9 (6.9%)	52 (40.0%)	* 0.022
	Contributed to stopping	39 (83.0%)	8 (17.0%)		8 (17.0%)	25 (53.2%)	3 (6.4%)	11 (23.4%)	
Not making enough milk for baby's needs	Did not contribute to stopping	56 (75.7%)	18 (24.3%)	0.692	18 (24.3%)	17 (23.0%)	3 (4.1%)	36 (48.6%)	* 0.004
	Contributed to stopping	79 (78.2%)	22 (21.8%)		22 (21.8%)	44 (43.6%)	9 (8.9%)	26 (25.7%)	
Had to return to work/school	Did not contribute to stopping	68 (70.8%)	28 (29.2%)	* 0.022	28 (29.2%)	28 (29.2%)	6 (6.3%)	34 (35.4%)	0.084
	Contributed to stopping	65 (85.5%)	11 (14.5%)		11 (14.5%)	33 (43.4%)	6 (7.9%)	26 (34.2%)	

* *p*-value based on the Chi-squared test, *p*-value less than 0.05 is significant.

The work environment was a major barrier to continued breastfeeding, as the majority of employed mothers (80.2%) reported that they had stopped breastfeeding. Additionally, 40.7% of employed mothers stopped breastfeeding when their infants were between 0 and 6 months of age, compared to 30% of housewives. With regard to family income, 43.3% of mothers who had a high income (more than 20,000 QR, approximately $5500) reported that they stopped breastfeeding when the infant was between 0 and 6 months of age. A higher proportion of mothers (38.1%) with a lower income stopped breastfeeding their infant before 12 months as compared to mothers with a higher income (29.9%).

The results showed that 84% of participants with two children had stopped breastfeeding. There was a significant association ($p = 0.025$) between the number of children and outcome 2 (infant age when BF was stopped); 49% of mothers with only one child stopped breastfeeding within the first 6 months and they were the least likely to continue breastfeeding their infants to 12 months or more (20.4%). The sex of the child could also play an important role in continued breastfeeding up to one year of age. Our results showed that 80.4% of mothers stopped breastfeeding their female child earlier than their male child. There was a slight significant association between the child's sex and outcome 2 (p-value = 0.059). In addition, 44.3% of mothers stopped breastfeeding their female infants between the ages of 0 and 6 months, while 40.5% of mothers reported that their infant males received breast milk for up to 12 months.

The results showed that mothers tended to stop breastfeeding despite good breastfeeding knowledge because of the influence of other individual, sociocultural, and environmental factors. The majority of women who had a negative attitude toward breastfeeding (42.1%) and disclosed non-optimal breastfeeding practices (87.9%) stated that they stopped breastfeeding between 0 and 6 months. Among mothers who had optimal practice, 26.5% of them were still breastfeeding their babies ($p = 0.001$) and (38.6%) of these mothers breastfed their children for 12 months or more.

The analysis showed that around 83% of the mothers stated that they stopped breastfeeding because they did not know how to breastfeed, and there was a statistically significant relationship between this barrier and outcome 2 ($p = 0.022$). Around 53% of mothers stopped breastfeeding their infant between the ages of 0 and 6 months because they did not know how to do it. Not making enough milk for the baby's needs was a barrier that many mothers faced. Around 78% of the respondents reported that they stopped breastfeeding due to this barrier and 43.6% of those stopped breastfeeding their infant between 0 and 6 months of age. There was a significant relationship between this barrier and outcome 2 ($p = 0.001$).

Considering the work environment, which acts as a huge barrier to breastfeeding for employed mothers, our results showed that there is a significant relationship between going back to work and outcome 1 (whether the mother had stopped breastfeeding) ($p = 0.022$). Around 86% of the respondents reported that they had stopped breastfeeding because they had to go back to work and 43.4% of those stopped breastfeeding between 0 and 6 months of age. Other barriers to continued breastfeeding were "disliking breastfeeding", preferring other methods (such as bottled milk), and mother's concerns about her figure. However, none of these factors showed a statistically significant relationship with the outcomes.

3.3. Multivariate Logistic Regression of Barriers by Outcome 1

The significant variables from the Chi-squared test were used to fit a model about the possible predictors of outcome 1 (whether the mother had stopped breastfeeding). The findings show that "Had to return to work/school" was the only significant predictor ($p = 0.021$), (odds ratio (OR) 2.698, 95% confidence interval (CI) 1.162, 6.267). Therefore, mothers who had to go back to work were more likely to stop breastfeeding because of the work environment was prohibitive to practicing breastfeeding (see Table 5).

Table 5. Association between significant predictors and breastfeeding.

Variable	OR (95% CI)	*p*-Value
Number of children	0.806 (0.493–1.320)	0.392
Sex of last child	1.602 (0.741–3.464)	0.231
Practice	0.468 (0.141–1.546)	0.213
I did not know how to breastfeed	1.356 (0.535–3.435)	0.521
I was not making enough milk for my baby's needs	0.782 (0.345–1.773)	0.556
I had to return to work/school	2.698 (1.162–6.267)	* 0.021

OR = odd ratio, CI = confidence interval, * *p*-value based on Chi-squared test, *p*-value less than 0.05 is significant.

3.4. Qualitative Analysis

A thematic analysis was conducted for participants' responses to an open-ended question about their recommendations to prolong breastfeeding duration. Most of the participants thought that raising awareness about the importance and benefits of breastfeeding for the mother and her child was necessary. This applied especially to new mothers and one of the participants suggested the provision of "... awareness lectures for mothers before and after giving birth about the importance of breastfeeding."

Many mothers suggested having professional support aimed at providing training courses/practical sessions for new mothers about the appropriate positions to breastfeed and providing health advice about suitable nutritional intake for mothers during breastfeeding. One of the participants stated that health professionals should: "explain to mothers the importance of skin-to-skin contact to increase the quality and quantity of the breast milk and to not use formula milk for the baby during the first months."

Finally, one of the recommendations was to have longer maternity leave, since working mothers face difficulties in balancing work and breastfeeding. Some of the participants mentioned that "Maternity leave is only 60 days, which is not enough to give baby breast milk" while another suggested extending "... maternal leave to 4–6 months so the mother will not stop breastfeeding and will not leave her child for long hours."

4. Discussion

The present study assessed selected factors and their association with continued breastfeeding at one year of age among mothers attending well-baby clinics at five primary health care in Qatar. Around 77% of the participants in our study reported that they had stopped breastfeeding and 42% of those had stopped within the infant's first year of life. Mothers in our study were more likely to stop breastfeeding early (0–6 months of infant's age) if they were between 21 to 25 years of age, had only one infant (first-time mothers), were employed, and had high incomes (more than 20,000 QR). Similar findings were reported in Saudi Arabia, where it was found that increased maternal age, lower levels of education, and low income contributed to longer duration of breastfeeding [20]. Therefore, it is crucial that these young women are targeted for breastfeeding educational campaigns to enhance their awareness of the importance of breastfeeding for them and their infants [23].

Culture and social norms play a role in influencing the duration of breastfeeding depending on the sex of the child. Our results showed that male infants were more likely to be breastfed for up to 12 months than female infants. This aligns with findings from Turkey, which showed that male infants are breastfed for one or two months longer than females [24]. In an Arab culture, mothers are always pleased if they have a baby boy and they do their best to raise a healthy man. As a result, these cultural values shape their breastfeeding practices and lead them to spend more time breastfeeding their male infants than females. Addressing religion when communicating to mothers, indicating that

Islam encourages mothers to breastfeed their infants for two years without preference for either sex, could help promote the duration of breastfeeding for both sexes.

At the individual level, we found that most of the participating mothers have adequate breastfeeding knowledge and a positive attitude. However, almost half of them stopped breastfeeding their infants before one year of age. These results are consistent with previous research in which having a high breastfeeding knowledge level did not enhance the rate of continued breastfeeding [25]. Other factors should thus be addressed to help explain why mothers stop breastfeeding, despite being aware of the benefits to them and their infants. Assessing practices followed by participants and other social and environmental factors could help explain what prohibits these mothers from continuing breastfeeding until the child is one year of age.

Participants reported following a variety of breastfeeding practices. Those who disclosed that they had good practices were more likely to breastfeed their children for 12 months or more, while others who had bad practices stopped breastfeeding after 0–6 months. Most of those who disclosed bad practices gave their infants formula or other milk between the first and the third month. Some mothers gave water to the child after every breastfeed and around half of the mothers used a pacifier after delivery, which may have accelerated the weaning process. Similar findings have been reported by previous research [26]. As a consequence, in our study only 10% of the participants exclusively breastfed their infants for the first six months, which is considered a low rate according to the WHO recommendations, but higher than exclusive breastfeeding rates from other regions. Kamudoni and colleagues (2007) reported that exclusive breastfeeding rates in Malawi at 2, 4, and 6 months of age were 39.1%, 27.5%, and 7.5%, respectively [27]. An explanation for these findings could be the lack of antenatal breastfeeding education and postnatal support provided by healthcare providers, which was strongly recommended by participants to enhance the duration of breastfeeding. Breastfeeding educators must contribute effectively to the promotion of breastfeeding and alleviate the current gap between knowledge and breastfeeding practice, so that it can be re-incorporated into the lives of Qatari women [11].

Other significant barriers to continued breastfeeding reported by participants were "not making enough milk for baby's needs" and "did not know how to breastfeed." These mothers were more likely to stop breastfeeding early, in the first 6 months. Our findings are consistent with previous research which showed that if women felt that their babies were not satisfied with breastfeeding, it might negatively influence breastfeeding duration [28]. Many women utilize infant satisfaction cues as their main indication of milk supply, since actual milk supply is difficult to measure [29,30]. A recent study conducted by Galipeau et al. has concluded that mother's perception of not having sufficient milk was not associated with an actual insufficiency of milk supply, as measured by the baby's weight loss or 24-h milk production. The authors found that factors associated with maternal perception versus actual insufficiency were different and therefore they recommended that interventions should be directed toward promoting early, optimal, and frequent feedings [31]. Training sessions about appropriate breastfeeding positions and practices to increase breastmilk should be incorporated into breastfeeding promotion campaigns. Another barrier to continued breastfeeding reported by the participants was feeling that "breastfeeding in public is uncomfortable." A study conducted in Saudi Arabia found that the chance of stopping breastfeeding increased among mothers who perceived lactation in public as a barrier [32].

In Qatar, one study found that women who practiced breastfeeding because they were aware of the benefits for them and their infants still struggle to commit to practice due to limited social support. Family has been recognized as a crucial context to promote breastfeeding duration by providing social support to mothers. It has been reported that mothers and mothers-in-law provide social support and encourage breastfeeding mothers to continue to one year of age [28]. These findings align with those of our study, which showed that mothers and mothers-in-law of the participants were the biggest providers of social support to continue breastfeeding for one year. In addition, partners provided less support. This indicates that various family members should be included in health education and promotion programs that aim to enhance the duration of breastfeeding among mothers in Qatar.

Multiple logistic regressions in our study showed that the most significant predictor of continued breastfeeding to one year was returning back to work or school. Mothers reported that if they had to go back to work, then they were more likely to stop breastfeeding their infants, which suggests that these women had difficulty combining work with breastfeeding. A Kuwaiti study disclosed work as a barrier to continued breastfeeding, with women reporting that they could not breastfeed and work. The Department of Health and Human Services in the US has claimed that returning to work is a barrier to continued breastfeeding, since mothers usually have less time and do not have an appropriate place to breastfeed at work. The creation of breastfeeding-conductive spaces in public and at work to increase social acceptability of breastfeeding and, as a consequence, enhance the duration of breastfeeding has been recognized by new initiatives in Gulf Cooperation Council (GCC) countries [30]. Additionally, participants in our study recommended increasing maternity leave to six months, which will enable them to spend more time with their infants and, therefore, enhance the probability of continued breastfeeding to one year.

Limitations in this study include the cross-sectional design, which limits the ability to infer the causation between the various factors and continued breastfeeding at one year. Using a self-administrated survey may lead to recall bias. The small sample size (this was a pilot study) limits the generalization to all mothers attending well-baby clinics at PHCCs in Qatar.

The current study provides baseline information and addresses a gap in the literature regarding factors influencing continued breastfeeding among mothers attending primary health care in Qatar. Understanding these factors will provide evidence for policy makers and breastfeeding educators to plan for effective health promotion programs that promote breastfeeding practices and prolong the duration, which align with the major goals of the national public health strategy in Qatar [33]. Improving the health and well-being of mothers and their infants will decrease the prevalence of major health issues the country is facing, including obesity and diabetes. Future research should focus on studying the factors and determinants associated with continued breastfeeding using a large, representative sample of mothers attending PHCCs in Qatar. More research is also needed to study actual breastfeeding practices in the country in relation to international recommendations.

5. Conclusions

Our study is the first of its kind in Qatar, assessing different factors on different levels and their association with continued breastfeeding at one year of age. Around 42% of the participants in our study had stopped breastfeeding within one year and only 10% of them did not use formula or other milk before six months of age. This is reflected in the low rate of exclusive breastfeeding in our sample. The findings suggested that continuation of breastfeeding is a process influenced by a variety of individual, sociocultural, and environmental factors which should be considered when planning for effective interventions to enhance continued breastfeeding until one year of age. First-time mothers, Qataris, and high-income mothers were more likely to stop breastfeeding when their child was between 0 and 6 months old. Working mothers and mothers who did not know how to effectively breastfeed their infants were also more likely to stop breastfeeding within one year.

Implementing the WHO and UNICEF (United Nations International Children's Emergency Fund) recommendations for breastfeeding-friendly hospitals in Qatar will improve continued breastfeeding to one year and beyond. Community-based interventions can facilitate the implementation of these recommendations and enhance exclusive and continued breastfeeding until one year of age. Breastfeeding educators and other healthcare providers can work with mothers to provide the skills needed for optimal breastfeeding practices, including appropriate breastfeeding positioning and practices that increase breastmilk. Educators can help mothers to seek family members for social support to enhance continued breastfeeding for at least one year and can help policy makers advocate for friendly breastfeeding work environments and longer maternity leave.

Author Contributions: This is a capstone project for undergraduate public health students focused on health education who conducted the research, performed the analysis, and wrote the paper. The first five authors are the students. The following two authors are two teaching assistants who helped in data entry, management, and analysis. The last author is the supervising professor for this project and the corresponding author for this manuscript.

Acknowledgments: We acknowledged the support provided by Primary Health Care Corporation in approving the data collection process from their centers.

References

1. World Health Organization: Exclusive Breastfeeding. Available online: http://www.who.int/nutrition/topics/exclusive_breastfeeding/en/ (accessed on 4 March 2017).
2. Qin, H.; Zhang, L.; Zhang, L.; Zhang, W.; Li, L.; Deng, X.; Tian, D.; Deng, J.; Hu, G. Prevalence of Breastfeeding: Findings from the First Health Service Household Interview in Hunan Province, China. *Int. J. Environ. Res. Public Health* **2017**, *14*, 150. [CrossRef] [PubMed]
3. UNICEF: Breastfeeding in Qatar. Available online: http://www.sidra.org/breastfeeding-in-qatar/ (accessed on 4 March 2017).
4. Stuebe, A. The risks of not breastfeeding for mothers and infants. *Rev. Obstet. Gynecol.* **2009**, *2*, 222–231. [PubMed]
5. International Diabetes Federation (IDF). *IDF Diabetes Atlas*, 6th ed.; IDF: Brussels, Belgium, 2013; ISBN 2-930229-85-3.
6. UNICEF. *Adopting Optimal Feeding Practices is Fundamental to a Child's Survival, Growth and Development, but Too Few Children Benefit*; UNICEF: New York, NY, USA, 2017. Available online: https://data.unicef.org/topic/nutrition/infant-and-young-child-feeding/# (accessed on 4 March 2017).
7. Multiple Indicator Cluster Survey (MICS), UNICEF. Available online: http://mics.unicef.org/surveys (accessed on 27 February 2017).
8. World Health Organization: Indicators for Accessing Breastfeeding Practices. Available online: http://apps.who.int/iris/bitstream/10665/62134/1/WHO_CDD_SER_91.14.pdf (accessed on 4 March 2017).
9. Al-Darweesh, F.; RaAl-Hendyani, R.; Al-Shatti, K.; Abdullah, A.; Taqi, M.; Abbas, A.; Mitra, A. Knowledge, Intention, Practice, and Perceived Barriers of Breastfeeding among Married Working Women in Kuwait. *Int. J. Community Fam. Med.* **2016**, *1*, IJCFM-108. [CrossRef] [PubMed]
10. Karimi, B.; Sani, M.Z.; Ghorbani, R.; Danai, N. The Pregnant Mothers' Knowledge about Breastfeeding in Semnan, Iran. *Middle East J. Rehabil. Health Stud.* **2014**, *1*, e20833. [CrossRef]
11. Nikaiin, B.B.; Nazir, N.; Mohammad, A.; Donnelly, T.; Dorri, R.A.; Petal, N. Contextual Factors Influencing Breastfeeding Practices Among Arab Women in the State of Qatar. *Qual. Sociol. Rev.* **2013**, *9*, 74–95.
12. Kornides, M.; Kitsantas, P. Evaluation of breastfeeding promotion, support, and knowledge of benefits on breastfeeding outcomes. *J. Child Health Care* **2013**, *17*, 264–273. [CrossRef] [PubMed]
13. Bertino, E.; Varalda, A.; Magnetti, F.; Di Nicola, P.; Cester, E.; Occhi, L.; Preathoner, C.; Soldi, A.; Prandi, G. Is breastfeeding duration influenced by maternal attitude and knowledge? A longitudinal study during the first year of life. *J. Matern. Fetal Neonatal Med.* **2012**, *25*, 32–36. [CrossRef] [PubMed]
14. Aghdas, K.; Talat, K.; Sepideh, B. Effect of immediate and continuous mother–infant skin-to-skin contact on breastfeeding self-efficacy of primiparous women: A randomized control trial. *Women Birth* **2014**, *27*, 37–40. [CrossRef] [PubMed]
15. Riva, E.; Banderali, G.; Agostoni, C.; Silano, M.; Radaelli, G.; Giovannini, M. Factors associated with initiation and duration of breastfeeding in Italy. *Acta Paediatr.* **1999**, *88*, 411–415. [CrossRef] [PubMed]
16. Al-Kohji, S.; Said, H.A.; Selim, N.A. Breastfeeding practice and determinants among Arab mothers in Qatar. *Saudi Med. J.* **2012**, *33*, 436–443. [PubMed]
17. Nassar, M.F.; Abdel-Kader, A.M.; Al-Refaee, F.A.; Mohammad, Y.A.; Al Dhafiri, S.; Gabr, S.; Al-Qattan, S. Breastfeeding practice in Kuwait: Determinants of success and reasons for failure/Pratique de l'allaitement maternel au Koweït: Déterminants de réussite et motifs d'échec. *East Mediterr. Health J.* **2014**, *20*, 409–415. [CrossRef] [PubMed]

18. Dashti, M.; Scott, J.A.; Edwards, C.A.; Al-Sughayer, M. Predictors of breastfeeding duration among women in Kuwait: Results of a prospective cohort study. *Nutrients* **2014**, *6*, 711–728. [CrossRef] [PubMed]
19. Al-Binali, A.M. Breastfeeding knowledge, attitude and practice among school teachers in Abha female educational district, southwestern Saudi Arabia. *Int. Breastfeed. J.* **2012**, *7*, 10. [CrossRef] [PubMed]
20. Al Juaid, D.A.; Binns, C.W.; Giglia, R.C. Breastfeeding in Saudi Arabia: A review. *Int. Breastfeed. J.* **2014**, *9*, 1. [CrossRef] [PubMed]
21. Begley, C. The National Infant Feeding Survey 2008/Prepared for the Health Service Executive by Cecily Begley (Rep.). Available online: http://hdl.handle.net/10147/118910 (accessed on 13 March 2017).
22. Schwager, H. Why Do Women Stop after Successfully Breastfeeding for 3 Months? (Rep.). Available online: https://hdl.handle.net/11244/9278 (accessed on 15 March 2017).
23. Radwan, H. Patterns and determinanats of breasfeeding and complementary feeding practices of Emirati mothers in the United Arab Emirates. *BMC Public Health* **2013**, *13*, 171. [CrossRef] [PubMed]
24. Hizel, S.; Ceyhun, G.; Tanzer, F.; Sanli, C. Traditional beliefs as forgotten influencing factors on breast-feeding performance in Turkey. *Saudi Med. J.* **2006**, *27*, 511–518. [PubMed]
25. Veghari, G.; Mansourian, A.; Abdollahi, A. Breastfeeding status and some related factors in Northern Iran. *Oman Med. J.* **2011**, *26*, 342–348. [CrossRef] [PubMed]
26. El Mouzan, M.I.; Al Omar, A.A.; Al Salloum, A.A.; Al Herbish, A.S.; Qurachi, M.M. Trends in infant nutrition in Saudi Arabia: Compliance with WHO recommendations. *Ann. Saudi Med.* **2009**, *29*, 20–23. [CrossRef] [PubMed]
27. Kamudoni, P.; Maleta, K.; Shi, Z.; Holmboe-Ottesen, G. Infant feeding practices in the first 6 months and associated factors in a rural and semiurban community in Manghotchi district, Malawi. *J. Hum. Lact.* **2007**, *23*, 325–332. [CrossRef] [PubMed]
28. Agunbiade, O.M.; Ogunleye, O.V. Constraints to exclusive breastfeeding practice among breastfeeding mothers in Southwest Nigeria: Implications for scaling up. *Int. Breastfeed. J.* **2012**, *7*, 5. [CrossRef] [PubMed]
29. Gatti, L. Maternal Perceptions of Insufficient Milk Supply in Breastfeeding. *J. Nurs. Scholarsh.* **2008**, *40*, 355–363. [CrossRef] [PubMed]
30. World Breastfeeding Trends Initiative. Saudi Arabia. 2012. Available online: www.wordbreastfeedingtrends.org/GenerateReports/report/WBTi-KSA-2012.pdf (accessed on 15 March 2017).
31. Galipeau, R.; Dumas, L.; Lepage, M. Perception of Not Having Enough Milk and Actual Milk Production of First-Time Breastfeeding Mothers: Is There a Difference? *Breastfeed. Med.* **2017**, *12*, 210–217. [CrossRef] [PubMed]
32. Saied, H.; Mohamed, A.; Suliman, A.; Al Anazi, W. Breastfeeding Knowledge, Attitude, and Barriers among Saudi Women in Riyadh. *J. Natural Sci. Res.* **2013**, *3*, 12.
33. National Health Strategy (NHS). Available online: http://www.nhsq.info/app/media/1541 (accessed on 4 May 2017).

11

Carbohydrates in Human Milk and Body Composition of Term Infants during the First 12 Months of Lactation

Zoya Gridneva [1,*], Alethea Rea [2], Wan Jun Tie [1], Ching Tat Lai [1], Sambavi Kugananthan [1,3], Leigh C. Ward [4], Kevin Murray [5], Peter E. Hartmann [1] and Donna T. Geddes [1]

1 School of Molecular Sciences, M310, The University of Western Australia, Crawley, Perth, WA 6009, Australia
2 Centre for Applied Statistics, The University of Western Australia, Crawley, Perth, WA 6009, Australia
3 School of Human Sciences, The University of Western Australia, Crawley, Perth, WA 6009, Australia
4 School of Chemistry and Molecular Biosciences, The University of Queensland, St. Lucia, Brisbane, QLD 4072, Australia
5 School of Population and Global Health, The University of Western Australia, Crawley, Perth, WA 6009, Australia
* Correspondence: zoya.gridneva@uwa.edu.au

Abstract: Human milk (HM) carbohydrates may affect infant appetite regulation, breastfeeding patterns, and body composition (BC). We investigated relationships between concentrations/calculated daily intakes (CDI) of HM carbohydrates in first year postpartum and maternal/term infant BC, as well as breastfeeding parameters. BC of dyads (n = 20) was determined at 2, 5, 9, and/or 12 months postpartum using ultrasound skinfolds (infants) and bioelectrical impedance spectroscopy (infants/mothers). Breastfeeding frequency, 24-h milk intake and total carbohydrates (TCH) and lactose were measured to calculate HM oligosaccharides (HMO) concentration and CDI of carbohydrates. Statistical analysis used linear regression/mixed effects models; results were adjusted for multiple comparisons. Higher TCH concentrations were associated with greater infant length, weight, fat-free mass (FFM), and FFM index (FFMI), and decreased fat mass (FM), FM index (FMI), %FM and FM/FFM ratio. Higher HMO concentrations were associated with greater infant FFM and FFMI, and decreased FMI, %FM, and FM/FFM ratio. Higher TCH CDI were associated with greater FM, FMI, %FM, and FM/FFM ratio, and decreased infant FFMI. Higher lactose CDI were associated with greater FM, FMI, %FM, and FM/FFM, ratio and decreased FFMI. Concentrations and intakes of HM carbohydrates differentially influence development of infant BC in the first 12 months postpartum, and may potentially influence risk of later obesity via modulation of BC.

Keywords: human milk carbohydrates; lactose; oligosaccharides; infant; body composition; lactation; daily intake; breastfeeding frequency; milk intake

---

1. Introduction

Nutrition [1] and development of infant body composition (BC) in the early months postpartum [2] are known to play a significant role in the programming of obesity. Breastfeeding and its duration are associated with reduced risk of developing obesity later in life [3]. These observations suggest a dose-dependent effect of breastfeeding on the development of infant BC, but the mechanisms of this effect are not fully elucidated. Although it is well established that added dietary sugar is a risk factor for obesity for children and adults [4] as well as infants [5] and contributes to metabolic diseases [6], little is known how human milk (HM) carbohydrates influence the development of BC during infancy and if they confer protection against the obesity.

The macronutrient composition of HM is remarkably conserved across populations appearing to be largely independent of geographic and ethnic factors [7], maternal nutritional status [8], and adiposity [9]. HM provides a constant supply of carbohydrates to the infant during early life, ensuring appropriate nutrition, maturation and development of their comparatively immature physiological systems. Considering that lactose, the principal carbohydrate, is important for maintenance of constant osmotic pressure in HM [10], it is unlikely that maternal adiposity would have a significant impact on lactose concentration, which is estimated to be approximately 60–78 g/L throughout the lactation, although lactose concentration is still variable between women [11]. As lactose synthesis results in water being drawn into the milk, the rate of lactose synthesis is a major controlling factor of milk production [12], and during the established lactation higher lactose concentration is associated with higher 24-h volumes [13] and higher breastfeeding frequency [14], which is also related to higher 24-h volumes [15].

HM carbohydrates also include small amounts of monosaccharides, such as glucose and galactose, as well as HM oligosaccharides (HMO). Nearly 200 unique oligosaccharides structures that vary from 2 to 22 sugars have been identified [16] and HMO composition and proportion varies between mothers [17], over the course of lactation [18] and is affected by parity, ethnicity, and place of residence, as well as breastfeeding exclusivity [19], and may exert different effects in the infant gut [20]. This suggests that HM carbohydrates may have a dose-dependent effect on infant growth and BC development.

Infant growth rate is associated with the volume of milk consumed [11] and lactose/carbohydrate intakes are lower in breastfed infants at 3 and 6 months compared to formula-fed infants and positively relate to weight and fat-free mass (FFM) but not fat mass (FM) gain [21]. Contradictory, studies of lactose concentration have reported either positive association of HM lactose with infant adiposity at 12 months [22] or no association with infant BC at 6 months [23]. Furthermore, there are differing associations for different HMO (16 HMO investigated) with infant BC, although total concentration was not analyzed [20]. In addition, concentrations of glucose are positively associated with relative weight and both fat and lean mass of breastfed infants [24]. The investigations in this area are extremely limited and need to discern the mechanisms by which HM carbohydrates, concentrations and intakes, may impact development of infant BC, allowing for future targeted interventions that may reduce risk of overweight and obesity later in life.

The purpose of this pilot longitudinal study was to assess the associations of concentration and daily intake of HM carbohydrates (total carbohydrates (TCH), lactose, and HMO) with anthropometric measurements and BC of healthy term infants breastfed on demand and their mothers during the first 12 months of lactation. Relationships of HM carbohydrates with infant 24-h milk intake and breastfeeding frequency were also investigated.

2. Materials and Methods

2.1. Study Overview

We curried out a longitudinal cohort study of mothers with milk supply within a normal range [25], and healthy term infants that were exclusively breastfed [26] at 2 and 5 months and continued breastfeeding on demand until 12 months postpartum without supplementation with formula. The study design, cohort characteristics, data collection procedures, and sample preparation have been described in detail previously, together with the methods for determining maternal and infant anthropometrics and BC [15,27,28], as well as infant 24-h milk intake [29] and breastfeeding frequency [25], and the relationships between the measured parameters.

Briefly, milk samples were collected and BC of healthy dyads (no suspected infectious illness, e.g., a cold or flu, at the time of study visit) was determined when the infants were two and/or five, nine, and 12 months-old utilising bioelectrical impedance spectroscopy (BIS; infants and mothers), and ultrasound for measurements of the skinfolds (ultrasound 2-skinfolds: triceps and subscapular; ultrasound 4-skinfolds: biceps, subscapular, suprailiac, and triceps; infants only) for use in the age and sex-specific equations [15,30]. Infant test-weighing before and after every breastfeeding from each breast over 24–26 h was conducted to measure infant 24-h milk intake and breastfeeding frequency between 2 and 5 months, when milk intake has been reported to be stable [27], and within two weeks of 9 and 12 months. Mothers also estimated and self-reported breastfeeding frequency at the study sessions as the current typical time (h) between the meals.

In addition to standard measured BC parameters (fat-free mass (FFM), fat mass (FM), and percentage FM (%FM)) we have calculated the height-normalized BC indices of mothers and infants: FFM index (FFMI) was calculated as FFM/length^2; FM index (FMI) was calculated as FM/length^2, both expressed as kg/m^2 [31]. The use of these BC indices is considered less statistically flawed than %FM [32], which includes a single variable (FM) in both numerator and denominator. Furthermore, the dyads' FM to FFM ratios (FM/FFM), which are emerging as values indicative of overall effects of BC (metabolic load and metabolic capacity) [33] were also calculated.

All mothers provided written informed consent for participation in the study, which was approved by the Human Research Ethics Committee of The University of Western Australia (RA/1/4253, RA/4/1/2639) and registered with the Australian New Zealand Clinical Trials Registry (ACTRN12616000368437).

2.2. Measurement of Human Milk Carbohydrates

Lactose concentration was measured in duplicate in pre- and postfeed samples using the enzymatic-spectrophotometric method [11] with recovery of 98.2 ± 4.1% ($n = 10$), detection limit of 30 mM and interassay coefficient of variation (CV) of 3.5%, and averaged for analysis.

Pre- and postfeed samples were pooled for measuring TCH. Skim HM was deproteinized with trichloroacetic acid [34] before dehydration by sulfuric acid [35]. TCH were analyzed in triplicate by UV spectrophotometry at 315nm. Recovery of added lactose was 101.4% ± 2.1% ($n = 7$) with a detection limit of 0.007 g/L and an interassay CV of 3.3% ($n = 7$).

The total HMO concentration (g/L) was estimated by deducting lactose concentration from TCH concentration. On two occasions, where the calculated HMO concentration was less than zero, it was taken to be zero. Glucose and galactose were not measured or accounted for in HMO concentration calculations, as their concentrations in HM are small and thus not detectable in these assays [36].

2.3. Calculated Daily Intakes of Carbohydrates

24-h milk intakes values measured during 24-h test-weighing, and HM carbohydrate concentrations measured in samples taken at the study sessions at corresponding time point were used for calculation of infant daily intakes (CDI). As there are no significant circadian [11] and short-term (weekly) [37] variations in HM carbohydrates concentration during the established lactation, these CDI were considered representative of a typical daily intake.

2.4. Statistical Analyses

This longitudinal study, the details of which, along with power calculation have been described previously [15,27,28], was analyzed using linear mixed models. Fitted models included (a) explanatory variable: maternal BC, responses: carbohydrate concentrations and CDI; (b) explanatory variables: carbohydrate concentration and CDI, response: infant BC; (c) explanatory variable: carbohydrate concentration, responses: breastfeeding parameters (24-h milk intake and breastfeeding frequency); and (d) explanatory variables: carbohydrate concentration, breastfeeding frequency, and 24-h milk intake, response: carbohydrate CDI. The fixed effects were infant age (as a categorical variable) included as an interaction with the explanatory variable and a random effect for each participant. The p-value associated with the interaction was examined and if it was below 0.05, the results were reported for a model with fixed effects for infant age and the explanatory variable of interest and a random effect for each participant. Where the interaction was not significant, results were reported for the same model fitted without the interaction.

The analyses for systematic differences between measured parameters at different months after birth used linear mixed model with age as effect factor and participant as a random factor. Differences between each month were analyzed using general linear hypothesis tests (Tukey's all pair comparisons).

Relationships between CDI of carbohydrates measured between 2 and 5, and at 9 and 12 months after birth and changes (Δ) in infant BC and anthropometric parameters between the time points were analyzed using linear regression models.

A false discovery rate (FDR) adjustment [38] was applied to the subgroupings of results to the interaction p-value if it was less than 0.05 or to the main effect p-value. The adjusted significance levels are reported in the tables or set at the 5% level otherwise. Descriptive statistics are reported as mean ± standard deviation (SD) and range; modeling results as parameters estimates ± standard error (SE). Missing data were dealt with using available case analysis. Statistical analysis and graphics were performed in R 3.1.2.

3. Results

3.1. Subjects

Participant demographic characteristics; determinants of maternal and infant BC, anthropometrics, and breastfeeding parameters (24-h milk intake, 24-h breastfeeding frequency, self-reported breastfeeding frequency); as well as participant attrition and missing data have been reported in detail previously [15,27,28]. The missing data in this analysis also included carbohydrates concentrations (from 80 expected measurements: TCH (n = 12); lactose (n = 14); HMO (n = 15)) and CDI (from 60 expected measurements: lactose (n = 27); TCH and HMO (n = 28)); missing data were distributed across the time points (Table 1). In addition to previously reported maternal and infant BC, the current analysis also included maternal and infant FM/FFM ratios (Table 1).

3.2. Changes in Body Composition and Human Milk Carbohydrates during First Year of Lactation

Description of the changes in infant and maternal BC and breastfeeding parameters (24-h milk intake, 24-h breastfeeding frequency, self-reported breastfeeding frequency) between 2 and 12 months of lactation have been reported previously [15]. Maternal and infant FM/FFM ratios as well as HM carbohydrates concentrations and CDI over the first year of lactation are detailed in Table 2.

Maternal FM/FFM decreased across the lactation. Infant FM/FFM measured with BIS initially increased and then decreased at the later months of lactation, while infant FM/FFM measured with either ultrasound 2-skinfolds or ultrasound 4-skinfolds did not differ (Table 2).

Concentrations of all, TCH, lactose and HMO did not differ between 2 and 12 months. CDI of TCH and lactose decreased across the lactation, while HMO CDI did not differ (Table 2).

3.3. Maternal Body Composition and Carbohydrates

No associations were seen between maternal BC and concentrations of carbohydrates (data not shown). No associations were seen between maternal BC and CDI of carbohydrates after adjusting for the FDR however, prior to the adjustment higher HMO CDI was associated with higher maternal %FM and FM/FFM between 2 and 5 months, and with lower maternal %FM and FM/FFM at 9 and 12 months (%FM: $p = 0.014$; FM/FFM: $p = 0.013$) (Table A1).

Table 1. Fat mass to fat-free mass ratios and concentrations and 24-h intakes of human milk carbohydrates during first 12 months of lactation.

Characteristics	2 Months	5 Months	9 Months	12 Months
	Mean ± SD (Min–Max)	**Mean ± SD (Min–Max)**	**Mean ± SD (Min–Max)**	**Mean ± SD (Min–Max)**
FM/FFM ratios	**(n = 14)**	**(n = 20)**	**(M = 18/I = 17)**	**(M = 17/I = 15)**
Maternal FM/FFM	0.56 ± 0.14 [a] (0.35–0.81)	0.51 ± 0.16 (0.30–0.89)	0.48 ± 0.16 (0.25–0.80)	0.43 ± 0.16 (0.24–0.80)
Infant FM/FFM with US 2SF	0.32 ± 0.04 (0.26–0.61)	0.37 ± 0.09 (0.24–0.64)	0.35 ± 0.08 (0.18–0.53)	0.34 ± 0.06 (0.22–0.45)
Infant FM/FFM with US 4SF	0.33 ± 0.05 (0.24–0.44)	0.36 ± 0.07 (0.26–0.56)	0.34 ± 0.07 (0.21–0.45)	0.31 ± 0.06 (0.21–0.41)
Infant FM/FFM with BIS	0.28 ± 0.04 (0.22–0.34)	0.41 ± 0.07 (0.28–0.56)	0.34 ± 0.08 (0.19–0.46)	0.33 ± 0.06 (0.24–0.44)
Concentrations	**(n = 15)**	**(n = 20)**	**(n = 19)**	**(n = 14)**
Total carbohydrates (g/L)	86.7 ± 9.2 (67.1–97.5)	80.7 ± 7.9 (69.3–94.1)	87.8 ± 11.1 (60.9–105.6)	88.4 ± 21.2 (56.9–126.9)
Lactose (g/L)	64.5 ± 4.1 (59.1–77.9)	64.3 ± 5.9 (53.5–70.6)	65.3 ± 5.3 (57.6–79.0)	66.9 ± 4.0 (60.1–79.3)
HMO (g/L)	22.3 ± 10.7 (0–35.8)	16.4 ± 9.9 (2.3–29.9)	22.5 ± 9.2 (0–36.9)	21.4 ± 22.3 (3.0–62.2)
CDI [b]	**n/a [b]**	**(n = 17)**	**(n = 8)**	**(n = 8)**
Total carbohydrates (g)	n/a	63.2 ± 15.0 (42.9–97.2)	44.8 ± 15.2 (21.2–69.6)	40.7 ± 29.8 (22.2–100.9)
Lactose (g)	n/a	51.2 ± 14.5 (32.6–83.6)	34.0 ± 11.0 (19.6–51.3)	28.7 ± 12.1 (18.0–51.4)
HMO (g)	n/a	12.0 ± 6.0 (2.0–21.6)	10.8 ± 5.4 (0–15.7)	12.0 ± 18.5 (1.5–49.5)

[a] Data are mean ± SD and ranges. [b] Daily intakes (CDI) of carbohydrates were calculated between 2 and 5 months (presented at 5 months here) and within 2 weeks of 9 and 12 months. BIS: bioelectrical impedance spectroscopy; CDI: calculated daily intakes; FFM: fat-free mass; FM: fat mass; FM/FFM: fat mass to fat-free mass ratio; HMO: human milk oligosaccharides; I: infants; M: mothers; n/a: not applicable; US 2SF: ultrasound 2-skinfolds; US 4SF: ultrasound 4-skinfolds.

3.4. *Infant Body Composition and Concentrations of Carbohydrates*

Higher TCH concentration was associated with increased infant length ($p < 0.001$), weight ($p = 0.003$), FFM (measured with BIS: $p < 0.001$; ultrasound 4-skinfolds: $p = 0.020$), and FFMI (BIS: $p = 0.002$). Higher TCH concentration was associated with an increase in adiposity measured with BIS (FM: $p = 0.016$; FMI: $p = 0.001$; %FM: $p = 0.001$; FM/FFM: $p = 0.003$) at 2 months and decrease at 5, 9, and 12 months (Table 3, Figure 1).

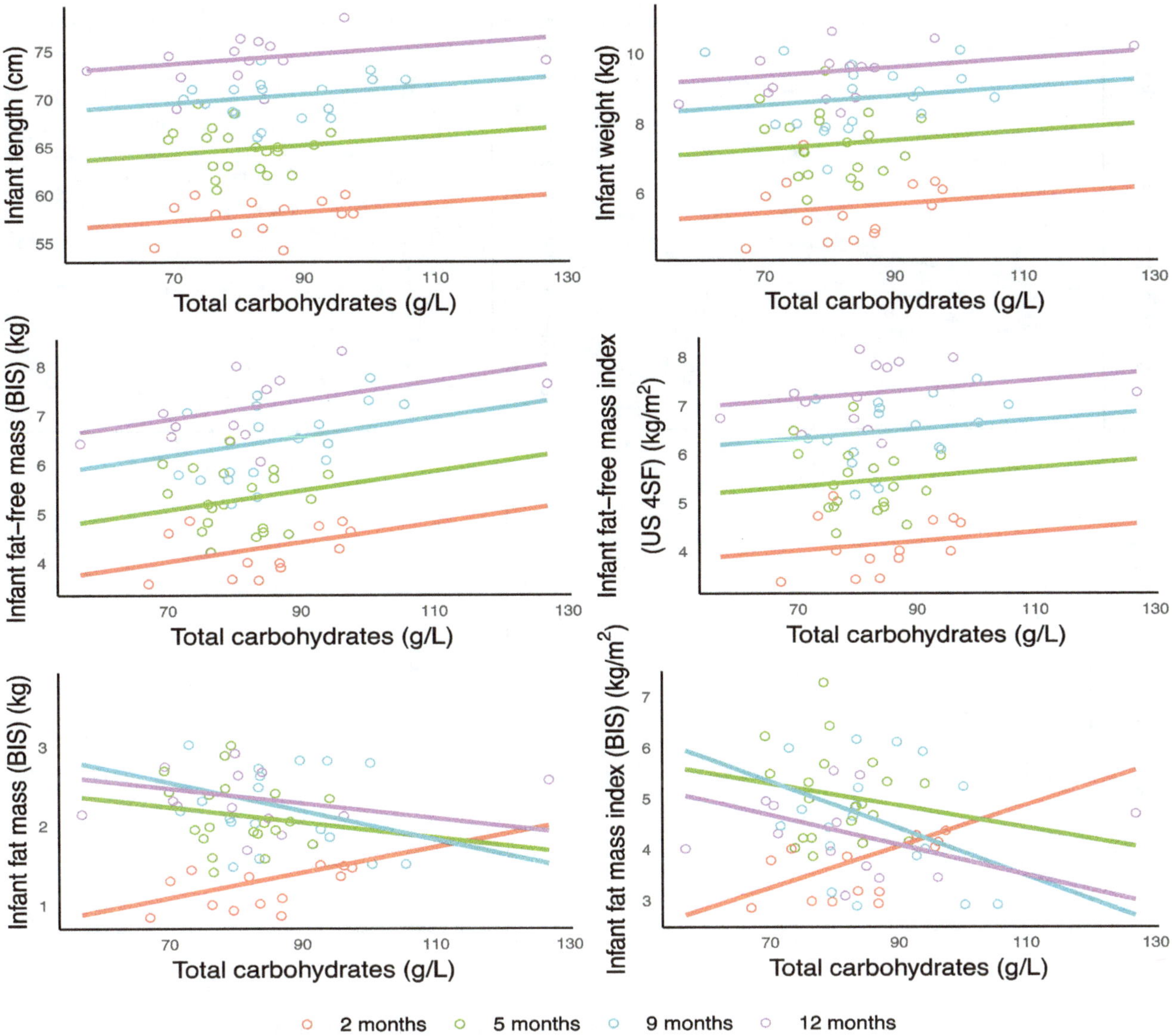

Figure 1. Significant associations between concentration of total carbohydrates and infant anthropometric and body composition measurements. Lines represent linear regression and grouped by the month of lactation. BIS: bioelectrical impedance spectroscopy; US 4SF: ultrasound 4-skinfolds.

Higher HMO concentration was associated with increased FFM (BIS: $p < 0.001$) and FFMI (BIS: $p = 0.008$). Higher HMO concentration was associated with an increase in adiposity measured with BIS (FMI: $p = 0.003$; %FM: $p = 0.005$; FM/FFM: $p = 0.006$) at 2 months and decrease at 5, 9 and 12 months (Table 3, Figure 2).

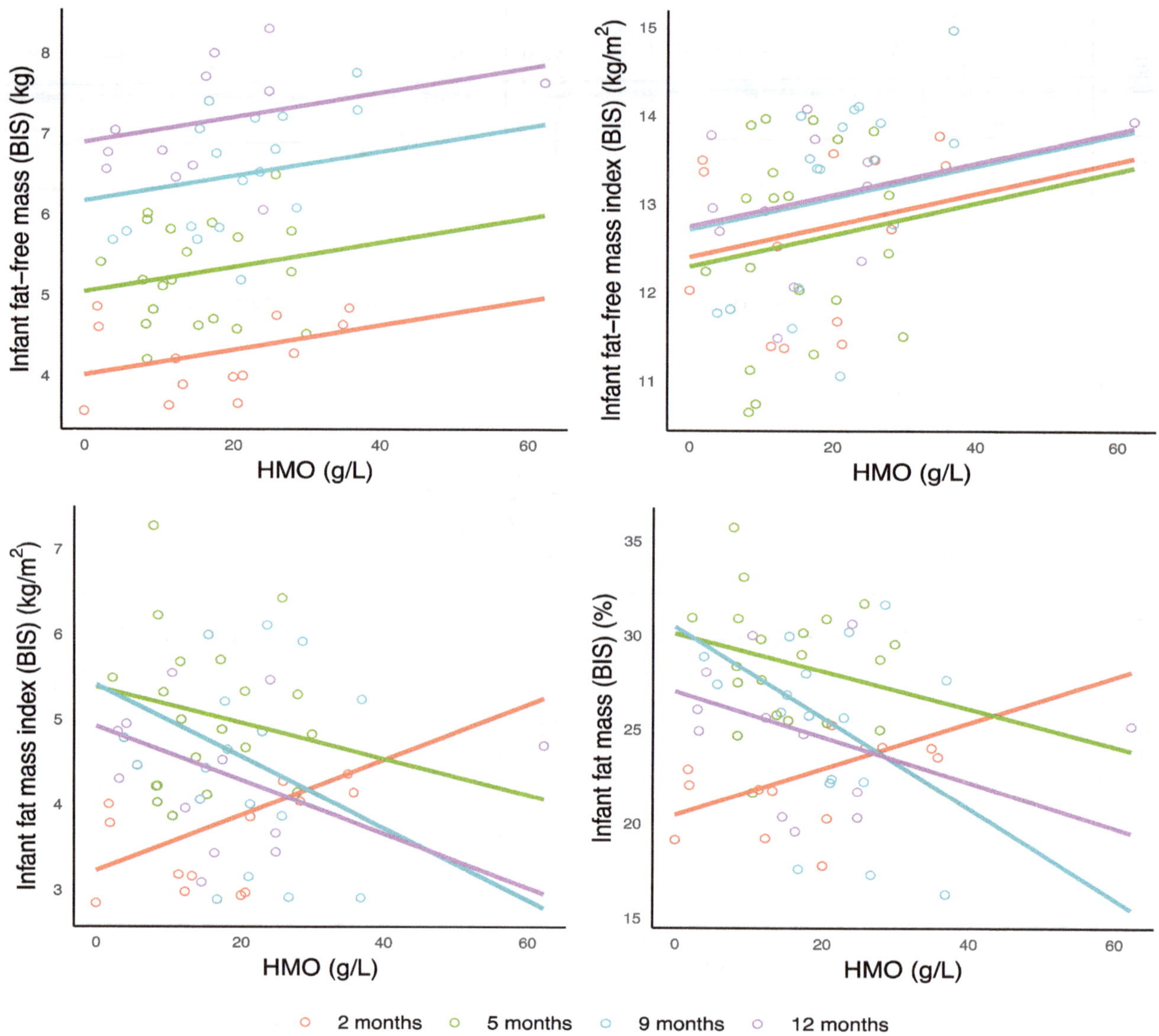

Figure 2. Significant associations between concentration of human milk oligosaccharides (HMO) and infant body composition parameters measured with bioelectrical impedance spectroscopy (BIS). Lines represent linear regression and grouped by the month of lactation.

No further associations were seen after adjusting for the FDR (Table 3).

3.5. Infant Body Composition and Daily Intakes of Carbohydrates

Higher TCH CDI was associated with increased infant FM (ultrasound 2-skinfolds: $p = 0.006$; ultrasound 4-skinfolds: $p < 0.001$), FMI (ultrasound 2-skinfolds: $p = 0.003$), %FM (ultrasound 2-skinfolds: $p = 0.005$), FM/FFM (ultrasound 2-skinfolds: $p = 0.004$), and decreased FFMI (ultrasound 4-skinfolds: $p < 0.001$); and also with BMI (an increase at 5 months and a decrease at 9 and 12 months, $p = 0.019$), and %FM ($p = 0.016$) and FM/FFM ($p = 0.007$) measured with ultrasound 4-skinfolds (an increase at 5 months and 12 months and a decrease at 9 months for both) (Table 4, Figure 3).

Table 2. Differences by infant age/lactation duration within fat mass to fat-free mass ratios and measured human milk carbohydrates [a].

Changes in Characteristics between Time Points	Months after Birth						
	5 and 2 Months	9 and 2 Months	12 and 2 Months	9 and 5 Months	12 and 5 Months	12 and 9 Months	Overall p Value
FM/FFM ratios	**(n = 14)**	**(n = 12)**	**(M = 11/I = 10)**	**(M = 18/I = 17)**	**(M = 18/I = 17)**	**(M = 16/I = 13)**	**(n = 20)**
Maternal FM/FFM	0.01 ± 0.01 [b] (0.98)	−0.02 ± 0.01 (0.63)	−0.04 ± 0.01 [d] (0.002)	−0.02 ± 0.01 (0.27)	−0.05 ± 0.01 [d] (<0.001)	−0.03 ± 0.01 [d] (0.042)	<0.001 [c,d]
Infant FM/FFM with ultrasound 2-skinfolds	0.03 ± 0.03 (0.69)	0.01 ± 0.03 (0.96)	−0.003 ± 0.03 (1.00)	−0.01 ± 0.02 (0.93)	−0.03 ± 0.02 (0.61)	−0.02 ± 0.03 (0.93)	0.59
Infant FM/FFM with ultrasound 4-skinfolds	0.02 ± 0.02 (0.86)	0.002 ± 0.02 (1.00)	−0.03 ± 0.02 (0.54)	−0.01 ± 0.02 (0.87)	−0.05 ± 0.02 (0.095)	−0.03 ± 0.02 (0.41)	0.16
Infant FM/FFM with BIS	**0.12 ± 0.02 (<0.001)**	**0.06 ± 0.02 (0.028)**	0.05 ± 0.02 (0.17)	**−0.06 ± 0.02 (0.006)**	**−0.07 ± 0.02 (0.002)**	−0.01 ± 0.02 (0.95)	**<0.001**
Concentrations	**(n = 15)**	**(n = 14)**	**(n = 8)**	**(n = 19)**	**(n = 14)**	**(n = 14)**	**(n = 20)**
Total carbohydrates (g/L)	−3.0 ± 3.7 (0.86)	1.4 ± 3.8 (0.98)	−1.2 ± 4.1 (0.99)	4.4 ± 3.5 (0.60)	1.8 ± 3.8 (0.97)	−2.6 ± 3.9 (0.91)	0.65
Lactose (g/L)	−1.3 ± 1.8 (0.89)	−1.1 ± 1.8 (0.93)	0.5 ± 1.9 (0.98)	0.2 ± 1.6 (1.00)	1.8 ± 1.8 (0.73)	1.6 ± 1.8 (0.80)	0.70
HMO (g/L)	−2.2 ± 3.9 (0.94)	2.2 ± 3.9 (0.95)	0.7 ± 4.3 (1.00)	4.3 ± 3.6 (0.63)	2.9 ± 3.9 (0.89)	−1.4 ± 4.0 (0.98)	0.69
CDI				**(n = 7)**	**(n = 6)**	**(n = 6)**	**(n = 9)**
Total carbohydrates (g) [e]	n/a [f]	n/a [f]	n/a [f]	**−21.0 ± 5.9 (0.001)**	**−24.7 ± 6.2 (<0.001)**	−3.7 ± 6.6 (0.84)	**0.003**
Lactose (g) [e]	n/a	n/a	n/a	**−19.4 ± 4.4 (<0.001)**	**−23.1 ± 4.4 (<0.001)**	−3.8 ± 4.8 (0.71)	**<0.001**
HMO (g) [e]	n/a	n/a	n/a	−1.4 ± 4.0 (0.94)	−1.5 ± 4.2 (0.94)	−0.05 ± 4.9 (1.00)	0.91

[a] Systematic differences in the measured variables between different months after birth were calculated using general linear hypothesis test (Tukey's all pair comparisons). [b] Data are parameter estimate ± SE of estimate and p-value (in parenthesis). [c] Overall p-value is associated with age as reported in linear mixed model. [d] Bold text indicates significant difference ($p < 0.05$) between two time points or overall. [e] 24-h milk intake and feeding frequency as meals per 24-h was measured at 24-h milk production and daily intakes (CDI) calculated between 2 and 5 months (n = 17) and within 2 weeks of 9 (n = 8) and 12 months (n = 8). [f] Results are not presented for impractical combinations. BIS: bioelectrical impedance spectroscopy; FFM: fat-free mass; FM: fat mass; FM/FFM: fat mass to fat-free mass ratio; HMO: human milk oligosaccharides; I: infants; M: mothers; n/a: not applicable.

Table 3. Associations between concentrations of human milk carbohydrates and infant characteristics.

Predictor (Concentration, g/L)	2 Months (n = 15)		5 Months (n = 20)		9 Months (n = 19)		12 Months (n = 14)		*P*-Value (n = 20)		
	Intercept (SE)	Slope (SE)	Intercept (SE)	Slope (SE)	Intercept (SE)	Slope (SE)	Intercept (SE)	Slope (SE)	Predictor	Infant Age (Months)	Interaction
Infant Length (cm)											
TCH	53.90 (1.22) [a]	0.047 (0.013)	60.90 (1.15)	0.047 (0.013)	66.20 (1.21)	0.047 (0.013)	70.40 (1.17)	0.047 (0.013)	**<0.001** [b]	<0.001	0.62 [c]
Lactose	53.60 (2.31)	0.065 (0.034)	60.50 (2.27)	0.065 (0.034)	66.10 (2.26)	0.065 (0.034)	70.0 (2.27)	0.065 (0.034)	0.047	<0.001	0.093
HMO	57.40 (0.62)	0.031 (0.014)	64.30 (0.55)	0.031 (0.014)	69.70 (0.60)	0.031 (0.014)	73.70 (0.60)	0.031 (0.014)	0.036	<0.001	0.67
Infant Weight (kg)											
TCH	4.55 (0.42)	0.013 (0.004)	6.39 (0.40)	0.013 (0.004)	7.65 (0.41)	0.013 (0.004)	8.47 (0.40)	0.013 (0.004)	**0.003**	<0.001	0.54
HMO	5.46 (0.22)	0.009 (0.004)	7.28 (0.21)	0.009 (0.004)	8.54 (0.21)	0.009 (0.004)	9.42 (0.22)	0.009 (0.004)	0.038	<0.001	0.17
Infant Body Mass Index (kg/m^2)											
TCH	11.30 (2.04)	0.063 (0.024)	18.20 (2.38)	−0.007 (0.029)	19.10 (1.83)	−0.016 (0.021)	18.30 (1.29)	−0.013 (0.015)	0.91	<0.001	0.044
HMO	15.70 (0.51)	0.049 (0.020)	17.80 (0.52)	−0.008 (0.026)	17.70 (0.59)	−0.001 (0.023)	17.90 (0.47)	−0.026 (0.016)	0.99	<0.001	0.027
Infant Fat-free Mass with Bioelectrical Impedance Spectroscopy (kg)											
TCH	2.63 (0.35)	0.020 (0.004)	3.69 (0.33)	0.020 (0.004)	4.78 (0.35)	0.020 (0.004)	5.53 (0.33)	0.020 (0.004)	**<0.001**	<0.001	0.28
HMO	4.02 (0.17)	0.015 (0.004)	5.05 (0.15)	0.015 (0.004)	6.17 (0.17)	0.015 (0.004)	6.90 (0.17)	0.015 (0.004)	**<0.001**	<0.001	0.069
Infant Fat-free Mass with Ultrasound 2-skinfolds (kg)											
TCH	3.41 (0.38)	0.009 (0.004)	4.66 (0.36)	0.009 (0.004)	5.63 (0.38)	0.009 (0.004)	6.32 (0.37)	0.009 (0.004)	0.032	<0.001	0.82
Infant Fat-free Mass with Ultrasound 4-skinfolds (kg)											
TCH	3.35 (0.38)	0.010 (0.004)	4.66 (0.36)	0.010 (0.004)	5.64 (0.38)	0.010 (0.004)	6.46 (0.36)	0.010 (0.004)	**0.020**	<0.001	0.86
Infant Fat-free Mass Index with Bioelectrical Impedance Spectroscopy (kg/m^2)											
TCH	10.90 (0.62)	0.022 (0.007)	10.80 (0.58)	0.022 (0.007)	11.20 (0.62)	0.022 (0.007)	11.20 (0.59)	0.022 (0.007)	**0.002**	0.054	0.83
HMO	12.40 (0.28)	0.018 (0.007)	12.30 (0.24)	0.018 (0.007)	12.70 (0.27)	0.018 (0.007)	12.80 (0.27)	0.018 (0.007)	**0.008**	0.030	0.30
Infant Fat Mass with Bioelectrical Impedance Spectroscopy (kg)											
TCH	−0.03 (0.71)	0.016 (0.008)	2.91 (0.83)	−0.010 (0.010)	3.81 (0.63)	−0.018 (0.007)	3.14 (0.44)	−0.010 (0.005)	0.051	<0.001	**0.016**
HMO	1.09 (0.17)	0.012 (0.007)	2.26 (0.17)	−0.009 (0.009)	2.56 (0.20)	−0.016 (0.008)	2.57 (0.15)	−0.011 (0.006)	0.11	<0.001	0.039
Infant Fat Mass with Bioelectrical Impedance Spectroscopy (%)											
TCH	9.84 (6.56)	0.154 (0.078)	37.20 (7.66)	−0.106 (0.010)	46.80 (5.87)	−0.244 (0.067)	35.60 (4.09)	−0.131 (0.049)	0.002	<0.001	**0.001**
HMO	20.50 (1.54)	0.122 (0.069)	30.10 (1.56)	−0.100 (0.087)	30.50 (1.87)	−0.241 (0.080)	27.00 (1.40)	−0.121 (0.055)	0.020	<0.001	**0.005**

Table 3. *Cont.*

Predictor (Concentration, g/L)	2 Months ($n = 15$)		5 Months ($n = 20$)		9 Months ($n = 19$)		12 Months ($n = 14$)		*P*-Value ($n = 20$)		
	Intercept (SE)	Slope (SE)	Intercept (SE)	Slope (SE)	Intercept (SE)	Slope (SE)	Intercept (SE)	Slope (SE)	Predictor	Infant Age (Months)	Interaction
Infant Fat Mass Index with Bioelectrical Impedance Spectroscopy (kg/m^2)											
TCH	0.40 (1.47)	0.041 (0.017)	6.81 (1.72)	−0.022 (0.021)	8.59 (1.32)	−0.046 (0.015)	6.72 (0.92)	−0.029 (0.011)	0.008	<0.001	**0.001**
HMO	3.23 (0.36)	0.033 (0.015)	5.39 (0.36)	−0.021 (0.019)	5.41 (0.43)	−0.042 (0.018)	4.93 (0.32)	−0.032 (0.012)	0.033	<0.001	**0.003**
Infant Fat Mass to Fat-free Mass Ratio with Bioelectrical Impedance Spectroscopy											
TCH	0.09 (0.12)	0.003 (0.001)	0.56 (0.14)	−0.002 (0.002)	0.70 (0.10)	−0.004 (0.001)	0.54 (0.07)	−0.003 (0.001)	0.001	<0.001	**0.003**
HMO	0.26 (0.03)	0.002 (0.001)	0.44 (0.03)	−0.002 (0.002)	0.44 (0.03)	−0.004 (0.001)	0.38 (0.03)	−0.002 (0.001)	0.027	<0.001	**0.006**

[a] Parameter estimate ± SE; effects of predictors taken from linear mixed effects models that accounted for month after birth and an interaction between month after birth and predictor with a random effect per participant; if the interaction is not significant parameter estimates are taken from a model with no interaction. [b,c] Results are presented only for interactions or predictors with raw *p*-values < 0.05; after the false discovery rate adjustment the interaction/predictor *p*-values were considered to be significant at <0.032 for total carbohydrates (TCH) concentration (indicated by the bold text), at <0.027 for human milk oligosaccharides (HMO) concentration (indicated by the bold text), and at <0.047 for lactose concentration (none are significant).

Table 4. Associations between calculated daily intakes of human milk carbohydrates and infant characteristics.

Predictor (CDI [d], g)	Between 2 and 5 Months ($n = 17$)		9 Months ($n = 8$)		12 Months ($n = 8$)		*P*-Value ($n = 18$)		
	Intercept (SE)	Slope (SE)	Intercept (SE)	Slope (SE)	Intercept (SE)	Slope (SE)	Predictor	Infant Age (Months)	Interaction
Infant Body Mass Index (kg/m^2)									
TCH	15.60 (1.30) [a]	0.033 (0.019)	18.60 (1.47)	−0.013 (0.029)	18.50 (0.72)	−0.018 (0.013)	0.65 [b]	0.77	**0.019** [c]
Lactose	15.70 (1.00)	0.038 (0.018)	17.90 (1.21)	0.0003 (0.032)	19.00 (0.88)	−0.040 (0.025)	0.38	0.59	**0.011**
Infant Fat-free Mass Index with Ultrasound 4-skinfolds (kg/m^2)									
TCH	15.20 (0.56)	−0.034 (0.007)	14.70 (0.47)	−0.034 (0.007)	15.10 (0.45)	−0.034 (0.007)	**<0.001**	0.035	0.37
Lactose	13.30 (0.73)	−0.006 (0.013)	12.90 (0.87)	0.003 (0.023)	15.40 (0.65)	−0.060 (0.018)	0.076	0.13	**0.015**
Infant Fat Mass with Ultrasound 2-skinfolds (kg)									
TCH	1.24 (0.29)	0.011 (0.004)	1.82 (0.25)	0.011 (0.004)	1.94 (0.23)	0.011 (0.004)	**0.006**	<0.001	0.29
Lactose	1.23 (0.31)	0.014 (0.006)	1.93 (0.24)	0.014 (0.006)	2.06 (0.21)	0.014 (0.006)	**0.008**	<0.001	0.19
Infant Fat Mass with Ultrasound 4-skinfolds (kg)									
TCH	1.09 (0.26)	0.014 (0.004)	1.73 (0.22)	0.014 (0.004)	1.64 (0.20)	0.014 (0.004)	**<0.001**	<0.001	0.16
Lactose	1.16 (0.30)	0.015 (0.005)	1.87 (0.23)	0.015 (0.005)	1.80 (0.21)	0.015 (0.005)	**0.004**	<0.001	0.21
HMO	1.73 (0.14)	0.020 (0.008)	2.13 (0.18)	0.020 (0.008)	1.99 (0.17)	0.020 (0.008)	0.010	0.061	0.77

Table 4. *Cont.*

Predictor (CDI [d], g)	Between 2 and 5 Months (*n* = 17)		9 Months (*n* = 8)		12 Months (*n* = 8)		*P*-Value (*n* = 18)		
	Intercept (SE)	Slope (SE)	Intercept (SE)	Slope (SE)	Intercept (SE)	Slope (SE)	Predictor	Infant Age (Months)	Interaction
Infant Fat Mass with Ultrasound 2-skinfolds (%)									
TCH	20.10 (2.51)	0.010 (0.036)	21.80 (2.15)	0.010 (0.036)	20.70 (1.98)	0.010 (0.036)	**0.005**	0.64	0.064
Lactose	19.80 (2.80)	0.128 (0.050)	22.30 (2.18)	0.128 (0.050)	21.60 (1.94)	0.128 (0.050)	**0.019**	0.59	0.11
Infant Fat Mass with Ultrasound 4-skinfolds (%)									
TCH	14.00 (2.91)	0.193 (0.043)	31.10 (4.47)	−0.083 (0.090)	18.80 (2.05)	0.103 (0.042)	<0.001	0.051	**0.016**
Lactose	18.30 (2.66)	0.156 (0.048)	21.60 (2.10)	0.156 (0.048)	18.70 (1.85)	0.156 (0.048)	**0.001**	0.079	0.069
HMO	24.60 (1.29)	0.168 (0.074)	25.10 (1.64)	0.168 (0.074)	21.30 (1.58)	0.168 (0.074)	0.025	0.095	0.51
Infant Fat Mass Index with Bioelectrical Impedance Spectroscopy (kg/m^2)									
Lactose	3.66 (0.74)	0.027 (0.013)	3.27 (0.58)	0.027 (0.013)	3.55 (0.53)	0.027 (0.013)	0.045	0.62	0.41
HMO	5.37 (0.32)	−0.024 (0.017)	4.51 (0.41)	−0.024 (0.017)	4.64 (0.40)	−0.024 (0.017)	0.049	0.013	0.18
Infant Fat Mass Index with Ultrasound 2-skinfolds (kg/m^2)									
TCH	3.10 (0.61)	0.025 (0.009)	3.64 (0.52)	0.025 (0.009)	3.36 (0.47)	0.025 (0.009)	**0.003**	0.32	0.10
Lactose	3.01 (0.67)	0.032 (0.012)	3.74 (0.51)	0.032 (0.012)	3.47 (0.47)	0.032 (0.012)	**0.005**	0.18	0.27
Infant Fat Mass Index with Ultrasound 4-skinfolds (kg/m^2)									
TCH	1.64 (0.74)	0.048 (0.011)	5.22 (1.12)	−0.007 (0.023)	3.21 (0.52)	0.020 (0.011)	<0.001	0.078	0.038
Lactose	2.72 (0.64)	0.038 (0.012)	3.52 (0.50)	0.038 (0.012)	2.84 (0.46)	0.038 (0.012)	**<0.001**	0.065	0.16
HMO	4.28 (0.32)	0.040 (0.018)	4.43 (0.41)	0.040 (0.018)	3.62 (0.39)	0.040 (0.018)	0.034	0.19	0.68
Infant Fat Mass to Fat-free Mass Ratio with Bioelectrical Impedance Spectroscopy									
HMO	0.43 (0.02)	−0.002 (0.001)	0.34 (0.03)	−0.002 (0.001)	0.36 (0.03)	−0.002 (0.001)	0.024	<0.001	0.095
Infant Fat Mass to Fat-free Mass Ratio with Ultrasound 2-skinfolds									
TCH	0.23 (0.05)	0.002 (0.001)	0.27 (0.04)	0.002 (0.001)	0.25 (0.04)	0.002 (0.001)	**0.004**	0.68	0.052
Lactose	0.22 (0.06)	0.003 (0.001)	0.28 (0.04)	0.003 (0.001)	0.27 (0.04)	0.003 (0.001)	**0.012**	0.50	0.14
Infant Fat Mass to Fat-free Mass Ratio with Ultrasound 4-skinfolds									
TCH	0.12 (0.05)	0.004 (0.001)	0.46 (0.08)	−0.002 (0.002)	0.23 (0.04)	0.002 (0.001)	<0.001	0.058	**0.007**
Lactose	0.21 (0.05)	0.003 (0.001)	0.27 (0.04)	0.003 (0.001)	0.22 (0.04)	0.003 (0.001)	**<0.001**	0.084	0.053
HMO	0.33 (0.02)	0.003 (0.001)	0.34 (0.03)	0.003 (0.001)	0.27 (0.03)	0.003 (0.001)	0.027	0.12	0.45

[a] Parameter estimate ± SE; effects of predictors taken from linear mixed effects models that accounted for month after birth and an interaction between month after birth and predictor with a random effect for participant; if the interaction is not significant parameter estimates are taken from a model with no interaction. [b,c] Results are presented only for interactions or predictors with raw *p*-values < 0.05; after the false discovery rate adjustment the interaction/predictor *p*-values were considered to be significant at <0.038 for calculated daily intake (CDI) of total carbohydrates (TCH) (indicated by the bold text), at <0.045 for lactose CDI (indicated by the bold text), and at <0.010 for human milk oligosaccharides (HMO) CDI (none are significant). [d] CDI were measured between 2 and 5 months and within 2 weeks of 9 and 12 months.

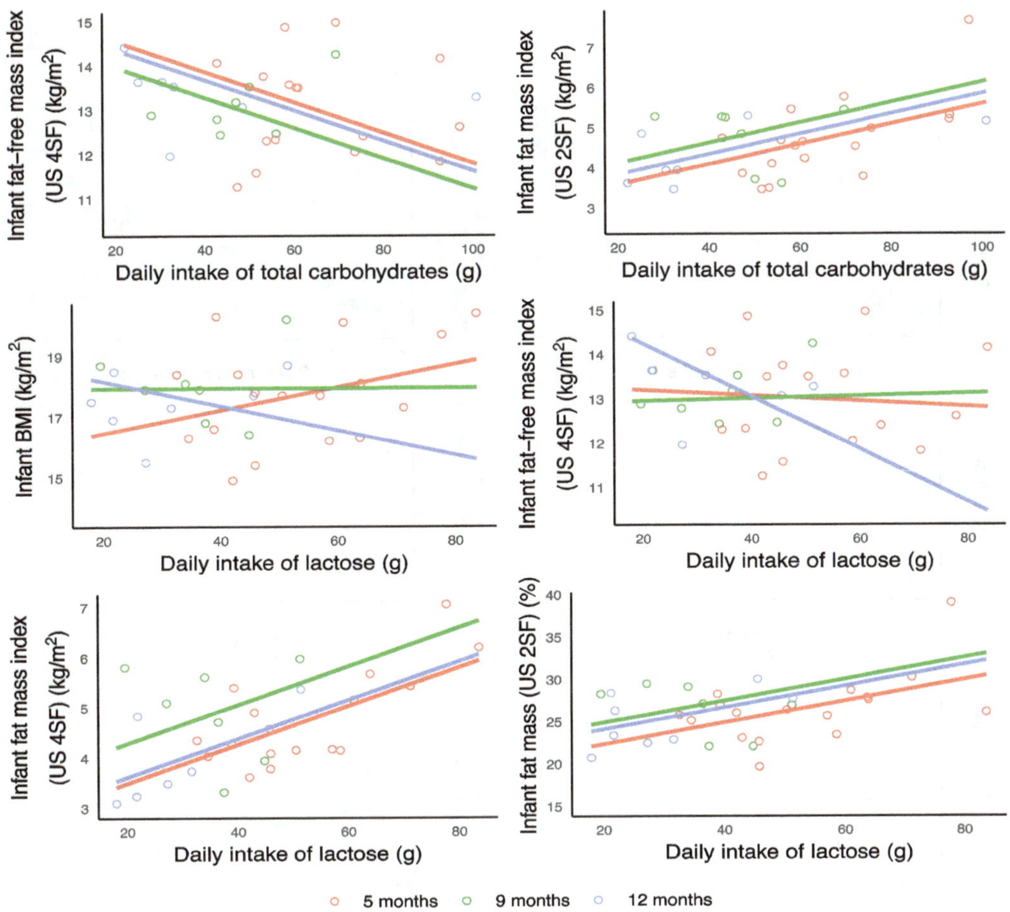

Figure 3. Significant associations between calculated daily intakes of carbohydrates and infant body composition measurements. Lines represent linear regression and grouped by the month of lactation. BMI: body mass index; BIS: US 2SF: ultrasound 2-skinfolds; US 4SF: ultrasound 4-skinfolds.

Higher lactose CDI was associated with increased FM (ultrasound 2-skinfolds: $p = 0.008$; ultrasound 4-skinfolds: $p = 0.004$), FMI (ultrasound 2-skinfolds: $p = 0.005$; ultrasound 4-skinfolds: $p < 0.001$), %FM (ultrasound 2-skinfolds: $p = 0.019$; ultrasound 4-skinfolds: $p = 0.001$), FM/FFM (ultrasound 2-skinfolds: $p = 0.012$; ultrasound 4-skinfolds: $p < 0.001$), and also with BMI (an increase at 5 months, no change at 9 months and a decrease at 12 months, $p = 0.011$) and FFMI (ultrasound 4-skinfolds: no change at 5 and 9 months and a decrease at 12 months, $p = 0.015$) (Table 4, Figure 3).

No further associations were found after adjusting for the FDR (Table 4).

3.6. Associations between Breastfeeding Parameters and Carbohydrates

No significant associations were found between carbohydrates concentrations and 24-h milk intake, 24-h breastfeeding frequency (meals per 24-h), and self-reported breastfeeding frequency (hours between feeds) (data not shown). Higher concentrations of TCH and HMO were associated with higher CDI of these carbohydrates, respectively (TCH: $p = 0.009$; HMO: $p = 0.014$), while no association was seen between lactose concentration and CDI (Table A2).

A higher 24-h milk intake was associated with higher CDI of all measured carbohydrates (TCH: $p < 0.001$; lactose: $p < 0.001$; HMO: $p = 0.016$).

Higher 24-h breastfeeding frequency and lower self-reported breastfeeding frequency were associated with higher CDI of TCH and lactose (24-h breastfeeding frequency: TCH, $p = 0.009$; lactose, $p < 0.001$; self-reported breastfeeding frequency: TCH, $p < 0.001$; lactose, $p = 0.006$) while no associations with HMO CDI were seen (Table A2, Figure 4).

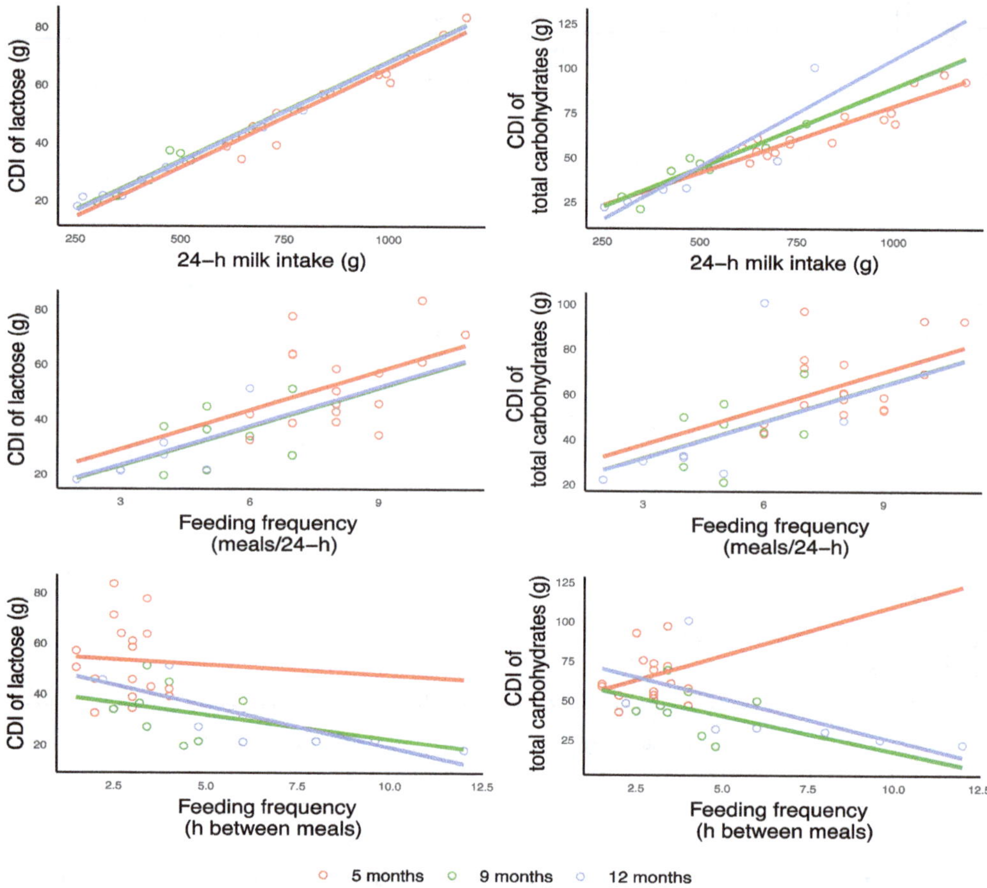

Figure 4. Significant associations between breastfeeding parameters and calculated daily intakes (CDI) of lactose and total carbohydrates measured during 24-h milk production. Lines represent linear regression and grouped by the month of lactation. Where is not seen, the linear regression line for 9 months (green) is under the 12 months line (blue) due to the similar intercept values.

3.7. Changes in Infant Body Composition and Calculated Daily Intakes of Carbohydrates

A significant association was found between changes in infant BC (Δ) between the time points and lactose CDI. Higher lactose CDI at 12 months was associated with greater decrease in FFMI (ultrasound 4-skinfolds: $p = 0.0004$) between 5 and 12 months (Table 5). No further significant associations were found at any time points between changes in infant BC (Δ) between the time points and CDI of both TCH and HMO after adjusting for the FDR (Tables 3 and 4).

Table 5. Associations of calculated daily intakes of lactose at the time points with changes in infant body composition between the time points.

Changes in Infant Characteristic (Response)	Months after Birth					
	5 and 2	9 and 2	12 and 2	9 and 5	12 and 5	12 and 9
	Lactose CDI (g) between 2 and 5 months (n = 17) [c]					
ΔLength (cm)	−0.019 (0.031) [a] 0.56 [b]	0.059 (0.032) 0.11	**0.100 (0.032)** [d] **0.016**	0.004 (0.026) 0.88	0.021 (0.034) 0.54	0.028 (0.033) 0.41
ΔBMI (kg/m²)	**0.049 (0.019)** **0.035**	0.015 (0.030) 0.63	−0.006 (0.038) 0.88	−0.015 (0.018) 0.44	−0.033 (0.023) 0.17	−0.017 (0.013) 0.23
ΔFFM with US 2SF (kg)	−0.013 (0.011) 0.27	**0.024 (0.009)** **0.029**	0.015 (0.014) 0.32	0.003 (0.008) 0.76	0.004 (0.010) 0.66	0.0002 (0.005) 0.96
ΔFFM with US 4SF (kg)	0.003 (0.013) 0.84	**0.043 (0.012)** **0.009**	0.044 (0.019) 0.052	0.005 (0.008) 0.51	0.008 (0.009) 0.41	0.004 (0.005) 0.44
ΔFFM with BIS (kg)	0.009 (0.005) 0.12	0.023 (0.016) 0.19	**0.035 (0.012)** **0.025**	0.004 (0.009) 0.63	0.011 (0.011) 0.32	0.012 (0.010) 0.24
ΔFFMI with US 4SF (kg/m²)	0.041 (0.023) 0.12	0.045 (0.026) 0.13	**0.088 (0.035)** **0.044**	0.006 (0.013) 0.64	−0.002 (0.018) 0.91	−0.004 (0.014) 0.77
ΔFM with US 2SF (kg)	**0.029 (0.010)** **0.014**	0.007 (0.010) 0.53	0.014 (0.015) 0.38	−0.004 (0.008) 0.68	−0.005 (0.008) 0.53	0.001 (0.004) 0.87
ΔFMI with US 2SF (kg/m²)	**0.057 (0.023)** **0.036**	−0.003 (0.022) 0.91	−0.009 (0.035) 0.80	−0.014 (0.018) 0.46	−0.025 (0.020) 0.23	−0.007 (0.008) 0.40
ΔFMI with BIS (kg/m²)	0.026 (0.015) 0.11	0.001 (0.029) 0.98	−0.020 (0.023) 0.42	−0.017 (0.017) 0.33	**−0.045 (0.017)** **0.023**	−0.026 (0.019) 0.19
ΔFM/FFM with US 2SF	**0.007 (0.003)** **0.036**	−0.001 (0.002) 0.60	−0.001 (0.005) 0.93	−0.002 (0.002) 0.35	−0.001 (0.001) 0.67	−0.0004 (0.001) 0.65
ΔFM/FFM with BIS	0.001 (0.001) 0.40	−0.001 (0.003) 0.80	**−0.006 (0.002)** **0.032**	−0.002 (0.001) 0.12	**−0.004 (0.002)** **0.034**	−0.002 (0.002) 0.32
	Lactose CDI (g) at 9 months (n = 8) [c]					
ΔFM with BIS (kg)	n/a [e]	0.053 (0.081) 0.58	−0.033 (0.062) 0.65	−0.020 (0.025) 0.46	**−0.037 (0.014)** **0.045**	−0.017 (0.018) 0.39
	Lactose CDI (g) at 12 months (n = 8) [c]					
ΔFFMI with US 2SF (kg/m²)	n/a [e]	n/a [e]	−0.082 (0.036) 0.15	n/a [e]	**−0.097 (0.018)** **0.003**	−0.041 (0.018) 0.072
ΔFFMI with US 4SF (kg/m²)	n/a	n/a	−0.075 (0.058) 0.33	n/a	**−0.080 (0.007)** **0.0004 *****	−0.042 (0.026) 0.17
ΔFM with US 2SF (kg)	n/a	n/a	**0.036 (0.010)** **0.032**	n/a	0.019 (0.011) 0.13	0.005 (0.006) 0.48

[a] Parameter estimate ± SE and [b] P-values for associations between [c] calculated daily intakes (CDI) of lactose (predictor) at given time points and the changes (Δ) in measured variables between different months after birth. [d] Results are presented only for variables with at least one significant raw P-value ($p < 0.05$, indicated by the bold text); after the false discovery rate adjustment, the predictor P-values were considered to be significant at <0.009 for CDI of lactose between 2 and 5 months (none are significant), at <0.045 for CDI at 9 months (none are significant) and at <0.003 for CDI at 12 months (indicated by the bold text and ***). [e] Results are not presented for impractical time combinations. BIS: bioelectrical impedance spectroscopy; BMI: body mass index; FFM: fat-free mass; FFMI: fat-free mass index; FM: fat mass; FM/FFM: fat mass to fat-free mass ratio; FMI: fat mass index; n/a: not applicable; US 2SF: ultrasound 2-skinfolds; US 4SF: ultrasound 4-skinfolds.

4. Discussion

This proof-of-concept longitudinal study elucidates some of the complex mechanisms by which breastfeeding and HM may affect the development of infant BC and possibly contribute to protection from obesity. Our findings are noteworthy, given the scarcity of data on the effect of HM components, specifically carbohydrates, on infant growth and development. In this study both, concentrations and, more importantly, daily intakes of HM carbohydrates have been found to associate with development of infant BC and are differentially related to infant anthropometry and BC (FM and FFM; Figure 5) throughout the first 12 months of lactation. Moreover, infant breastfeeding frequency was associated with CDI of TCH and lactose, highlighting the important role of breastfeeding in programming of infant appetite regulation and BC in the first year of life.

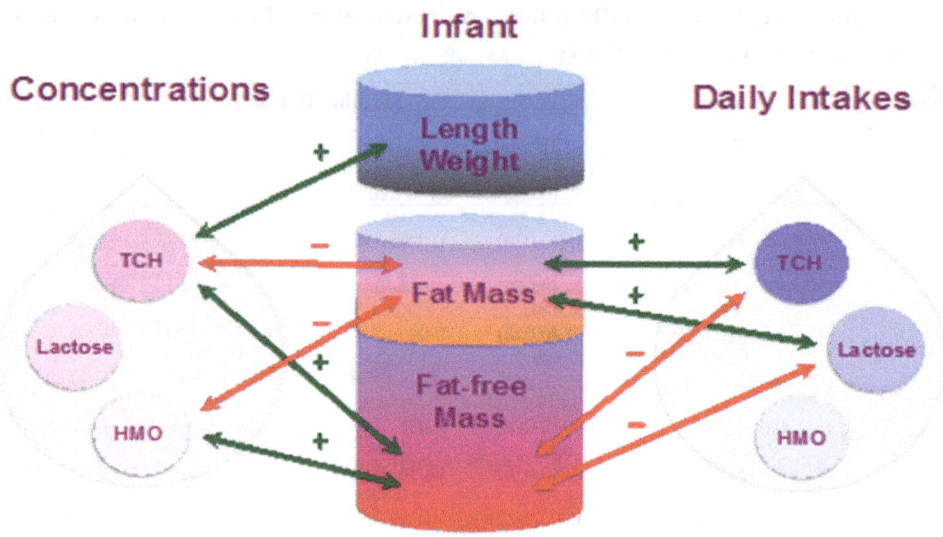

Figure 5. Suggested lactocrine programming of the infant body composition during first 12 months of life. Green arrows indicate positive associations of human milk carbohydrates (concentrations and calculated daily intakes) with infant body composition parameters and red arrows—negative associations. HMO: human milk oligosaccharides; TCH: total carbohydrates.

HM carbohydrates are a major macronutrient which contributes over 40% of energy of the HM [39], predominantly from lactose, and may have greater biological significance compared with other components; thus, it is not surprising that we have established multiple strong associations with infant BC. What is interesting is that the directions of the associations with infant BC were not uniform for the concentration and CDI of the same measured component. This is due to the lack of association between CDI and concentration of lactose, and differences in CDI of TCH and lactose, but not in CDI of HMO, across the time.

Within the normal developmental context of breastfeeding we established that the concentration of lactose, the principal HM carbohydrate, was not related to infant BC or anthropometrics during the first 12 months of lactation (Table 3). Although added dietary sugars have been shown to promote excess adiposity in infants [5], studies of the effect of HM lactose on infant BC are rare. While there has been increased interest in HMO, the importance of lactose for infant development and digestive issues, such as lactose intolerance and malabsorption, is still not well understood. Two recent observational studies found higher HM lactose concentration was related to greater infant weight gain. The first study confirmed a positive association between HM lactose concentration (2–4 weeks lactation) and weight-to-length *z*-score of 6-month-old infants of mothers with excess weight and obesity [40]. The second study also showed that increased HM lactose concentration (4–8 weeks lactation) was related to increased infant weight gain, BMI, and adiposity (skinfolds) at 12 months [22]. Our contrasting results are likely due to the mixed feeding present in both of the previous studies particularly in the first 5 months, and pooling of HM samples over two weeks in one study [22]. On the other hand, our findings are similar to two studies that reported no relationship of lactose concentration with BC of 6-month-old exclusively breastfed infants [23] and infant growth rate (1–6 months) of exclusively breastfed infants (4 or more months) [11], supporting the notion that exclusivity in the first 4–6 months of life may be important. Alternatively, the lack of associations of lactose concentration could be due to its role in maintaining a constant osmotic pressure [10], and thus being one of the least variable HM components [11,14] during the established lactation.

To account for variation in infant 24-h milk intake, which is known to contribute to infant growth [11], we calculated the CDI of carbohydrates and observed that the absence of associations of lactose concentration with infant BC was mediated by daily intakes. CDI of lactose was positively associated with infant adiposity and negatively with lean body mass (Table 4). Furthermore, lactose CDI at 12 months was associated with a decrease in infant FFMI between 5 and 12 months (Table 5).

Previously daily lactose intake has not been shown to be related to the growth rate of the 4-month-old breastfed infants [11], however the study sample size was very small ($n = 6$). Another study found contradictory results to ours with higher daily intakes of HM lactose being related to increased weight and lean mass gain but not FM in 3–6 months-old breastfed infants [21]. The hypothesis of the growth regulating effect of lactose is supported by porcine studies that show increased weight gain with administered lactose [41], which has been attributed to the prebiotic effect on gut microbiome resulting in growth of lactobacilli and bifidobacteria, improved intestinal health and better minerals absorption. Further, one in vitro HM study reported that in colonic epithelial cells HM lactose induces the gene (*CAMP*) that encodes an antimicrobial peptide, human cathelicidin LL-37, in both a dose- and time-dependent manner [42]. Furthermore, the *CAMP*-inducing capacity of HM lactose increased with time postpartum, while no *CAMP*-inducing effect was found for lactose in commercial formulas. Authors have speculated that small amount of lactose may not be absorbed and, via the *CAMP*-induction, contribute to infant gut homeostasis, protection against pathogens and regulation of gut microbiome [42], which has been implicated in the development of infant weight gain and obesity [43].

The measured HM concentrations of lactose or TCH in our cohort were not related to maternal adiposity, similar to previous findings in a larger cohort [9]. Given that lactose is important for maintaining a constant osmotic pressure in HM [10], maternal adiposity was not expected to have a significant impact on lactose concentration, although negative associations between the lactose concentration and maternal BMI but not %FM have been reported [44]. In contrast, one longitudinal study found positive association between maternal BMI and TCH concentration [45], however this was in a cohort of women with high milk supply which may have influenced the relationship.

Lactose accounts for approximately 85% of the total HM carbohydrates [46] and is often considered akin to TCH despite the significant presence of other carbohydrates. HMO is the third most plentiful component of HM, the amount of which often exceeds total amount of protein [17], while monosaccharides (glucose and galactose) are present in HM in very small quantities [36]. We have used the technique that reliably estimates concentrations and carbon content for monosaccharides, disaccharides as well as polysaccharides with very high molecular weight [34,35] and found that higher concentrations of TCH were associated with greater infant length, weight and lean body mass and decreased adiposity (Table 3). However, TCH CDI was associated with increased infant adiposity and reduced lean mass (Table 4), similar to lactose CDI. Comparable to our findings for TCH, higher concentrations of glucose have been reported to associate with higher relative weight and BMI of 1-month-old breastfed infants [24], while concentration of fructose, thought to be present in HM from maternal diet, was positively associated with weight and lean mass in 6-month-old exclusively breastfed infants [23]. Although present in HM in much lower quantities, together with lactose these small carbohydrates may have a synergistic effect, as previously seen in an in vitro study where stimulation of colonic epithelial cells with combinations of various mono- and disaccharides produced enhanced *CAMP* gene expression compared with the individual effects [42], implying potential roles of multiple HM carbohydrates in infant gut homeostasis in addition to HMO.

Our estimations of HMO also resulted in associations with infant BC. HMO concentration was positively associated with infant lean mass and negatively with adiposity (Table 3), and not HMO CDI (Table 4). Our results are consistent with HMO effects seen in the study of 6-month-old breastfed infants, where concentrations of 16 detected HMO displayed various associations with infant BC, and higher HMO diversity and evenness were associated with lower FM and %FM at 1 month postpartum [20]. Importantly, when examined collectively, the concentration of several HMO in that study explained 33% more of variance in infant adiposity than maternal pre-pregnancy BMI, weight gain during pregnancy or infant sex and age alone. There were discrepancies between HMO concentrations though, with the sum of the 16 individual HMO concentrations (11 g/L at 1 month; 10 g/L at 6 months) [20] being a half of our estimated total HMO concentration at all time points, which could be explained partially by the methodology, with the sulfuric acid–UV method detecting saccharides usually excluded from measurement with HPLC technique, such as acidic oligosaccharides, large oligosaccharides with a degree of polymerization, and small amounts of unidentified saccharides [18].

Other studies of concentrations of individual HMO (2′fucosyllactose) have shown no relationships [47]. Further, a study where 2′fucosyllactose and lacto-N-neotetraose were added to formula showed no relationships with infant anthropometrics over the first year of life [48]. Our results indicate that total HMO as opposed to individual HMO are important, and indeed it has been shown that specific bacteria differentially consume specific HMO [49], with a mixture of HMO feeding the whole microbiome. Thus, HMO likely have an indirect effect on BC by enhancing the growth of beneficial gut bacteria and altering the structure or function of the gut microbiome during the critical periods for the development of obesity [43,50]. Directly measuring the wider variety of HMO would be an advantage in the future research.

The recommendations for breastfeeding are to feed on demand. While we have not seen any associations between concentrations of HM carbohydrates and breastfeeding parameters, we found that infants who fed more frequently and had a higher 24-h milk intake consumed higher daily doses (CDI) of lactose and TCH (Table A2). We have previously reported that frequent feeders consume more milk and have lower FFM and higher FM [15], although the order of the relationship is not clear. Further, lactose is also implicated in gastric emptying of breastfed infants, with higher volumes of higher lactose concentration emptying faster compared to lower volumes of lower concentration [51], supported by previous findings in the group that higher lactose concentration is associated with increased breastfeeding frequency [14]. All of these multiple associations culminate in relationships to infant adiposity and highlight the complexity of pathways by which HM components and the dose that the infant receives impact infant development. In contrast, HMO CDI was not associated with breastfeeding frequency in this study, nor were any strong associations previously seen between total HMO concentration/single dose and gastric emptying of breastfed infants [51], indicating the absence of short-term response to total HMO and their target being the small intestine rather than the stomach.

Before the FDR adjustment, we established that HMO CDI was associated with maternal adiposity (%FM and FM/FFM, Table A1), and associations were contrasting at different stages of lactation; during the exclusive breastfeeding period the relationship was positive, but at 9 and 12 months it was negative. This is in agreement with a study that found negative associations between BMI/adiposity and individual HMO concentrations in maternal serum during pregnancy [52], and with two HM studies, which reported positive and negative correlations between maternal BMI and individual HMO [19,53], indicating maternal factors may contribute to total HMO content. It is plausible that relationships of HMO with maternal adiposity may change when mother returns to pre-pregnancy adiposity, or indicate a possible shift in HMO profile later in lactation when volume of milk produced declines. While the total proportion of HMO has been reported to decline during lactation [18], we did not see the decline in total HMO concentrations over the 12 months of lactation. This emphasizes the importance of HMO for the infant development and accounting for the dose of these carbohydrates.

These findings highlight pitfalls in HM research, with HM components concentrations being the major factor measured with respect to various infant outcomes. Pointedly we see none or opposite relationships for these components when analyzing both, raw concentrations and intakes, rising a question if concentration is a dependable measure. When it comes to HM, concentration of component does not necessarily reflect the dose of the component, considering the variability in volumes of HM consumed, duration of exclusive breastfeeding, as well as in breastfeeding patterns and mixed feeding. When examining the nutritional physiology of the breastfed infant CDI may be a more relevant to understanding the development of BC than concentrations.

Our proof-of-concept study concentrated on women that breastfed on demand for 12 months (exclusively to 5 months and without formula use thereafter), and therefore is more indicative of normative development of BC of the breastfed infant as well as lactation. The strengths of this study also include the longitudinal assessment of HM composition and BC of dyads, the broad variation of maternal adiposity and the analysis of TCH along with lactose. The study limitations are the modest number of dyads related to the multiple measurement time points; the small number of 24-h milk productions at the later months of lactation; an estimation of the total HMO concentration, notwithstanding the technical difficulties with accounting for all HMO. We were unable to collect infant dietary intake data after 5 months, yet it is introduction of and duration of use of formula that alters the BC of breastfed infants, not introduction of solids [21]. Our sample was relatively homogenous (primarily Caucasian term healthy fully-breastfed singletons from mothers of higher social-economic status), thus our results may not be transferable to more diverse populations.

5. Conclusions

This pilot study has provided the methods and design to identify relationships between the maternal BC, HM carbohydrates, 24-h milk intake, breastfeeding frequency, and infant BC. Our results point to a differential effect of concentrations and daily intakes of HM carbohydrates on development of infant lean mass and adiposity during this early time, indicating a potential to improve infant outcome through continuation of breastfeeding during the first 12 months and beyond, which could promote appropriate developmental programming and impact future metabolic health.

Author Contributions: Conceptualization, Z.G., L.C.W., K.M., P.E.H., and D.T.G.; Data curation, Z.G.; Formal analysis, Z.G., A.R., and K.M.; Funding acquisition, D.G.; Investigation, Z.G., W.J.T., C.T.L., S.K., and D.T.G.; Methodology, C.T.L., L.C.W., and D.T.G.; Resources, D.T.G.; Supervision, C.T.L., L.C.W., K.M., P.E.H., and D.T.G.; Visualization, Z.G., A.R., and K.M.; Writing—original draft, Z.G., A.R., and D.T.G.; Writing—review & editing, W.J.T., C.T.L., S.K., L.C.W., K.M., and P.E.H.

Acknowledgments: The authors are thankful to all the mothers and infants who participated in this study and Anna R. Hepworth for consultation on research design and assistance with data analyses.

Appendix A

Table A1. Associations between maternal characteristics and calculated daily intakes of human milk oligosaccharides.

Maternal Predictor	Between 2 and 5 Months ($n = 17$)		9 Months ($n = 7$)		12 Months ($n = 7$)		p-Value ($n = 18$)		
	Intercept (SE)	Slope (SE)	Intercept (SE)	Slope (SE)	Intercept (SE)	Slope (SE)	Predictor	Infant Age (Months)	Interaction
Calculated daily intake of human milk oligosaccharides (g)									
Fat mass (%)	1.64 (10.50) [a]	0.322 (0.315)	18.60 (16.00)	−0.209 (0.525)	64.80 (20.10)	−2.01 (0.735)	0.80 [b]	0.90	**0.014** [c]
FM/FFM	6.25 (6.75)	11.80 (12.80)	16.30 (10.80)	−9.10 (23.70)	52.40 (15.40)	−112.0 (40.30)	0.93	0.92	**0.013**

[a] Parameter estimate ± SE; effects of predictors taken from linear mixed effects models that accounted for month after birth and an interaction between month after birth and predictor with a random effect per participant; if the interaction is not significant parameter estimates are taken from a model with no interaction. [b,c] Results are presented only for interactions or predictors with raw p-values < 0.05 (indicated by the bold text); after the false discovery rate adjustment, the interaction/predictor p-values were considered to be significant at <0.013 for human milk oligosaccharides (none are significant). FF/FFM, fat mass to fat-free mass ratio.

Table A2. Associations of daily intakes of human milk carbohydrates with concentrations and breastfeeding parameters.

Predictor	Between 2 and 5 Months ($n = 17$)		9 Months ($n = 8$)		12 Months ($n = 8$)		*P*-Value ($n = 18$)		
	Intercept (SE)	Slope (SE)	Intercept (SE)	Slope (SE)	Intercept (SE)	Slope (SE)	Predictor	Infant Age (Months)	Interaction
CDI of TCH (g) [d]									
Concentration of TCH (g)	21.80 (17.10) [a]	0.544 (0.207)	−4.05 (19.30)	0.544 (0.207)	−5.47 (18.60)	0.544 (0.207)	**0.009** [b]	<0.001	0.50 [c]
24-h milk intake (g) [d]	−5.84 (7.05)	0.087 (0.008)	0.92 (5.13)	0.087 (0.008)	0.70 (5.05)	0.087 (0.008)	**<0.001**	0.22	0.059
Feeding frequency (24-h MP) [d]	21.80 (17.30)	5.39 (2.07)	15.80 (12.30)	5.39 (2.07)	15.80 (11.20)	5.39 (2.07)	**0.009**	0.69	0.13
Feeding frequency (SR) [d]	77.30 (5.65)	−4.25 (1.35)	60.50 (7.32)	−4.25 (1.35)	68.40 (10.40)	−4.25 (1.35)	**<0.001**	<0.001	0.052
CDI of lactose (g) [d]									
Concentration of lactose (g)	17.80 (24.00)	0.551 (0.366)	−3.56 (25.40)	0.551 (0.366)	−7.77 (25.70)	0.551 (0.366)	0.14	<0.001	0.31
24-h milk intake (g)	−2.80 (2.54)	0.069 (0.003)	−0.50 (1.86)	0.069 (0.003)	−0.78 (1.72)	0.069 (0.003)	**<0.001**	0.33	0.29
Feeding frequency (24-h MP)	15.10 (11.90)	4.74 (1.42)	8.98 (8.45)	4.74 (1.42)	9.29 (7.38)	4.74 (1.42)	**<0.001**	0.51	0.12
Feeding frequency (SR)	62.00 (4.26)	−3.04 (1.04)	45.70 (5.60)	−3.04 (1.04)	49.80 (7.71)	−3.04 (1.04)	**0.006**	<0.001	0.78
CDI of HMO (g) [d]									
Concentration of HMO (g)	2.62 (1.87)	0.612 (0.105)	2.47 (2.96)	0.388 (0.125)	−4.50 (1.91)	0.799 (0.071)	<0.001	0.001	**0.014**
24-h milk intake (g)	10.00 (8.24)	0.003 (0.010)	−0.04 (10.00)	0.022 (0.019)	−16.10 (8.20)	0.057 (0.016)	0.020	0.50	**0.016**
Feeding frequency (24-h MP)	0.42 (9.60)	1.45 (1.15)	3.00 (6.99)	1.45 (1.15)	4.12 (6.32)	1.45 (1.15)	0.22	0.82	0.76
Feeding frequency (SR)	15.30 (3.62)	−1.10 (1.00)	15.10 (5.16)	−1.10 (1.00)	18.10 (7.54)	−1.10 (1.00)	0.29	0.87	0.36

[a] Parameter estimate ± standard error (SE); effects of predictors taken from linear mixed effects models that accounted for month after birth and an interaction between month after birth and predictor with a random effect per participant; if the interaction is not significant parameter estimates are taken from a model with no interaction. [b,c] After the false discovery rate adjustment, the interaction/predictor *p*-values were considered to be significant at <0.05 for all predictors (indicated by the bold text). [d] 24-h milk intake and breastfeeding frequency as meals per 24-h were measured at 24-h MP; current breastfeeding frequency was also self-reported by mothers at the session as typical hours between meals; CDI were calculated between 2 and 5 months and within 2 weeks of 9 and 12 months.

Table 3. Associations of calculated daily intakes of total carbohydrates at the time points with changes in infant body composition between the time points.

Changes in Infant Characteristic (Response)	Months after Birth					
	5 and 2	9 and 2	12 and 2	9 and 5	12 and 5	12 and 9
Total carbohydrates CDI (g) between 2 and 5 months (n = 17) [c]						
ΔLength (cm)	−0.006 (0.026) [a] 0.83 [b]	0.041 (0.028) 0.18	**0.074 (0.026)** [d] **0.023**	0.003 (0.024) 0.91	0.013 (0.030) 0.67	0.016 (0.030) 0.59
ΔWeight (kg)	**0.018 (0.008)** **0.039**	0.025 (0.012) 0.067	0.025 (0.014) 0.11	0.002 (0.007) 0.81	−0.0002 (0.009) 0.98	−0.001 (0.003) 0.81
ΔBMI (kg/m^2)	**0.040 (0.016)** **0.037**	0.013 (0.025) 0.61	−0.008 (0.029) 0.79	−0.009 (0.017) 0.59	−0.022 (0.021) 0.30	−0.013 (0.012) 0.31
ΔFFM with US 4SF (kg)	0.013 (0.012) 0.30	**0.034 (0.013)** **0.038**	**0.045 (0.016)** **0.024**	0.004 (0.007) 0.57	0.007 (0.008) 0.39	0.004 (0.004) 0.33
ΔFFM with BIS (kg)	**0.009 (0.004)** **0.045**	0.021 (0.013) 0.16	0.024 (0.010) 0.051	0.003 (0.008) 0.67	0.006 (0.010) 0.55	0.006 (0.009) 0.54
ΔFM with US 2SF (kg)	**0.024 (0.008)** **0.019**	0.007 (0.008) 0.41	0.011 (0.013) 0.42	−0.003 (0.008) 0.72	−0.003 (0.007) 0.65	0.001 (0.003) 0.85
ΔFMI with US 2SF (kg/m^2)	**0.050 (0.018)** **0.022**	0.001 (0.018) 0.94	−0.004 (0.027) 0.88	−0.013 (0.017) 0.46	−0.020 (0.018) 0.28	−0.006 (0.007) 0.44
ΔFMI with US 4SF (kg/m^2)	0.006 (0.015) 0.73	−0.043 (0.030) 0.19	−0.064 (0.033) 0.10	−0.014 (0.017) 0.41	−0.029 (0.014) 0.071	**−0.015 (0.006)** **0.031**
ΔFM with US 4SF (%)	−0.037 (0.092) 0.70	−0.247 (0.136) 0.11	**−0.371 (0.139)** **0.032**	−0.058 (0.075) 0.45	−0.115 (0.063) 0.089	−0.060 (0.036) 0.12
ΔFM/FFM with US 4SF	−0.0004 (0.002) 0.83	−0.004 (0.002) 0.12	**−0.007 (0.003)** **0.034**	−0.002 (0.002) 0.13	−0.002 (0.001) 0.26	−0.001 (0.001) 0.31
ΔFM/FFM with BIS	0.001 (0.001) 0.37	−0.001 (0.002) 0.71	**−0.005 (0.002)** **0.040**	−0.002 (0.001) 0.14	−0.003 (0.002) 0.15	−0.001 (0.002) 0.58
Total carbohydrates CDI (g) at 9 months (n = 8) [c]						
ΔBMI (kg/m^2)	n/a [e]	−0.198 (0.272) 0.54	−0.009 (0.238) 0.97	−0.062 (0.037) 0.16	**−0.081 (0.029)** **0.037**	−0.019 (0.028) 0.52
ΔFFM with US 2SF (kg)	n/a	**0.107 (0.021)** **0.037**	−0.011 (0.032) 0.76	−0.006 (0.017) 0.75	0.002 (0.019) 0.92	−0.008 (0.014) 0.62
ΔFM with BIS (kg)	n/a	−0.029 (0.122) 0.84	−0.095 (0.062) 0.27	−0.022 (0.019) 0.30	**−0.033 (0.010)** **0.018**	−0.011 (0.015) 0.50
ΔFMI with BIS (kg/m^2)	n/a	−0.114 (0.315) 0.75	−0.181 (0.194) 0.45	−0.051 (0.041) 0.27	**−0.077 (0.028)** **0.040**	−0.027 (0.037) 0.51
Total carbohydrates CDI (g) at 12 months (n = 8) [c]						
ΔFFMI with US 2SF (kg/m^2)	n/a [e]	n/a [e]	−0.093 (0.030) 0.092	n/a [e]	**−0.038 (0.014)** **0.038**	**−0.021 (0.007)** **0.033**
ΔFFMI with US 4SF (kg/m^2)	n/a	n/a	−0.089 (0.055) 0.25	n/a	**−0.031 (0.009)** **0.029**	−0.022 (0.011) 0.11

[a] Parameter estimate ± SE of estimate and [b] P-values for associations between [c] calculated daily intakes (CDI) of total carbohydrates (predictor) at given time points and the changes (Δ) in measured variables between different months after birth. [d] Results are presented only for variables with at least one significant raw p-value ($p < 0.05$, indicated by the bold text); after the FDR adjustment, the predictor p-values were considered to be significant at <0.019 for CDI of total carbohydrates between 2 and 5 months, at <0.018 for CDI at 9 months and at <0.029 for CDI at 12 months (none are significant). [e] Results are not presented for impractical time combinations. BIS: bioelectrical impedance spectroscopy; BMI: body mass index; FFM: fat-free mass; FFMI: fat-free mass index; FM: fat mass; FM/FFM: fat mass to fat-free mass ratio; FMI: fat mass index; n/a: not applicable; SE: US 2SF: ultrasound 2-skinfolds; US 4SF: ultrasound 4-skinfolds.

Table 4. Associations of calculated daily intakes of total carbohydrates at the time points with changes in infant body composition between the time points.

Changes in Infant Characteristic (Response)	Months after Birth					
	5 and 2	9 and 2	12 and 2	9 and 5	12 and 5	12 and 9
HMO CDI (g) between 2 and 5 months (n = 17) [c]						
ΔHead circumference (cm)	0.083 (0.054) [a] 0.16 [b]	−0.007 (0.075) 0.93	0.087 (0.063) 0.21	−0.010 (0.030) 0.74	**0.047 (0.018)** **0.023**	0.047 (0.028) 0.12
HMO CDI (g) at 9 months (n = 8) [c]						
ΔBMI (kg/m^2)	n/a [e]	−0.425 (0.231) 0.21	**−0.401 (0.082)** [d] **0.040**	−0.247 (0.129) 0.11	**−0.361 (0.053)** **0.001**	−0.114 (0.096) 0.29
ΔFFMI with US 4SF (kg/m^2)	n/a	−0.130 (0.208) 0.60	−0.211 (0.295) 0.55	−0.024 (0.094) 0.81	−0.185 (0.119) 0.20	**−0.169 (0.058)** **0.032**
ΔFM with BIS [5] (kg)	n/a	−0.200 (0.058) 0.075	−0.048 (0.108) 0.70	−0.115 (0.060) 0.12	**−0.110 (0.043)** **0.049**	0.005 (0.059) 0.94
ΔFMI with BIS (kg/m^2)	n/a	−0.513 (0.176) 0.10	−0.186 (0.257) 0.55	−0.274 (0.119) 0.069	**−0.294 (0.097)** **0.029**	−0.019 (0.143) 0.90

Table 4. *Cont.*

Changes in Infant Characteristic (Response)	Months after Birth					
	5 and 2	9 and 2	12 and 2	9 and 5	12 and 5	12 and 9
	HMO CDI (g) at 12 months (n = 8) [c]					
ΔFMI with BIS (kg/m^2)	n/a [e]	n/a [e]	−0.336 (0.327) 0.41	n/a [e]	**−0.052 (0.017) 0.032**	−0.037 (0.024) 0.17
ΔFM with BIS (%)	n/a	n/a	−1.488 (1.901) 0.52	n/a	**−0.184 (0.070) 0.047**	−0.157 (0.124) 0.26
ΔFM/FFM with BIS	n/a	n/a	−0.024 (0.032) 0.53	n/a	**−0.004 (0.001) 0.021**	−0.003 (0.002) 0.24

[a] Parameter estimate ± standard errors of estimate and [b] P-values for associations between [c] calculated daily intakes (CDI) of human milk oligosaccharides (predictor) at given time points and the changes (Δ) in measured variables between different months after birth. [d] Results are presented only for variables with at least one significant raw p-value ($p < 0.05$, indicated by the bold text); after the false discovery rate adjustment, the predictor p-values were considered to be significant at <0.023 for CDI of human milk oligosaccharides (HMO) between 2 and 5 months, at <0.001 for CDI at 9 months and at <0.021 for CDI at 12 months (none are significant). [e] Results are not presented for impractical time combinations. BIS: bioelectrical impedance spectroscopy; BMI: body mass index; FFM: fat-free mass; FFMI: fat-free mass index; FM: fat mass; FM/FFM: fat mass to fat-free mass ratio; FMI: fat mass index; n/a: not applicable; US 4SF: ultrasound 4-skinfolds.

References

1. Koletzko, B.; Brands, B.; Chourdakis, M.; Cramer, S.; Grote, V.; Hellmuth, C.; Kirchberg, F.; Prell, C.; Rzehak, P.; Uhl, O.; et al. The power of programming and the EarlyNutrition project: Opportunities for health promotion by nutrition during the first thousand days of life and beyond. *Ann. Nutr. Metab.* **2014**, *64*, 187–196. [CrossRef] [PubMed]
2. Wells, J.C.; Chomoto, S.; Fewtrell, M.S. Programming of body composition by early growth and nutrition. *Proc. Nutr. Soc.* **2007**, *66*, 423–434. [CrossRef] [PubMed]
3. Victora, C.G.; Bahl, R.; Barros, A.J.D.; Franca, G.V.A.; Horton, S.; Krasevec, J.; Murch, S.; Sankar, M.J.; Walker, N.; Rollins, N.C.; et al. Breastfeeding in the 21st century: Epidemiology, mechanisms, and lifelong effect. *Lancet* **2016**, *387*, 475–490. [CrossRef]
4. Malik, V.S.; Pan, A.; Willett, W.C.; Hu, F.B. Sugar-sweetened beverages and weight gain in children and adults: A systematic review and meta-analysis. *Am. J. Clin. Nutr.* **2013**, *98*, 1084–1102. [CrossRef] [PubMed]
5. Pan, L.; Li, R.; Park, S.; Galuska, D.A.; Sherry, B.; Freedman, D.S. A longitudinal analysis of sugar-sweetened beverage intake in infancy and obesity at 6 years. *Pediatrics* **2014**, *134*, S29–S35. [CrossRef] [PubMed]
6. Stanhope, K.L. Sugar consumption, metabolic disease and obesity: The state of the controversy. *Crit. Rev. Clin. Lab. Sci.* **2016**, *53*, 52–67. [CrossRef] [PubMed]
7. Butts, C.A.; Hedderley, D.I.; Herath, T.D.; Paturi, G.; Glyn-Jones, S.; Wiens, F.; Stahl, B.; Gopal, P. Human milk composition and dietary intakes of breastfeeding women of different ethnicity from the Manawatu-Wanganui region of New Zealand. *Nutrients* **2018**, *10*, 1231. [CrossRef] [PubMed]
8. Prentice, A. Regional variations in the composition of human milk. In *Handbook of Milk Composition*; Jensen, R.G., Ed.; Academic Press, Inc.: San Diego, CA, USA, 1995; p. 919.
9. Kugananthan, S.; Gridneva, Z.; Lai, C.T.; Hepworth, A.R.; Mark, P.J.; Kakulas, F.; Geddes, D.T. Associations between maternal body composition and appetite hormones and macronutrients in human milk. *Nutrients* **2017**, *9*, 252. [CrossRef] [PubMed]
10. Martin, C.R.; Ling, P.R.; Blackburn, G.L. Review of infant feeding: Key features of breast milk and infant formula. *Nutrients* **2016**, *8*, 279. [CrossRef] [PubMed]
11. Mitoulas, L.R.; Kent, J.C.; Cox, D.B.; Owens, R.A.; Sherriff, J.L.; Hartmann, P.E. Variation in fat, lactose and protein in human milk over 24 h and throughout the first year of lactation. *Br. J. Nutr.* **2002**, *88*, 29–37. [CrossRef] [PubMed]
12. Arthur, P.G.; Smith, M.; Hartmann, P.E. Milk lactose, citrate, and glucose as markers of lactogenesis in normal and diabetic women. *J. Pediatr. Gastroenterol. Nutr.* **1989**, *9*, 488–496. [CrossRef] [PubMed]
13. Nommsen, L.A.; Lovelady, C.A.; Heinig, M.; Lonnerdal, B.; Dewey, K.G. Determinants of energy, protein, lipid, and lactose concentrations in human milk during the first 12 mo of lactation: The Darling study. *Am. J. Clin. Nutr.* **1991**, *53*, 457–465. [CrossRef] [PubMed]

14. Khan, S.; Hepworth, A.R.; Prime, D.K.; Lai, C.T.; Trengove, N.J.; Hartmann, P.E. Variation in fat, lactose, and protein composition in breast milk over 24 hours: Associations with infant feeding patterns. *J. Hum. Lact.* **2013**, *29*, 81–89. [CrossRef] [PubMed]
15. Gridneva, Z.; Rea, A.; Hepworth, A.R.; Ward, L.C.; Lai, C.T.; Hartmann, P.E.; Geddes, D.T. Relationships between breastfeeding patterns and maternal and infant body composition over the first 12 months of lactation. *Nutrients* **2018**, *10*, 45. [CrossRef] [PubMed]
16. Ninonuevo, M.R.; Park, Y.; Yin, H.; Zhang, J.; Ward, R.E.; Clowers, B.H.; German, J.B.; Freeman, S.L.; Killeen, K.; Grimm, R.; et al. A strategy for annotating the human milk glycome. *J. Agric. Food Chem.* **2006**, *54*, 7471–7480. [CrossRef] [PubMed]
17. Bode, L. The functional biology of human milk oligosaccharides. *Early Hum. Dev.* **2015**, *91*, 619–622. [CrossRef] [PubMed]
18. Chaturvedi, P.; Warren, C.D.; Altaye, M.; Morrow, A.L.; Ruiz-Palacios, G.; Pickering, L.K.; Newburg, D.S. Fucosylated human milk oligosaccharides vary between individuals and over the course of lactation. *Glycobiology* **2001**, *11*, 365–372. [CrossRef] [PubMed]
19. Azad, M.B.; Robertson, B.; Atakora, F.; Becker, A.B.; Subbarao, P.; Moraes, T.J.; Mandhane, P.J.; Turvey, S.E.; Lefebvre, D.L.; Sears, M.R.; et al. Human milk oligosaccharide concentrations are associated with multiple fixed and modifiable maternal characteristics, environmental factors, and feeding practices. *J. Nutr.* **2018**, *148*, 1733–1742. [CrossRef] [PubMed]
20. Alderete, T.A.; Autran, C.; Brekke, B.E.; Knight, R.; Bode, L.; Goran, M.; Fields, D. Associations between human milk oligosaccharides and infant body composition in the first 6 mo of life. *Am. J. Clin. Nutr.* **2015**, *102*, 1381–1388. [CrossRef] [PubMed]
21. Butte, N.; Wong, W.; Hopkinson, J.; Smith, E.; Ellis, K. Infant feeding mode affects early growth and body composition. *Pediatrics* **2000**, *16*, 1355–1366. [CrossRef] [PubMed]
22. Prentice, P.; Ong, K.K.; Schoemaker, M.H.; van Tol, E.A.F.; Vervoort, J.; Hughes, I.A.; Acerini, C.L. Breast milk nutrient content and infancy growth. *Acta Paediatr.* **2016**, *105*, 641–647. [CrossRef] [PubMed]
23. Goran, M.I.; Martin, A.A.; Alderete, T.A.; Fujiwara, H.; Fields, D. Fructose in breast milk is positively associated with infant body composition at 6 months of age. *Nutrients* **2017**, *9*, 146. [CrossRef] [PubMed]
24. Fields, D.; Demerath, E. Relationship of insulin, glucose, leptin, IL-6 and TNF-a in human breast milk with infant growth and body composition. *Pediatr. Obes.* **2012**, *7*, 304–312. [CrossRef] [PubMed]
25. Kent, J.C.; Mitoulas, L.R.; Cregan, M.D.; Ramsay, D.T.; Doherty, D.A.; Hartmann, P.E. Volume and frequency of breastfeedings and fat content of breast milk throughout the day. *Pediatrics* **2006**, *117*, e387–e395. [CrossRef] [PubMed]
26. Binns, C.W.; Fraser, M.L.; Lee, A.H.; Scott, J. Defining exclusive breastfeeding in Australia. *J. Paediatr. Child Health* **2009**, *45*, 174–180. [CrossRef] [PubMed]
27. Gridneva, Z.; Kugananthan, S.; Rea, A.; Lai, C.T.; Ward, L.C.; Murray, K.; Hartmann, P.E.; Geddes, D.T. Human milk adiponectin and leptin and infant body composition over the first 12 months of lactation. *Nutrients* **2018**, *10*, 1125. [CrossRef] [PubMed]
28. Gridneva, Z.; Tie, W.J.; Rea, A.; Lai, C.T.; Ward, L.C.; Murray, K.; Hartmann, P.E.; Geddes, D.T. Human milk casein and whey protein and infant body composition over the first 12 months of lactation. *Nutrients* **2018**, *10*, 1332. [CrossRef]
29. Arthur, P.; Hartmann, P.; Smith, M. Measurement of the milk intake of breast-fed infants. *J. Pediatr. Gastroenterol. Nutr.* **1987**, *6*, 758–763. [CrossRef]
30. Gridneva, Z.; Hepworth, A.R.; Ward, L.C.; Lai, C.T.; Hartmann, P.E.; Geddes, D.T. Determinants of body composition in breastfed infants using bioimpedance spectroscopy and ultrasound skinfolds-Methods comparison. *Pediatr. Res.* **2016**, *81*, 423–433. [CrossRef]
31. Van Itallie, T.B.; Yang, M.U.; Heymsfield, S.B.; Funk, R.C.; Boileau, R.A. Height-normalized indices of the body's fat-free mass and fat mass: Potentially useful indicators of nutritional status. *Am. J. Clin. Nutr.* **1990**, *52*, 953–959. [CrossRef]
32. Wells, J.C.K.; Cole, T.J. Adjustment of fat-free mass and fat mass for height in children aged 8 y. *Int. J. Obes.* **2002**, *26*, 947–952. [CrossRef] [PubMed]
33. Xiao, J.; Purcell, S.A.; Prado, C.M.; Gonzalez, M.C. Fat mass to fat-free mass ratio reference values from NHANES III using bioelectrical impedance analysis. *Clin. Nutr.* **2018**, *37*, 2284–2287. [CrossRef] [PubMed]

34. Euber, J.; Brunner, J. Determination of lactose in milk products by high-performance liquid chromatography. *J. Dairy Sci.* **1979**, *62*, 685–690. [CrossRef]
35. Albalasmeh, A.; Berhe, A.; Ghezzehei, T. A new method for rapid determination of carbohydrate and total carbon concentrations using UV spectrophotometry. *Carbohydr. Polym.* **2013**, *97*, 253–261. [CrossRef] [PubMed]
36. Newburg, D.; Neubauer, S. Carbohydrates in milks: Analysis, quantities, and significance. In *Handbook of Milk Composition*; Jensen, R., Ed.; Academic Press, Inc.: San Diego, CA, USA, 1995; pp. 273–349.
37. Khan, S.; Prime, D.K.; Hepworth, A.R.; Lai, C.T.; Trengove, N.J.; Hartmann, P.E. Investigation of short-term variations in term breast milk composition during repeated breast expression sessions. *J. Hum. Lact.* **2013**, *29*, 196–204. [CrossRef] [PubMed]
38. Curran-Everett, D. Multiple comparisons: Philosophies and illustrations. *Am. J. Physiol. Regul. Integr. Comp. Physiol.* **2000**, *279*, R1–R8. [CrossRef] [PubMed]
39. Hambraeus, L. Human milk composition. *Nutr. Abstr. Rev. Clin. Nutr.* **1984**, *54*, 219–236.
40. Young, B.E.; Patinkin, Z.W.; Pyle, L.; de la Houssaye, B.; Davidson, B.S.; Geraghty, S.; Morrow, A.L.; Krebs, N. Markers of oxidative stress in human milk do not differ by maternal BMI but are related to infant growth trajectories. *Matern. Child Health J.* **2017**, *21*, 1367–1376. [CrossRef] [PubMed]
41. Pierce, K.; Callan, J.; McCarthy, P.; O'Doherty, J. Effects of high dietary concentration of lactose and increased soyabean meal inclusion in starter diets for piglets. *Anim. Sci.* **2004**, *79*, 445–452. [CrossRef]
42. Cederlund, A.; Kai-Larsen, Y.; Printz, G.; Yoshio, H.; Alvelius, G.; Lagercrantz, H.; Strömberg, R.; Jörnvall, H.; Gudmundsson, G.H.; Agerberth, B. Lactose in human breast milk, an inducer of innate immunity with implications for a role in intestinal homeostasis. *PLoS ONE* **2013**, *8*, e53876:1–e53876:12. [CrossRef]
43. Koleva, P.T.; Bridgman, S.L.; Kozyrskyj, A.L. The infant gut microbiome: Evidence for obesity risk and dietary intervention. *Nutrients* **2015**, *7*, 2237–2260. [CrossRef] [PubMed]
44. Quinn, E.A.; Largado, F.; Power, M.; Kuzawa, C.W. Predictors of breast milk macronutrient composition in Filipino mothers. *Am. J. Hum. Biol.* **2012**, *24*, 533–540. [CrossRef] [PubMed]
45. Michaelsen, K.F.; Skafte, L.; Badsberg, J.H.; Jorgensen, M. Variation in macronutrients in human bank milk: Influencing factors and implications for human milk banking. *J. Pediatr. Gastroenterol. Nutr.* **1990**, *11*, 229–239. [CrossRef] [PubMed]
46. Coppa, G.V.; Gabrielli, O.; Pierani, P.; Catassi, C.; Carlucci, A.; Giorgi, P.L. Changes in carbohydrate composition in human milk over 4 months of lactation. *Pediatrics* **1993**, *91*, 637–641. [PubMed]
47. Sprenger, N.; Lee, L.Y.; De Castro, C.A.; Steenhout, P.; Thakkar, S.K. Longitudinal change of selected human milk oligosaccharides and association to infants' growth, an observatory, single center, longitudinal cohort study. *PLoS ONE* **2017**, *12*, e0171814:1–e0171814:15. [CrossRef] [PubMed]
48. Puccio, G.; Alliet, P.; Cajozzo, C.; Janssens, E.; Corsello, G.; Sprenger, N.; Wernimont, S.; Egli, D.; Gosoniu, L.; Steenhout, P. Effects of infant formula with human milk oligosaccharides on growth and morbidity: A randomized multicenter trial. *J. Pediatr. Gastroenterol. Nutr.* **2017**, *64*, 624–631. [CrossRef] [PubMed]
49. Yu, Z.-T.; Chen, C.; Newburg, D.S. Utilization of major fucosylated and sialylated human milk oligosaccharides by isolated human gut microbes. *Glycobiology* **2013**, *23*, 1281–1292. [CrossRef] [PubMed]
50. Bode, L. Human milk oligosaccharides: Every baby needs a sugar mama. *Glycobiology* **2012**, *22*, 1147–1162. [CrossRef]
51. Gridneva, Z.; Kugananthan, S.; Hepworth, A.R.; Tie, W.J.; Lai, C.T.; Ward, L.C.; Hartmann, P.E.; Geddes, D.T. Effect of human milk appetite hormones, macronutrients, and infant characteristics on gastric emptying and breastfeeding patterns of term fully breastfed infants. *Nutrients* **2017**, *9*, 15. [CrossRef]
52. Jantscher-Krenn, E.; Aigner, J.; Reiter, B.; Köfeler, H.; Csapo, B.; Desoye, G.; Bode, L.; van Poppel, M.N.M. Evidence of human milk oligosaccharides in maternal circulation already during pregnancy—A pilot study. *Am. J. Physiol. Endocrinol. Metab.* **2019**, *316*, E347–E357. [CrossRef]
53. McGuire, M.K.; Meehan, C.L.; McGuire, M.A.; Williams, J.E.; Foster, J.; Sellen, D.W.; Kamau-Mbuthia, E.W.; Kamundia, E.W.; Mbugua, S.; Moore, S.E.; et al. What's normal? Oligosaccharide concentrations and profiles in milk produced by healthy women vary geographically. *Am. J. Clin. Nutr.* **2017**, *105*, 1086–1100. [CrossRef] [PubMed]

12

Longitudinal Changes of Mineral Concentrations in Preterm and Term Human Milk from Lactating Swiss Women

Magalie Sabatier [1,*], Clara L. Garcia-Rodenas [1], Carlos A. De Castro [2], Peter Kastenmayer [1], Mario Vigo [1], Stéphane Dubascoux [1], Daniel Andrey [1], Marine Nicolas [1], Janique Richoz Payot [1], Valentine Bordier [1], Sagar K. Thakkar [2], Lydie Beauport [3], Jean-François Tolsa [3], Céline J. Fischer Fumeaux [3] and Michael Affolter [1]

1 Nestlé Research, Société des Produits Nestlé SA, 1000 Lausanne, Switzerland
2 Nestle Research Singapore Hub, Société des Produits Nestlé SA, 29 Quality Road, Singapore 618802, Singapore
3 Clinic of Neonatology, Department Woman Mother Child, University Hospital of Lausanne, 1011 Lausanne, Switzerland
* Correspondence: magalie.sabatier@rdls.nestle.com

Abstract: An adequate mineral supply to preterm infants is essential for normal growth and development. This study aimed to compare the mineral contents of human milk (HM) from healthy mothers of preterm (28–32 weeks) and full term (>37 weeks) infants. Samples were collected weekly for eight weeks for the term group (n = 34) and, biweekly up to 16 weeks for the preterm group (n = 27). Iron, zinc, selenium, copper, iodine, calcium, magnesium, phosphorus, potassium, and sodium were quantitatively analyzed by Inductively Coupled Plasma-Mass Spectrometry. The mineral contents of both HM showed parallel compositional changes over the period of lactation, with occasional significant differences when compared at the same postpartum age. However, when the comparisons were performed at an equivalent postmenstrual age, preterm HM contained less zinc and copper from week 39 to 48 ($p < 0.002$) and less selenium from week 39 to 44 ($p < 0.002$) than term HM. This translates into ranges of differences (min–max) of 53% to 78%, 30% to 72%, and 11% to 33%lower for zinc, copper, and selenium, respectively. These data provide comprehensive information on the temporal changes of ten minerals in preterm HM and may help to increase the accuracy of the mineral fortification of milk for preterm consumption.

Keywords: human milk; term; preterm; calcium; phosphorus; magnesium; zinc; iron; copper; iodine; selenium; potassium; sodium

1. Introduction

An estimated 15 million babies are born preterm (i.e., born before 37 weeks of gestation) worldwide every year, with the incidence ranging from 5% to 18% of births according to the area [1]. Very preterm infants (i.e., born before 32 weeks of gestation) represent a highly vulnerable population with complications that can lead to growth failure, lifetime disability including learning difficulties, visual and hearing impairments, or even death. This population requires a high level of medical care, including nutritional support, to offset the risk of nutritional deficiencies and associated adverse health outcomes. Indeed, term infants are generally born with adequate stores of minerals, the accrual of which occurs during the third trimester of pregnancy. A consequence of being born before term is a high risk of mineral shortfalls due to the limited stores, but also to the rapid postnatal growth, immature gastrointestinal tracts, high endogenous losses, and variable intakes [2]. Due to their essentiality, minerals need to be provided at a level to meet the in utero accretion rates to favor catch-up growth and to not compromise long-term neuronal and cognitive development [3]. The essential minerals or trace elements include iron, zinc, copper, iodine, selenium, calcium, phosphorus, and magnesium, but also potassium and sodium (non-exhaustive list). Among other physiological roles in humans, iron, zinc, copper, and iodine are essential for optimal brain development [4]; calcium, phosphorus, and magnesium are required for adequate bone health [5]; selenium, zinc, and iodine play a crucial role in thyroid hormone metabolism [2]; and potassium and sodium are key electrolytes involved in water fluxes and enzymatic functions [6]. Breastfeeding is the gold standard source of nutrition for term infants and is also highly recommended for preterm infants, as it is protective against several complications of preterm birth [7,8]. However, because of the risk of inadequate nutrient intakes, the fortification of mothers' own milk or donor human milk (HM) is generally prescribed for very preterm infants to enhance the protein, energy, and micronutrients intake [7–9]. Fortification is often recommended to be continued until a postconceptional age of 40 weeks, but possibly until about 52 weeks if infants are discharged with a suboptimal weight for a postconceptional age [3]. Nevertheless, there is no consensus on nutrition after discharge from the neonatal intensive care unit (NICU) [10]. However, it may be assumed that to support adequate growth and development, breastfed preterm infants should have, at the minimum, a similar mineral intake to breastfed term infants of an equivalent developmental stage [11].

Optimal HM mineral fortification during an NICU stay and, potentially, after discharge, requires a precise understanding of HM mineral content and its potential sources of variability. Although decades of research have been allocated to HM mineral concentrations, most of the research has been performed on HM of mothers delivering at term, and for some elements, there are a limited number of reports on preterm HM. When available, comparisons between term HM and preterm HM have been performed at an equivalent postpartum age (i.e., lactation stage), but, to our knowledge, there is no evaluation of differences at the same postmenstrual age (i.e., infant developmental stage). As concentrations of several minerals and trace elements in milk change over lactation [12], the assumption was that the comparison by postmenstrual age could reveal unexplored differences between both groups of HM in the period that surrounds preterm infant discharge from NICU. Therefore, the objectives of the present study were (i) to precisely describe the concentration of zinc, copper, iodine, selenium, iron, calcium, phosphorus, magnesium, potassium, and sodium in HM from mothers of preterm (28–32 weeks of gestation) infants over a period of 16 weeks; (ii) to compare preterm HM mineral content with that of milk from mothers of full term (>37 weeks of gestation) infants at equivalent infant postpartum and postmenstrual ages.

2. Materials and Methods

2.1. Subjects

The aim of the study was to characterize the nutritional composition of preterm and term HM. The study design (monocentric, prospective cohort) and characteristics of the subjects were already reported elsewhere [13], with the results on longitudinal changes for other nutrients (i.e., macronutrients [14], proteins [13], lipids [15], and human milk oligosaccharide [16]). In brief, the study was conducted at the University Hospital in Lausanne (CHUV), Switzerland, between October 2013 and July 2014. The study included women older than 18 years of age and intending to breastfeed their infants for a minimum of 4 months. The preterm group included infants with a gestational age from 28 0/7 to 32 6/7 weeks and the full-term group referred to infants with a gestational age of 37 0/7 to 41 6/7 weeks. The exclusion criteria included any counter-indication to breastfeeding, the mother having been diagnosed with diabetes (type I or II) before pregnancy, alcohol or drugs consumption during pregnancy, and/or mothers having insufficient French language skills to follow the study guidelines.

Mothers who participated in the study were followed until postpartum week 16 for the preterm group, and week 8 for the term group, or until lactation discontinuation (whatever came first), by a dedicated research nurse who was qualified as a lactation consultant (International Board of Lactation Consultant, IBCLC).

The study protocol was established following the Declaration of Helsinki's guidelines and was approved by the local Ethical Committee (Commission cantonale d'éthique de la recherche sur l'être humain du Canton de Vaud, Switzerland; Protocol 69/13, clinical study 11.39.NRC) on April 9, 2013. All the subjects participating in the study signed an inform consent before the enrollment. Registration of this trial was completed at ClinicalTrials.gov under NCT02052245.

2.2. Data Collection

Neonatal demographic and delivery data were prospectively collected and recorded in electronic case report forms. The following infant characteristics were collected: single or multiple gestation, mode of delivery, sex, weight, length, head circumference, and gestational age at birth. Birth weight was monitored with an electronic scale accurate to the nearest 5 g, crown-heel length with a height gauge, and head circumference with a tape. An electronic scale was used to measure the maternal weight at delivery, whereas the maternal age, height, and weight before pregnancy were self-reported and completed during face-to-face interviews between mothers and the research nurse, and were verified by one of the two referent pediatricians (LB, CJFF).

2.3. Human Milk Sampling and Processing

A schematic representation of the HM sampling and processing has already been published previously [16]. Preterm HM samples were collected every 7 days ± 1 day during the first 8 weeks and then every 14 days ± 1 day during the following 8 weeks, which yielded a total of 12 samples during the 16 weeks. For term HM, a total of 8 samples were collected every 7 days ± 1 day for 8 weeks.

Full HM expression from a single breast was performed between 6 am and noon (i.e., corresponding to first morning expression) using an electric breast pump (Symphony®, Medela, 6340 Baar, Switzerland). After full milk collection, the milk was homogenized. A maximum volume of 10 mL milk was reserved for analysis. Lower volumes were collected for the two first time points in the preterm group (i.e., max 5 mL). The remaining HM volumes were provided to the infant for feeding. Samples of HM for analysis were transferred by the mothers into 15 mL polypropylene tubes (Falcon™, Fisher Scientific, Reinach, Switzerland), previously labelled with the subject number and collection information, and stored at −18 °C in the home freezer until being transferred to the hospital. Samples were temporarily kept at −80 °C at the hospital before shipment to the Nestlé Research Centre (Lausanne, Switzerland). To avoid multiple thawing/freezing cycles, HM samples were thawed once for splitting into 15 aliquots before storage at −80 °C until analysis.

2.4. Mineral Quantification

Quantification of minerals was realized using Inductively Coupled Plasma Mass Spectrometry (ICP-MS, Nexion 300-D, PerkinElmer, SCIEX, Norwalk, CT, USA). For sodium, magnesium, phosphorous, potassium, calcium, iron, copper, zinc, and selenium, 0.7 mL of human breast milk was transferred into perfluoroalkoxy alkane vessels and mineralized in a MARS XPress microwave digestion system (CEM® Corp., Matthews, NC, USA) using HNO_3/H_2O_2. Mineralized samples were transferred to PE tubes, diluted with Milli Q water and germanium and tellurium were added as internal standards. Quantification was realized by ICP-MS using helium or CH_4 as a collision or reaction gas. For iodine, 1 mL of human breast milk was treated with 1 mL tetramethylammonium hydroxide (25%) and 4.5 mL of Milli Q water in a drying oven at 90 °C for 3 h. Sample solutions were diluted to 15 mL and centrifuged at 1730 *g* for 15 min. Quantification was realized using ICP-MS in normal mode using germanium as the internal standard. Certified Reference Materials (CRM) were added to all analytical series to control the quality of the quantification.

2.5. Statistics

Statistical analyses were done using SAS (version 9.3, SAS Institute Inc., Cary, NC, USA, 2013) and R (version 3.2.1, R Foundation for Statistical Computing, Vienna, Austria). The longitudinal changes of mineral contents were compared in preterm HM and term HM at equivalent infant (1) postpartum ages and (2) postmenstrual ages. Mixed linear models were used for both comparisons to estimate the differences between the groups. The models used age (either postpartum or postmenstrual), term/preterm status, interaction between age and term/preterm status, sex of infant, and mode of delivery as fixed effects as follows: concentration = visit × term_status + child_sex + delivery + twin_type. There was only one case of mixed sex twins out of six "sets". Since the milk samples analyses were conducted according to the mothers and not the infants, the statistical models used the mother as an individual and the sex of the infant was chosen as the sex of the first child (for twins). This entails that one mother is represented as having a male infant where indeed she has both (because of twins). Within-subject variability was accounted for by declaring the subject ID as a random effect. Contrast estimates of the model were calculated by comparing preterm and term HM groups at each time point. No imputation method was applied for missing data (both in between visits and loss to follow up) as the method used is adapted to handle incomplete data. A conventional two-sided test with a 5% error rate was used without adjusting for multiplicity. Mixed linear models were produced using the package nlme and contrast estimates were made with contrast package. R graphs were created using the package ggplot2.

3. Results

3.1. General Characteristics of the Subjects

The subjects' characteristics were reported elsewhere [13,16] and are summarized in Table 1. In brief, 27 mothers having delivered 33 preterm infants and 34 mothers having delivered 34 term infants were included. In the respective groups, two (7.4% for preterm) and six (17.4% for term) mothers dropped out the study. In total, 473 HM samples, 257 from preterm and 216 from full-term infant mothers, were available for mineral analyses. Except for the rate of Caesarean delivery being higher in the preterm mothers than in the term ones, none of the baseline characteristics were significantly different between the two groups of mothers. Regarding the infants' characteristics, thirty-six percent of the preterm births were twins. As expected, the weight, height, and head circumference were statistically significantly lower in the preterm group than in the term group, but not the sex distribution.

Table 1. General characteristics of the two groups of mothers and infants.

Study Population	Preterm	Term	p-Value *
Mothers (drop outs)	N = 27 (2)	N = 34 (2)	
Age (years)	32.4 ± 5.6	31.2 ± 4.2	0.3173
BMI before pregnancy (Kg/m^2)	22.8 ± 3.3	23.2 ± 4.9	0.6990
BMI at child birth (Kg/m^2)	25.8 ± 3.7	26.9 ± 4.7	0.3141
Delivery type: caesarean (%)	63	23.5	0.0019
Infants	N = 33	N = 34	
Gestational age at birth (weeks)	30.8 ± 1.4	39.5 ± 1.0	<0.0001
Males (%)	54.5	52.9	0.8952
Twins (%)	36.4	0.0	0.0001
Height (cm)	40.4 ± 3.2	49.4 ± 1.7	<0.0001
Weight (g)	1421.4 ± 372.8	3277.6 ± 353.6	<0.0001
Head circumference (cm)	27.8 ± 2.1	34.4 ± 1.5	<0.0001

* t-test and Fisher test of proportions were used for the comparison of continuous and discrete variables, respectively.

3.2. Mineral Concentration and Longitudinal Change in Preterm and Term Human Milk at the Same Postpartum Age

A summary of the results i.e., mean ± SD and median (min-max) for each mineral, is provided in Table 2 along with the range of values reported in the literature. The most concentrated element in both HMs was found to be potassium, followed by, in order of decreasing concentrations, calcium, sodium, phosphorus, magnesium, zinc, iron, copper, iodine, and selenium. The longitudinal concentrations (mean ± SD) of minerals in preterm and term HM per visit at equivalent postpartum ages are reported in Supplementary Table S1. As depicted in Figure 1, in preterm and term HM, the changes in concentration over the 4-month period of sample collection converge into three main patterns. First, the mineral concentrations were observed to increase during the first week postpartum and then to decline during the lactation, like for phosphorus and copper. Secondly, the concentrations were highest in the first week and then either decreased quickly (i.e., zinc, potassium), or gradually (i.e., calcium, selenium, sodium) over the lactation, or remained stable in mature milk (i.e., iodine, iron). Finally, for magnesium, the concentrations remained fairly stable during the course of lactation.

Table 2. Summary of mineral concentrations (i.e., mean ± SD and median (min-max)) in preterm (from sample collection from postpartum week 1 to 16) and term human milk (as collected over 8 weeks postpartum). Retrieved published ranges of mineral concentration in human milk * are also provided for comparison.

Minerals	Statistic	Preterm Milk	Term Milk	Literature Range
(mg/L)				
Potassium	Mean	578 ± 107	575 ± 92	515$ [17], 688$ [18]
	Median	569 (209–907)	562 (308–908)	-
Calcium	Mean	281 ± 51	286 ± 47	-
	Median	282 (145–459)	287 (136–433)	252 (84–462)# [19]
Sodium	Mean	205 ± 177	235 ± 237	135–371# [20]
	Median	160 (54–1577)	170 (84–1969)	-
Phosphorus	Mean	145 ± 32	148 ± 30	-
	Median	145 (48–225)	146 (45–257)	143 (17–278)# [19]
Magnesium	Mean	37 ± 9	32 ± 7	-
	Median	36 (12–70)	33 (17–53)	31 (15–64)# [21]
Zinc	Mean	2.4 ± 1.7	3.2 ± 1.9	2.2–2.5; 2.9–3.9; 1.7–5.3# [22]
	Median	2.1 (0.2–15.5)	2.7 (0.4–11.9)	-
Iron	Mean	0.36 ± 0.23	0.44 ± 0.26	-
	Median	0.32 (0.13–2.78)	0.36 (0.13–1.8)	0.47 (0.04–1.92)# [23]
Copper	Mean	0.36 ± 0.16	0.44 ± 0.15	-
	Median	0.35 (0.06–1.1)	0.42 (0.13–1.0)	0.33 (0.03–2.19)# [23]
(µg/L)				
Iodine	Mean	92 ± 67	87 ± 41	15–150# [20]
	Median	76 (2–422)	76 (18–228)	62 (5.4–2170)# [24]
Selenium	Mean	14.3 ± 4.7	15.0 ± 4.2	11$ [25]–28$ [26]
	Median	13 (4–45)	14 (6–34)	-

* Published median (min-max) value where preferred for reporting. # indicates that values were calculated from term human milk (HM); $ corresponds to data calculated from preterm HM.

No statistical difference was found in mineral concentrations between preterm and term HM at the same postpartum age, except at a few time points. The phosphorus concentration was higher in preterm HM than in term HM at week 1 ($p = 0.024$). The same direction of difference was observed for magnesium at week 4 ($p = 0.027$), week 6 ($p = 0.0357$), and week 7 ($p = 0.047$). Inversely, the sodium and copper concentrations were lower in preterm HM than in term HM at week 2 ($p = 0.032$ and $p = 0.024$, respectively). The calcium to phosphorus mass ratios were found to range between 1.57 and 2.32 in preterm HM, and between 1.84 and 2.22 in term HM, with a statistically significant difference between groups found at week 1 ($p = 0.042$; preterm HM < term HM) and at week 2 ($p = 0.018$, preterm HM < term HM). The zinc to copper molar ratio ranged between 20.6 (at week 1) and 5.2 in preterm HM, and between 29.8 (at week 1) and 5.6 in term HM, with no significant difference between the two HMs.

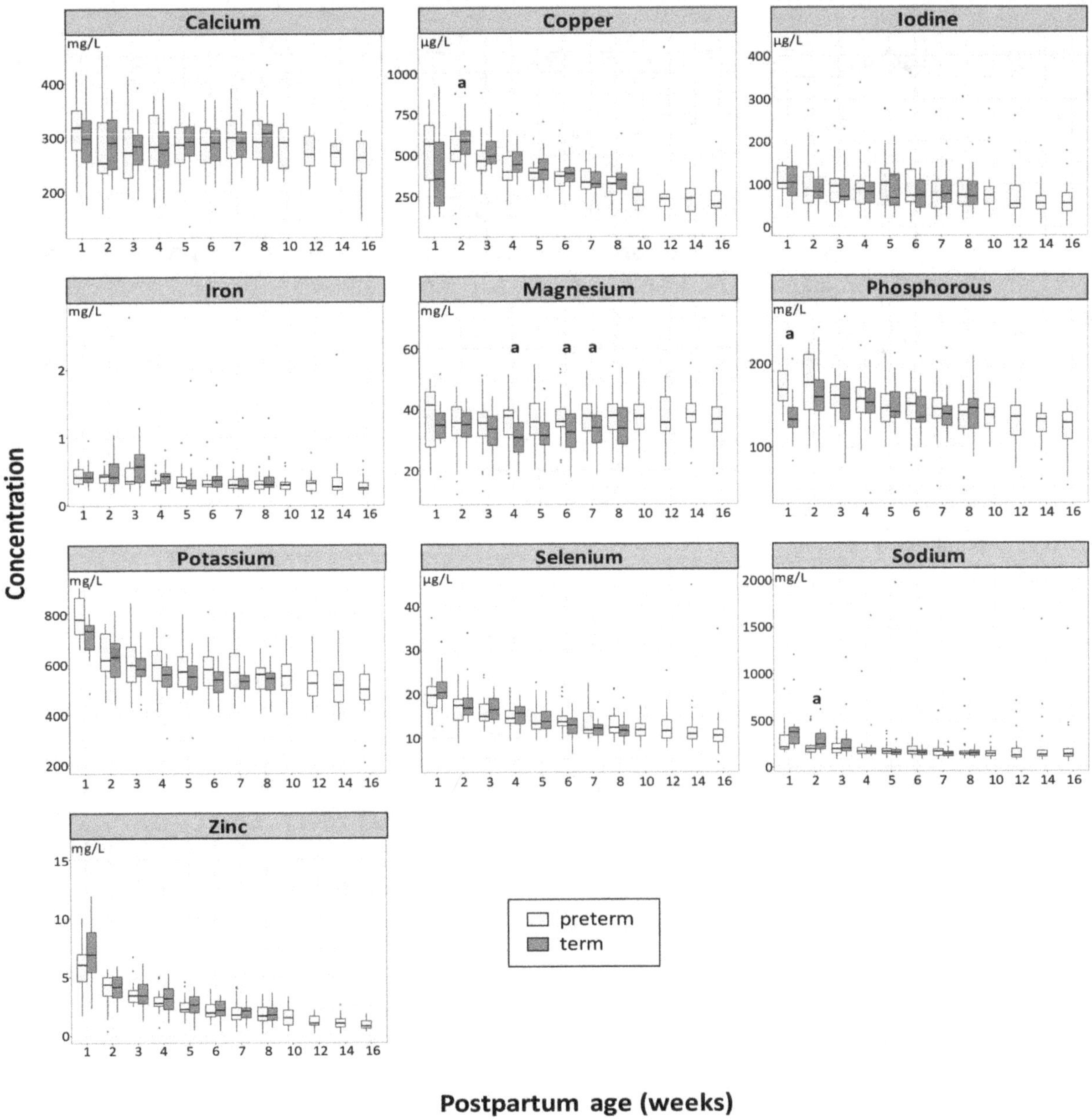

Figure 1. Longitudinal changes of mineral concentration (means) in term (dark grey) and preterm (light grey) human milk (HM) at an equivalent postpartum age. The letter (a) indicates if differences between term and preterm are significant $p < 0.05$. Box plots represent medians with 25th and 75th percentile, min-max range and outliers.

No significant differences were found when comparing mineral concentrations by sex, mode of delivery, or twin/single delivery.

3.3. Longitudinal Changes of Mineral Concentration in Term and Preterm Human Milk at an Equivalent Postmenstrual Age

When the HM from mothers of preterm and full term infants was compared at an equivalent postmenstrual age, the main significant differences were observed for zinc, copper, selenium, and magnesium. As depicted in Figure 2, zinc and copper concentrations in term HM were significantly higher than in preterm HM from week 39 to 48 of postmenstrual age ($p < 0.002$). Similar observations were made for selenium, with significant differences being found at week 39 to 44 ($p < 0.002$). In comparison to term HM, preterm HM contained 53% to 78% (average 62%), 30% to 72% (average 44%), and 11% to 33% (average 24%) less zinc, copper, and selenium, respectively.

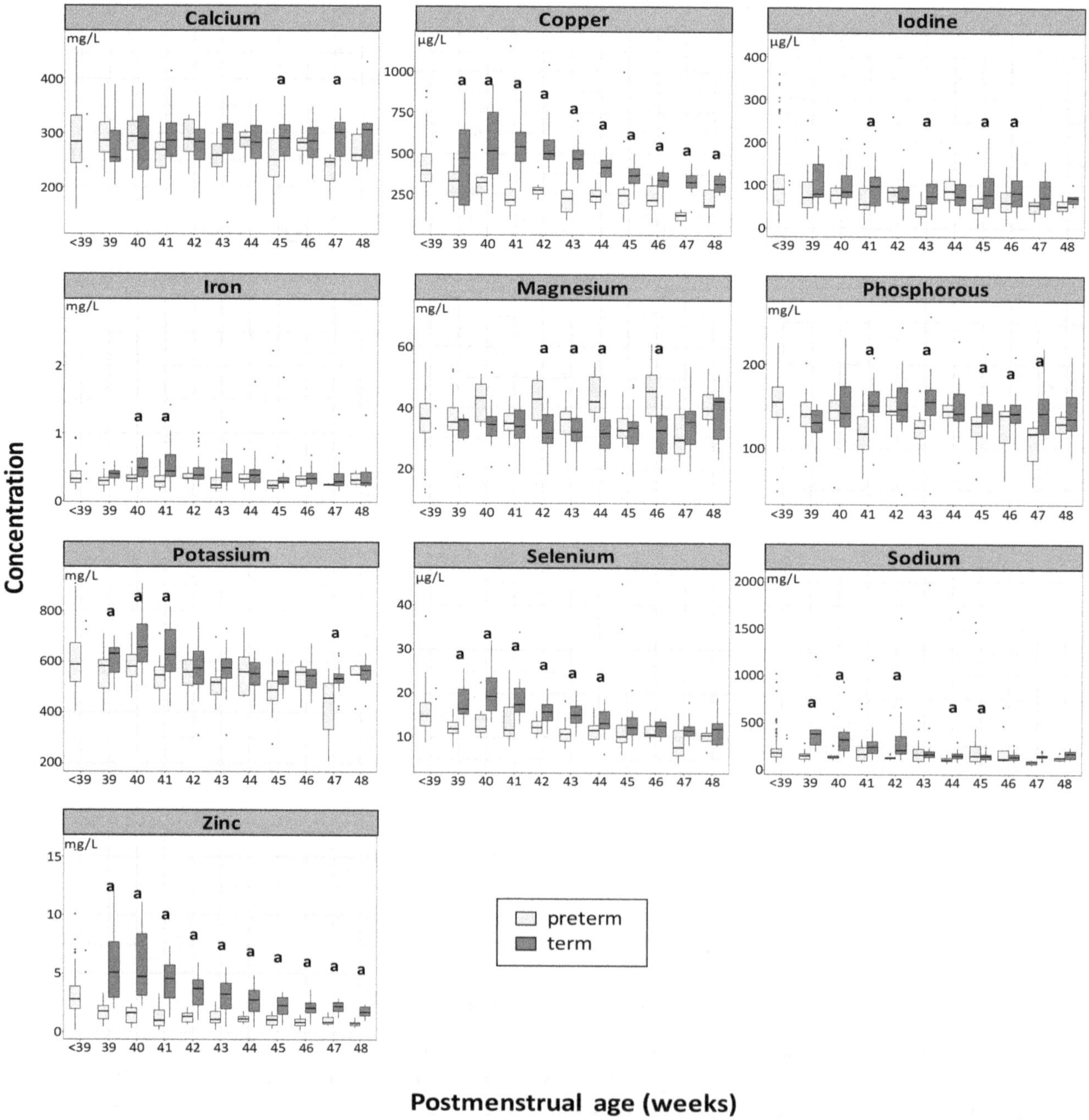

Figure 2. Longitudinal changes of mineral concentration (means) in term (dark grey) and preterm (light grey) human milk (HM) at an equivalent postmenstrual age. The letter (a) indicates if differences between term and preterm are significant $p < 0.05$. Box plots represent medians with 25th and 75th percentile, min-max range and outliers.

Magnesium is the only element for which the concentration in preterm HM was found to be statistically significantly higher than in term HM from weeks 42 to 44 and week 46 ($p < 0.05$). The differences between preterm HM and term HM per postmenstrual age ranged from minus 17% to plus 39% (average + 12%).

Statistically significant differences were also found for sodium, potassium, phosphorus, iron, iodine, and calcium at scattered postmenstrual weeks, with higher values in favor of term HM. The sodium concentration in preterm HM was significantly lower at weeks 39, 40, and 42, and weeks 44 to 45 ($p < 0.01$). The potassium concentration was significantly lower at week 39 to 41 ($p < 0.006$); for phosphorus, at week 41, 43, 45, and 47 ($p < 0.05$); for iodine, at week 41, 43, 45, and 46; for iron, at week 40 and 41 ($p < 0.002$); and for calcium, at week 45 and 47 ($p < 0.05$). The longitudinal concentrations (mean ± SD) of minerals in preterm and term HM per visit at equivalent postmenstrual ages are reported in Supplementary Table S2.

4. Discussion

We have reported a comprehensive longitudinal overview of the content of 10 minerals in 500 HM samples from women delivering before term or at term. The study design enabled the comparison of preterm and term HM mineral contents at the same postpartum weeks (i.e., same lactation stages) and at equivalent postmenstrual weeks (i.e., equivalent infant developmental stages).

4.1. Mineral Concentration and Longitudinal Change in Preterm and Term Human Milk at the Same Postpartum Age

To our knowledge, the results of our study represent the first set of mineral analyses from breast milk in apparently healthy Swiss mothers of preterm and term infants. As illustrated in Table 2, the mean and median concentration determined for each individual element in preterm HM over the period of sample collection was found to be in the range of retrieved published values for HM [17–28]. These ranges can be wide and this variability is mainly due to the stage of lactation and to the intra and intersubject variability, including the circadian rhythm [12,29]. The presented result is in line with previous research performed in HM from a well-nourished population which showed, for several minerals, that their diet, status, or supplementation have a limited or no impact on their milk concentration. That is, for instance, the case for iron, copper, zinc, and magnesium [12], and to some extent, for phosphorus, potassium, and sodium [30–32]. Inversely, the calcium, iodine, and selenium concentration in HM can be impacted by the diet of the mother, and therefore, except for calcium, by the use of dietary supplements [12]. In the present study, the dietary intakes of the mother were not recorded, and no recent survey on either dietary intakes or mineral status in Swiss pregnant or lactating women was retrieved for these three elements. Nevertheless, data on iodine intake in the general Swiss population was classified as sufficient by the Iodine Global Network (http://www.ign.org/scorecard.htm). In our study, this is reflected by an iodine median concentration in milk above the published median value of 62 μg/L [24]. A similar observation is made for calcium, despite the results of a Swiss cross-sectional study showing that in 28% of subjects following an omnivore diet, calcium intake does not reach the corresponding nutritional recommendation [33]. No recent data on the prevalence of intake inadequacy or deficiency was retrieved for selenium, but the rather low levels in milk observed in our study may indicate a need for a higher selenium intake in Swiss lactating women, as underlined in a review published earlier for the Swiss population [34]. This may help to increase the selenium milk content. In any case, even if dietary intakes of the mother do not influence their milk mineral concentration, they should give particular attention to the mineral density of their diet to match their own increased requirements if adaptation of the mechanism of absorption is not enough to avoid putting themselves at risk of mineral deficiencies.

The comparison of concentration at the same postpartum age shows no statistically significant difference between preterm HM and term HM for six minerals, i.e., potassium, zinc, iodine, selenium, iron, and calcium. These data are in agreement with previous published results for potassium [17,18,28,35,36], zinc [22,37,38], iodine [24,39], and selenium [26,40]. Few papers have reported higher levels of iron in preterm HM during the early lactation period [28,41,42], but some others [43,44] and a more recent one [45], failed to observe any differences. In HM, 2% to 9% of iron is linked to lactoferrin [45] and our iron content results correlate with the results of lactoferrin analyzed from the same set of samples [13]. Only minor and scattered differences between preterm HM and term HM have previously been reported for calcium. A recent systematic review and meta-analysis performed with 11 studies showed no differences from day 1 to week 12 postpartum, except at week 7 to 9, where a statistically significant difference of 15% was reported (preterm HM > term HM) [46]. Calcium along with phosphorus are the two main minerals required for the multifaceted mechanisms of bone metabolism [47]. Therefore, the meta-analysis was also performed for phosphorus from eight independent studies, and showed that the phosphorus concentration in preterm HM was not statistically different than in term HM, except between week 3 and 4 and week 5 to 6, with reported differences of 14% and 16%, respectively (preterm HM < term HM) [46]. In our study, a significant difference was only found at week 1 for this mineral in the opposite direction (preterm HM > term HM). We also found a higher concentration in preterm HM than in term HM for magnesium and only at three time points during the transitional phase (i.e., week 1 to 4). These differences were below 20%. In the literature, only one study out of 16 reported a similar difference [21,48]. In addition, we found lower concentrations of copper and sodium in preterm HM than in term HM, but only at postpartum week 2. Like for iron, inconsistent results were retrieved for copper in the literature [23]. Preterm HM copper concentrations were reported to be significantly lower [42,44], higher [41], or no different from the concentrations of term HM [44,49,50]. Except for one study [17], the sodium concentration in preterm HM is consistently reported as higher in preterm HM than in term HM, at the very early stage of lactation [18,51]. Our result goes in an opposite direction, but only at week 2. These discrepancies are most probably due to the difference in the timing of sample collection and comparison that, in most studies, started at day 1 postpartum versus day 7 in the present report. Other analytical reasons may be the differences in the number of samples, the collection method (e.g., foremilk vs. hindmilk as compared to full-breast expression in our study), and the storage procedures [45]. Beside this reading, although it is well-established that the levels of minerals in preterm HM are not sufficient to meet the needs of the preterm infant, it is not unusual to read that when higher concentrations are found in preterm HM than in term HM, it could be due to a physiological adaption to meet the increased requirement of the preterm infants [28,41,42,51]. This explanation goes along with the hypothesis of a reduced blood flow to the mammary gland and thus milk volume, and the immaturity of the gland (i.e., incomplete differentiation of epithelial cells, and the absence of tight junctions between the cells) [52]. However, some authors reported no difference in milk volumes produced by both preterm and term mothers, stressing that understanding of the physiological processes responsible for the micronutrient composition in human milk still requires investigation [17]. Some authors also report that it is likely that these discrepancies are due to differences in hormonal balance and metabolic regulation due to the shorter gestational period [17,53,54].

Overall, in agreement with previous reports, the present results show parallel compositional changes in the mineral content of milk from mothers of preterm and term infants throughout the 8 postpartum weeks of common sample collection. While breastfeeding is the gold standard for term and preterm feeding, for the latter, it is prescribed that human milk should be fortified with nutrients in short supply [7–9]. Despite the punctual differences described above, when comparing the median of values for each individual element to the recommendations by the ESPGHAN [9], it appeared that, except for iodine and potassium, none of the concentrations reached the minimum recommended level [9] (results presented in Supplementary Figure S1). This emphasizes the need for fortifying with only those minerals whose content in HM is lower than the recommended levels, in order to avoid overloads of those minerals that are present in HM at sufficient levels.

4.2. Longitudinal Changes of Mineral Concentration in Term and Preterm Human Milk at an Equivalent Postmenstrual Age

Fortification of human milk is recommended up to preterm infant discharge from the neonatal care unit, to address the mismatch between its content and the nutritional recommendations for optimal growth and development. However, there is a lack of consensus about the need to fortify human milk after discharge (usually occurring at around term corrected age) [10]. Considering that the references for an optimal growth of preterm infants after they reach the term corrected age are calibrated against the standards of infants born at term, we assumed that the preterm infant nutritional requirements during this period would be at least the same as those of their term counterparts. Therefore, the mineral contents of preterm HM were compared to those of term HM at the same postmenstrual ages (i.e., from postmenstrual weeks 39 to 48). This comparison showed highly significant differences for zinc, copper, and selenium, with a lower concentration in preterm HM than in term HM. Zinc and copper contribute to many cellular and molecular processes and therefore are essential for growth, the immune response, and cognitive function [4]. The serum zinc concentration in term and preterm infants is reported to be high at birth and then to progressively decrease, which was correlated with normal growth [55]. Selenium is an important factor for optimal function of the antioxidant systems and its serum concentration has been showed to increase in healthy term breastfed infants after birth [56]. Therefore, the observed differences of concentrations of these three trace elements in preterm HM and term HM at the same postmenstrual age may be physiologically relevant and require further investigation.

4.3. Strengths and Limitations of the Study

This study has some limitations. First, the samples were collected at only one time of the day. As the fluctuation of mineral concentration in milk has been previously observed over the day [29], one may argue that the data are not representative of the whole day concentration. Nevertheless, the sampling time was standardized and it allowed us to perform a comparison of the HM of the two infant populations at a postpartum and postmenstrual age. Finally, the number of subjects was limited in both groups, reducing the power of the study and limiting the number of association analyses.

5. Conclusions

This study represents the first set of simultaneous analyses of ten minerals in human term and preterm milk comprehensively covering the period of 2 months postpartum. It confirms previous observations of concentrations and temporal changes, as well as the global similarity in the composition of term and preterm milk when compared at the same lactation stage. Interestingly, zinc, copper, and selenium contents were found to be consistently lower in preterm milk than in term milk when compared at an equivalent infant developmental stage. The relevance of the observed differences to the health, growth, and development of preterm infants, as well as the impact on fortification practices, remain to be further investigated.

Supplementary Materials:
Table S1: Concentration of human milk minerals and trace elements in term or preterm milk at different weeks postpartum; Table S2: Concentration of human milk minerals and trace elements in term or preterm milk at equivalent postmenstrual ages; Figure S1: Longitudinal changes of mineral concentration (means) in term (dark grey) and preterm (light grey) human milk (HM) at an equivalent postmenstrual age, with dotted lines representing the range of recommended intakes (converted in mg/L, using measured energy density of preterm HM), as provided by ESPGHAN [3].

Author Contributions: Conceptualization: C.L.G.-R., M.A., L.B., J.-F.T., and C.J.F.F.; investigation: L.B., J.-F.T., and C.J.F.F.; analysis: ICP-MS: P.K., M.V., S.D., D.A., M.N., and J.R.P.; statistics: C.A.D.C.; results interpretation: M.S., C.L.G.R., M.A., and V.B.; writing—original draft: M.S. and M.A.; writing—review and editing: M.S., C.A.D.C., M.A., C.L.G.-R., S.D.; L.B., J.-F.T., S.K.T., and C.J.F.F.; visualization: C.A.D.C. and M.A.; supervision: C.L.G.-R., M.A., and C.J.F.F.; project administration: M.A.; funding acquisition: C.L.G.-R. and M.A.

Acknowledgments: Sincere thanks to all mothers who enthusiastically participated in this study; to Nassima Grari, the study lactation nurse who admirably cared about all mothers during the full study duration; and to Céline Romagny and Emilie Darcillon, who managed the organizational and operational part of the clinical study and the data management.

References

1. March of Dimes; PMNCH; Save the Children; WHO. *Born Too Soon: The Global Action Report on Preterm Birth*; World Health Organization: Geneva, Switzerland, 2012.
2. Finch, C.W. Review of trace mineral requirements for preterm infants: What are the current recommendations for clinical practice? *Nutr. Clin. Pract.* **2015**, *30*, 44–58. [CrossRef] [PubMed]
3. Aggett, P.J.; Agostoni, C.; Axelsson, I.; De Curtis, M.; Goulet, O.; Hernell, O.; Koletzko, B.; Lafeber, H.N.; Michaelsen, K.F.; Puntis, J.W.; et al. Feeding preterm infants after hospital discharge: A commentary by the espghan committee on nutrition. *J. Pediatr. Gastroenterol. Nutr.* **2006**, *42*, 596–603. [CrossRef] [PubMed]
4. Ramel, S.E.; Georgieff, M.K. Preterm nutrition and the brain. *World Rev. Nutr. Diet.* **2014**, *110*, 190–200. [PubMed]
5. Mimouni, F.B.; Mandel, D.; Lubetzky, R.; Senterre, T. Calcium, phosphorus, magnesium and vitamin d requirements of the preterm infant. *World Rev. Nutr. Diet.* **2014**, *110*, 140–151. [PubMed]
6. Fusch, C.; Jochum, F. Water, sodium, potassium and chloride. *World Rev. Nutr. Diet.* **2014**, *110*, 99–120. [PubMed]
7. Patel, P.; Bhatia, J. Human milk: The prefered firts food for premature infants. *J. Hum. Nutr. Food Sci.* **2016**, *4*.
8. Tudehope, D.I. Human milk and the nutritional needs of preterm infants. *J. Pediatr.* **2013**, *162*, S17–S25. [CrossRef]
9. Agostoni, C.; Buonocore, G.; Carnielli, V.P.; De Curtis, M.; Darmaun, D.; Decsi, T.; Domellof, M.; Embleton, N.D.; Fusch, C.; Genzel-Boroviczeny, O.; et al. Enteral nutrient supply for preterm infants: Commentary from the european society of paediatric gastroenterology, hepatology and nutrition committee on nutrition. *J. Pediatr. Gastroenterol. Nutr.* **2010**, *50*, 85–91. [CrossRef]
10. Arslanoglu, S.; Boquien, C.Y.; King, C.; Lamireau, D.; Tonetto, P.; Barnett, D.; Bertino, E.; Gaya, A.; Gebauer, C.; Grovslien, A.; et al. Fortification of human milk for preterm infants: Update and recommendations of the european milk bank association (emba) working group on human milk fortification. *Front. Pediatr.* **2019**, *7*, 76. [CrossRef]
11. van de Lagemaat, M.; Rotteveel, J.; van Weissenbruch, M.M.; Lafeber, H.N. Increased gain in bone mineral content of preterm infants fed an isocaloric, protein-, and mineral-enriched postdischarge formula. *Eur. J. Nutr.* **2013**, *52*, 1781–1785. [CrossRef]
12. Dror, D.K.; Allen, L.H. Overview of nutrients in human milk. *Adv. Nutr.* **2018**, *9*, 278S–294S. [CrossRef] [PubMed]
13. Garcia-Rodenas, C.L.; De Castro, C.A.; Jenni, R.; Thakkar, S.K.; Beauport, L.; Tolsa, J.F.; Fischer-Fumeaux, C.J.; Affolter, M. Temporal changes of major protein concentrations in preterm and term human milk. A prospective cohort study. *Clin. Nutr.* **2018**. [CrossRef] [PubMed]
14. Fischer Fumeaux, C.J.; Garcia-Rodenas, C.L.; De Castro, C.A.; Courtet-Compondu, M.C.; Thakkar, S.K.; Beauport, L.; Tolsa, J.F.; Affolter, M. Longitudinal analysis of macronutrient composition in preterm and term human milk: A prospective cohort study. *Nutrients* **2019**, *11*, 1525. [CrossRef] [PubMed]
15. Thakkar, S.K.; De Castro, C.A.; Beauport, L.; Tolsa, J.F.; Fischer Fumeaux, C.J.; Affolter, M.; Giuffrida, F. Temporal progression of fatty acids in preterm and term human milk of mothers from switzerland. *Nutrients* **2019**, *11*, 112. [CrossRef] [PubMed]
16. Austin, S.; De Castro, C.A.; Sprenger, N.; Binia, A.; Affolter, M.; Garcia-Rodenas, C.L.; Beauport, L. Human milk oligosaccharides in the milk of mothers delivering term versus preterm infants. *Nutrients* **2019**, *11*, 1282. [CrossRef] [PubMed]
17. Bauer, J.; Gerss, J. Longitudinal analysis of macronutrients and minerals in human milk produced by mothers of preterm infants. *Clin. Nutr.* **2011**, *30*, 215–220. [CrossRef] [PubMed]
18. Gross, S.J.; David, R.J.; Bauman, L.; Tomarelli, R.M. Nutritional composition of milk produced by mothers delivering preterm. *J. Pediatr.* **1980**, *96*, 641–644. [CrossRef]

19. Dorea, J.G. Breast milk calcium and phosphorus concentrations. *Nutrition* **2000**, *16*, 146–147. [CrossRef]
20. Salamon, S.; Csapó, J. Composition of mother's milk iii. Macroand microelements contents. A review. *Acta Univ. Sapiente. Alimentaria* **2009**, *2*, 235–275.
21. Dorea, J.G. Magnesium in human milk. *J. Am. Coll. Nutr.* **2000**, *19*, 210–219. [CrossRef]
22. Dorea, J.G. Zinc and copper concentrations in breastmilk. *Indian Pediatr.* **2012**, *49*, 592. [CrossRef] [PubMed]
23. Dorea, J.G. Iron and copper in human milk. *Nutrition* **2000**, *16*, 209–220. [CrossRef]
24. Dorea, J.G. Iodine nutrition and breast feeding. *J. Trace Elem. Med. Biol.* **2002**, *16*, 207–220. [CrossRef]
25. Kim, S.Y.; Park, J.H.; Kim, E.A.; Lee-Kim, Y.C. Longitudinal study on trace mineral compositions (selenium, zinc, copper, manganese) in korean human preterm milk. *J. Korean Med. Sci.* **2012**, *27*, 532–536. [CrossRef] [PubMed]
26. Ellis, L.; Picciano, M.F.; Smith, A.M.; Hamosh, M.; Mehta, N.R. The impact of gestational length on human milk selenium concentration and glutathione peroxidase activity. *Pediatr. Res.* **1990**, *27*, 32–35. [CrossRef] [PubMed]
27. Dutta, S.; Saini, S.; Prasad, R. Changes in preterm human milk composition with particular reference to introduction of mixed feeding. *Indian Pediatr.* **2014**, *51*, 997–999. [CrossRef]
28. Lemons, J.A.; Moye, L.; Hall, D.; Simmons, M. Differences in the composition of preterm and term human milk during early lactation. *Pediatr. Res.* **1982**, *16*, 113–117. [CrossRef]
29. Picciano, M.F.; Guthrie, H.A. Copper, iron, and zinc contents of mature human milk. *Am. J. Clin. Nutr.* **1976**, *29*, 242–254. [CrossRef]
30. Zhao, A.; Ning, Y.; Zhang, Y.; Yang, X.; Wang, J.; Li, W.; Wang, P. Mineral compositions in breast milk of healthy chinese lactating women in urban areas and its associated factors. *Chin. Med. J. (Engl.)* **2014**, *127*, 2643–2648.
31. Ereman, R.R.; Lonnerdal, B.; Dewey, K.G. Maternal sodium intake does not affect postprandial sodium concentrations in human milk. *J. Nutr.* **1987**, *117*, 1154–1157. [CrossRef]
32. Finley, D.A.; Lonnerdal, B.; Dewey, K.G.; Grivetti, L.E. Inorganic constituents of breast milk from vegetarian and nonvegetarian women: Relationships with each other and with organic constituents. *J. Nutr.* **1985**, *115*, 772–781. [CrossRef] [PubMed]
33. Schupbach, R.; Wegmuller, R.; Berguerand, C.; Bui, M.; Herter-Aeberli, I. Micronutrient status and intake in omnivores, vegetarians and vegans in switzerland. *Eur. J. Nutr.* **2017**, *56*, 283–293. [CrossRef] [PubMed]
34. Berger, M.M. Oligoéléments en suisse et en europe. *Rev. Med. Suisse* **2012**, *8*, 2078–2084. [PubMed]
35. Atkinson, S.A.; Radde, I.C.; Chance, G.W.; Bryan, M.H.; Anderson, G.H. Macro-mineral content of milk obtained during early lactation from mothers of premature infants. *Early Hum. Dev.* **1980**, *4*, 5–14. [CrossRef]
36. Grumach, A.S.; Jeronimo, S.E.; Hage, M.; Carneiro-Sampaio, M.M. Nutritional factors in milk from brazilian mothers delivering small for gestational age neonates. *Rev. Saude Publica* **1993**, *27*, 455–462. [CrossRef] [PubMed]
37. De Figueiredo, C.S.; Palhares, D.B.; Melnikov, P.; Moura, A.J.; dos Santos, S.C. Zinc and copper concentrations in human preterm milk. *Biol. Trace Elem. Res.* **2010**, *136*, 1–7. [CrossRef]
38. Fernandez-Menendez, S.; Fernandez-Sanchez, M.L.; Fernandez-Colomer, B.; de la Flor St Remy, R.R.; Cotallo, G.D.; Freire, A.S.; Braz, B.F.; Santelli, R.E.; Sanz-Medel, A. Total zinc quantification by inductively coupled plasma-mass spectrometry and its speciation by size exclusion chromatography-inductively coupled plasma-mass spectrometry in human milk and commercial formulas: Importance in infant nutrition. *J. Chromatogr. A.* **2016**, *1428*, 246–254. [CrossRef] [PubMed]
39. Ares, S.; Quero, J.; Duran, S.; Presas, M.J.; Herruzo, R.; Morreale de Escobar, G. Iodine content of infant formulas and iodine intake of premature babies: High risk of iodine deficiency. *Arch Dis. Child. Fetal Neonatal Ed.* **1994**, *71*, F184–F191. [CrossRef]
40. Hunt, C.D.; Friel, J.K.; Johnson, L.K. Boron concentrations in milk from mothers of full-term and premature infants. *Am. J. Clin. Nutr.* **2004**, *80*, 1327–1333. [CrossRef]
41. Atinmo, T.; Omololu, A. Trace element content of breastmilk from mothers of preterm infants in nigeria. *Early Hum. Dev.* **1982**, *6*, 309–313. [CrossRef]
42. Perrone, L.; Di Palma, L.; Di Toro, R.; Gialanella, G.; Moro, R. Interaction of trace elements in a longitudinal study of human milk from full-term and preterm mothers. *Biol. Trace Elem. Res.* **1994**, *41*, 321–330. [CrossRef]

43. Trugo, N.M.; Donangelo, C.M.; Koury, J.C.; Silva, M.I.; Freitas, L.A. Concentration and distribution pattern of selected micronutrients in preterm and term milk from urban brazilian mothers during early lactation. *Eur. J. Clin. Nutr.* **1988**, *42*, 497–507.
44. Mendelson, R.A.; Anderson, G.H.; Bryan, M.H. Zinc, copper and iron content of milk from mothers of preterm and full-term infants. *Early Hum. Dev.* **1982**, *6*, 145–151. [CrossRef]
45. Fernández-Sánchez, M.L.; De la Flor St. Remy, R.; González Iglesias, H.; López-Sastre, J.B.; Fernández-Colomer, B.; Pérez-Solís, D.; Sanz-Medel, A. Iron content and its speciation in human milk from mothers of preterm and full-term infants at early stages of lactation: A comparison with commercial infant milk formulas. *Microchem. J.* **2012**, *105*, 108–114.
46. Gidrewicz, D.A.; Fenton, T.R. A systematic review and meta-analysis of the nutrient content of preterm and term breast milk. *BMC Pediatr.* **2014**, *14*, 216. [CrossRef]
47. Rigo, J.; Pieltain, C.; Salle, B.; Senterre, J. Enteral calcium, phosphate and vitamin d requirements and bone mineralization in preterm infants. *Acta Paediatr.* **2007**, *96*, 969–974. [CrossRef]
48. Butte, N.F.; Garza, C.; Johnson, C.A.; Smith, E.O.; Nichols, B.L. Longitudinal changes in milk composition of mothers delivering preterm and term infants. *Early Hum. Dev.* **1984**, *9*, 153–162. [CrossRef]
49. Aquilio, E.; Spagnoli, R.; Seri, S.; Bottone, G.; Spennati, G. Trace element content in human milk during lactation of preterm newborns. *Biol. Trace Elem. Res.* **1996**, *51*, 63–70. [CrossRef]
50. Sann, L.; Bienvenu, F.; Lahet, C.; Bienvenu, J.; Bethenod, M. Comparison of the composition of breast milk from mothers of term and preterm infants. *Acta Paediatr. Scand.* **1981**, *70*, 115–116. [CrossRef]
51. Koo, W.W.; Gupta, J.M. Breast milk sodium. *Arch Dis. Child.* **1982**, *57*, 500–502. [CrossRef]
52. Anderson, G.H. The effect of prematurity on milk composition and its physiological basis. *Fed. Proc.* **1984**, *43*, 2438–2442.
53. Chatterton, R.T., Jr.; Hill, P.D.; Aldag, J.C.; Hodges, K.R.; Belknap, S.M.; Zinaman, M.J. Relation of plasma oxytocin and prolactin concentrations to milk production in mothers of preterm infants: Influence of stress. *J. Clin. Endocrinol. Metab.* **2000**, *85*, 3661–3668. [CrossRef] [PubMed]
54. Hill, P.D.; Aldag, J.C.; Demirtas, H.; Naeem, V.; Parker, N.P.; Zinaman, M.J.; Chatterton, R.T., Jr. Association of serum prolactin and oxytocin with milk production in mothers of preterm and term infants. *Biol. Res. Nurs.* **2009**, *10*, 340–349. [CrossRef] [PubMed]
55. Ackland, M.L.; Michalczyk, A.A. Zinc and infant nutrition. *Arch Biochem. Biophys.* **2016**, *611*, 51–57. [CrossRef] [PubMed]
56. Tindell, R.; Tipple, T. Selenium: Implications for outcomes in extremely preterm infants. *J. Perinatol.* **2018**, *38*, 197–202. [CrossRef] [PubMed]

13

Comparison of Inductively Coupled Plasma Optical Emission Spectrometry with an Ion Selective Electrode to Determine Sodium and Potassium Levels in Human Milk

Ching Tat Lai *, Hazel Gardner and Donna Geddes

School of Molecular Sciences, University of Western Australia, 35 Stirling Highway, Crawley, 6009 WA, Australia; hazel.gardner@uwa.edu.au (H.G.); donna.geddes@uwa.edu.au (D.G.)

* Correspondence: ching-tat.lai@uwa.edu.au

Abstract: Sodium (Na), potassium (K), and the ratio Na:K in human milk (HM) may be useful biomarkers to indicate secretory activation or inflammation in the breast. Previously, these elements have been measured in a laboratory setting requiring expensive equipment and relatively large amounts of HM. The aim of this study was to compare measurements of Na and K in HM using inductively coupled plasma optical emission spectrometry (ICP-OES) with small portable ion selective electrode probes for Na and K. Sixty-five lactating women donated 5 mL samples of HM. Samples were analyzed with two ion selective probes (Na and K) and also ICP-OES. The data were analyzed using paired *t*-test and Bland–Altman plots. Na concentrations were not significantly different when measured with ion selective electrode (6.18 ± 2.47mM; range: 3.59–19.8) and ICP-OES (5.91 ± 3.37 mM; range: 2.59–21.5) ($p = 0.20$). K concentrations measured using the ion selective electrode (11.7 ± 2.21 mM: range: 7.69–18.1) and ICP-OES (11.1 ± 1.55 mM: range: 7.91–15.2) were significantly different ($p = 0.01$). However, the mean differences of 0.65 mM would not be clinically relevant when testing at point of care. Compared to ICP-OES, ion selective electrode is sufficiently accurate to detect changes in concentrations of Na and K in HM associated with secretory activation and inflammation in the mammary gland.

Keywords: human milk; potassium; sodium; ICP-OES; ion selective electrode

1. Introduction

Human milk (HM) sodium (Na) and potassium (K) concentrations change dramatically during the first week postpartum at the onset of secretory activation. Sodium, in particular, follows a rapid downward trajectory after birth as a result of tight junction closure, which is essential for secretory activation of the onset of copious milk production [1]. It has been reported that human milk sodium drops from 60 mM to 10 mM between days 1 and 5 postpartum, this precipitous drop reflects tight junction closure [2]. Delayed onset of secretory activation is established as a risk factor for poor lactation outcomes [3] with high sodium concentrations at day 7 considered a risk factor for the cessation of breastfeeding [4].

The Na:K ratio is another marker that has been historically used to define secretory activation. The Na:K ratio is greater than 2.0 after birth and then declines as sodium concentrations decline with closure of the tight junctions. The Na:K ratio has been used to biochemically define lactation stages as follows: $\geq$2 colostral milk, <2 transitional milk, and <0.6 mature milk [1,5]. This is mirrored by changes in the human milk transcriptome during this period and is therefore considered more accurate than using time postpartum to define lactation stage [5]. Changes in the Na:K ratio form a continuum over the first week postpartum, with a high Na:K ratio on day 7 (>0.8) [4] indicative of suboptimal milk supply or feeding problems and consequently a higher risk of breastfeeding cessation. An elevated ratio on day 7 is associated with 3.3 times greater odds of stopping breastfeeding in mothers reporting concerns about milk supply [4].

A high Na:K ratio is also indicative of the increased mammary epithelial permeability associated with breast inflammation, breast engorgement or mastitis [4,6–8]. The Na:K ratio is viewed as superior to sodium alone as it negates the variation found in proportions of aqueous and fat layers of the milk which occur when different sampling methods are used. Interestingly, the Na:K ratio has been found to be positively associated with the inflammatory chemokine interleukin-8 concentrations suggesting that this ratio is also a marker for inflammation of the mammary epithelium [7].

Immediate measurement of HM sodium and potassium concentrations would be advantageous in situations of suspected delayed secretory activation and mammary infection allowing rapid intervention. Currently these components are measured with instruments such as flame photometry [4], atomic absorption spectroscopy [7], ion chromatography, inductively coupled plasma optical emission spectroscopy (ICP-OES), and inductively coupled plasma mass spectroscopy (ICP-MS). All of these techniques, which require hazardous chemicals, laboratory facilities, and highly skilled operators, are not immediate and are also costly. Alternatively, the ion selective electrode (ISE) is easy to use, portable, and provides immediate results and therefore has potential as a point of care device for screening of high-risk lactating women. Ion specific electrodes have been used previously, but have not been compared directly to other methods to determine their accuracy [9].

The objective of this study was to compare the accuracy of the sodium and potassium ion selective electrodes against inductively coupled plasma optical emission spectrometry (ICP-OES).

2. Materials and Methods

2.1. Biochemical Analysis

Sixty-five preterm/term mothers provided written informed consent to participate in the study, which was approved by the Human Ethics Committee at the University of Western Australia (RA/4/1/2369). Five mothers who participated in this study had a premature delivery (<37 weeks gestation). Each participant completed a 24 h milk profile using the test weighing method [10]. Mothers were issued with a set of baby weigh scales (Medela AG, Baar, Switzerland). Samples were collected in 5 mL polypropylene tubes (P5016SL, Techno Plas Pty Ltd, St Marys, SA, Australia) before and after each feed or breast expression. Milk samples collected from the 24 h milk production were then pooled and approximately 5 mL of the pooled samples were used in this study.

2.1.1. Ion Selective Electrode Measurement of HM Na and K

Concentrations of sodium and potassium in the milk samples were determined by ion selective electrodes (Sodium: B-722; potassium: B-731; Horiba, Japan). Calibration of the electrodes was conducted according to the manufacturer's recommendations. The calibration range for both Na and K electrodes were set between 150 to 2000 ppm according to the manufacturer's instructions. For each assay, the whole milk samples were thawed at 37 °C for 1 h. Prior to the measurement, the milk samples were shaken with an Intelli-mixer (RM-2, ELMI Ltd, Riga, Latvia) using tube stand mode for 15 s at 50 rpm followed by 3 inversions. Three hundred microliters of the mixed milk was pipetted onto the electrode sensor. The sample was allowed to stabilize for 15 s before the reading was taken. After each measurement, the milk sample was removed from the sensor and returned to the storage tube. The sensor was then rinsed with double deionized water and wiped with KimWipes (Kimberly-Clark Worldwide, Irving, TX, USA) prior to the next measurement. All samples were analyzed together, in duplicate. The same procedures were applied to both electrodes. The results of Na and K obtained from the electrodes were averaged and were converted from ppm to mM using the molecular weight of Na and K (23 and 39 g/mol, respectively).

2.1.2. Inductively Coupled Plasma Optical Emission Spectrometry (ICP-OES) Measurement of HM Na and K Reagents

Standard solutions of Na and K (High Purity Standard, USA, 1000 μg/mL) were in the range of 50–500 μg/mL. Yittrium and scandium were used as internal standards (1000 μg/mL) from Sigma Aldrich (Castle Hill, NSW, Australia). All standards were diluted with 18.2 MΩ water.

Sample Preparation and Measurement

Whole milk or standard solution (200 μL) was mixed with 300 μL of nitric acid (65%, Suprapur®, Merck, Kenilworth, NJ, USA) into disposable borosilicate glass tubes (10 × 75 mM, Kimble Chase, Rockwood, TN, USA). The tubes were placed into a dry heating block (DBH40D, Ratek, Boronia, Victoria, Australia) and a dry acid washed marble was placed on top of the tube. The tubes were incubated at 110 °C for 1 h to allow for the completion of acid digestion. The hot tubes were allowed to cool down in an ice bath before adding the internal standard (2.1 μg/mL) and topped up to 2 mL with 18.2 MΩ water. The concentrations of Na and K in the digested milk samples were determined in triplicate by ICP-OES (5100, Agilent technologies, Santa Clara, CA, USA). Na and K were detected and measured at 568.263 nm and 568.821 nm for Na; and 766.491 mM and 769.897 mM for K. The results of Na and K obtained from those specific wavelengths were averaged and were converted from μg/mL to mM using the molecular weight of Na and K (23 and 39 g/mol, respectively).

2.1.3. Validation of Analytical Methods

Both methods were validated using a spike/recovery assay. In each set of recovery assay, there was 3 tubes: (a) known standard solution + milk; (b) water + milk; (c) known standard solution + water. The mixture in each tube was 1:1 (v:v). The concentrations of Na or K in the tubes were measured and the following formula was applied: ((a)−(b))/(c) × 100% to obtain the recovery (%) for the set. Five sets were measured for each method to ensure the recovery was between 95–105% with a coefficient of variation (CV) <10%. The recovery (%) for the electrode method was 95 ± 4.1 for Na and 99 ± 3.9% for K with a CV of 4.1% and 3.9%, respectively (n = 5), and for ICP-OES was 99.0 ± 9.9 for Na and 99 ± 9.3% for K with a CV of 9.9% and 9.4%, respectively (n = 5).

2.2. Statistical Analysis

Statistical analyses were carried out using R 3.4.4 [11] and R Studio 1.1.419 [12] with package Lattice [13] for Bland–Altman plots. A paired sample t-test was used the compare the Na or K concentrations between the two methods. The limits of agreement and the precision of the estimated limits of agreement between the two measuring methods were calculated [14]. Bland–Altman plots were created to illustrate the limits of agreement. Pearson correlation was used to determine the correlation between concentrations of Na or K measured by the two methods. Boxplots were used to illustrate the medians, quartiles, and the 5th and 95th percentiles. The results were expressed as mean ± standard deviation (SD) unless stated otherwise. Differences were considered significant if $p < 0.05$.

3. Results

Sixty-five participants were recruited to include a range of lactation stages and milk productions as shown in Table 1.

The correlation coefficient (r^2) of the Na measurement between the ISE and ICP-OES was 0.76, $p < 0.001$ (Figure 1A). The mean difference in the Na measurement between ISE and ICP-OES was within ±2 standard derivations (SD) (Figure 1B). There was no significant difference between the measurement of Na between the ISE and ICP-OES (p = 0.20, Figure 1C).

Table 1. Participant Characteristics.

$n = 65$	Mean	Standard Deviation	Range
Maternal age (years)	34	4	24–43
Length of gestation (weeks)	39	2	30–41
Stage of lactation (weeks)	10	5	0.5–27
24 h milk production (millilitres)	780	318	36–1932

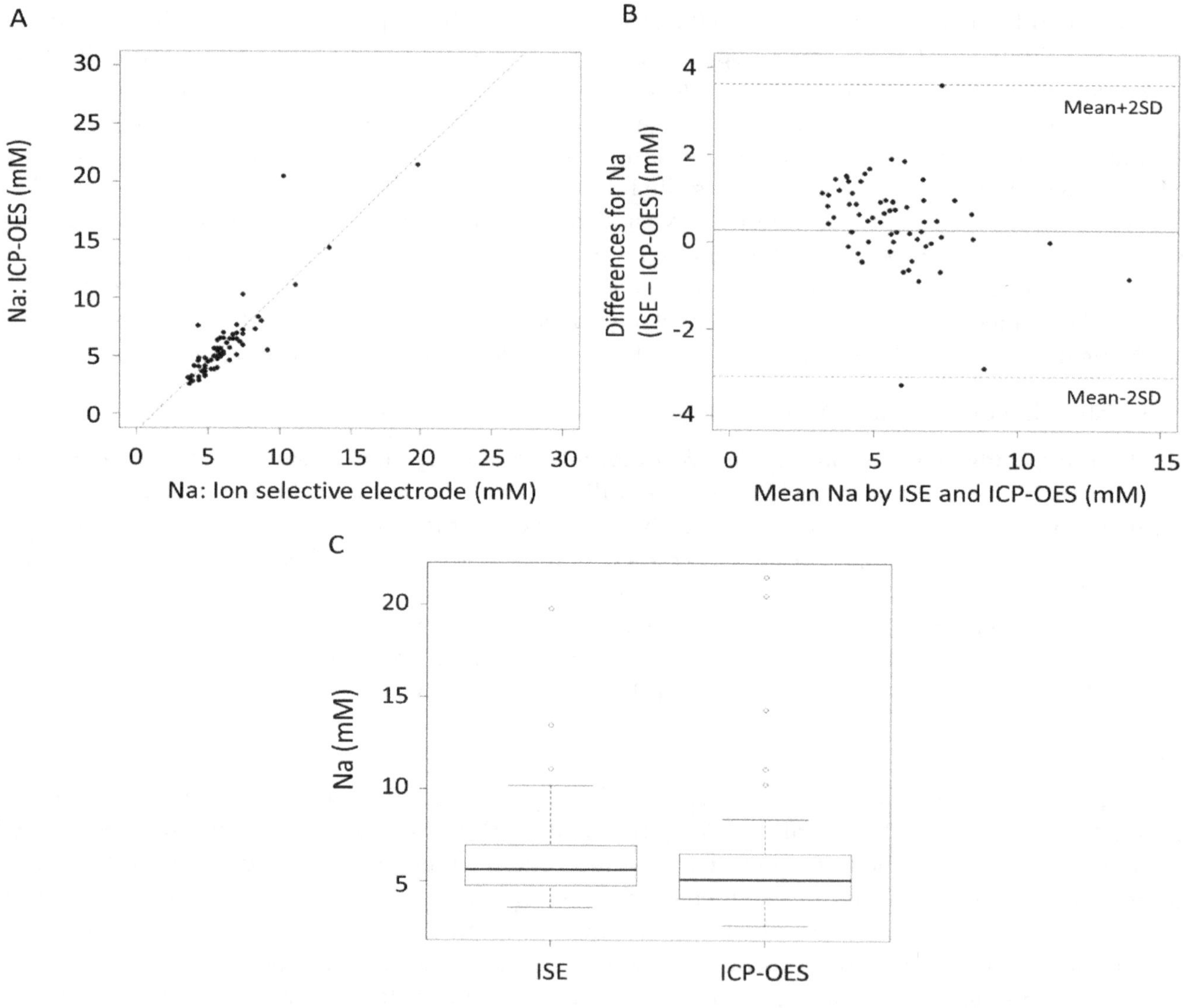

Figure 1. (**A**) Correlation of Na concentrations as measured by the ion selective electrode and inductively coupled plasma optical emission spectrometry (ICP-OES), $r^2 = 0.76$, $p < 0.001$. (**B**) Bland–Altman plot showing the mean differences and limits of agreement. (**C**) Boxplot of Na concentrations, ion selective electrode (ISE).

The correlation coefficient (r^2) of the K measurement between ISE and ICP-OES was 0.26, $p < 0.001$ (Figure 2A). The mean difference in the K measurement between ISE and ICP-OES was within ± 2 standard deviations (SD) (Figure 2B). Measurement of K by the K ISE was significantly higher than ICP-OES ($p = 0.01$, Figure 2C).

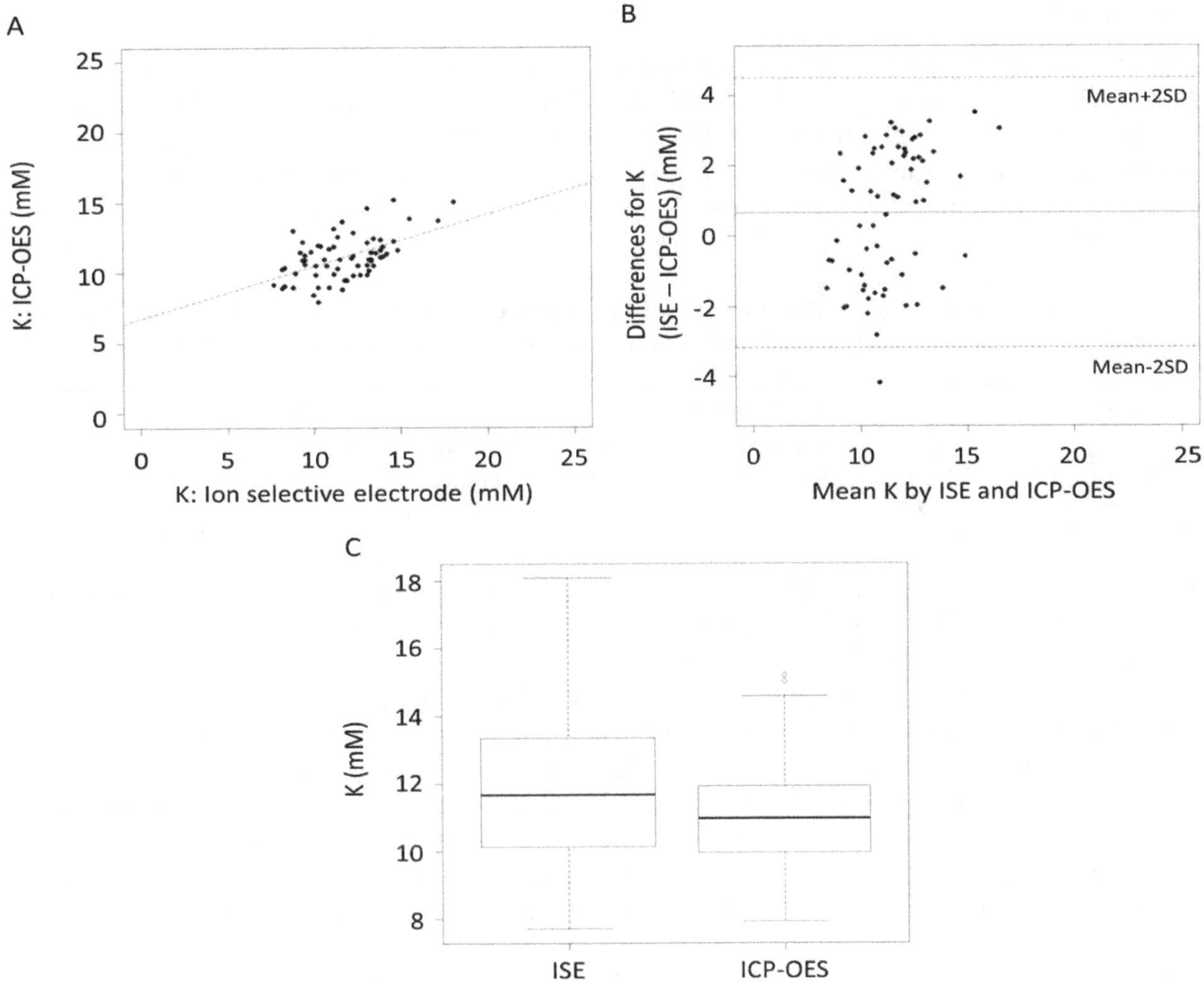

Figure 2. (**A**) Correlation of K concentrations as measured by the ion selective electrode and ICP-OES, $r^2 = 0.26$, $p < 0.001$. (**B**) Bland-Altman plot showing the mean differences and limits of agreement. (**C**) Boxplot of K concentrations.

Twelve scenarios were considered (high to low measures for both Na and K) to evaluate the impact of the change in the measurement of K on the Na:K ratio as shown in Table 2. In all 12 scenarios a movement equivalent to the mean difference in K is not enough to move the Na:K ratio over either the 0.8 or 2 thresholds.

Table 2. Calculated Na:K ratio with or without the mean difference of K measurement between ISE and ICP-OES.

	Na (mM)	K (mM)	K + 0.65 mM	Na:K Ratio	Na:K + 0.65 mM Ratio
Low K	60	4	4.65	15.00	12.90
	40	4	4.65	10.00	8.60
	20	4	4.65	5.00	4.30
	12	4	4.65	3.00	2.58
Medium K	60	12	12.65	5.00	4.74
	40	12	12.65	3.33	3.16
	20	12	12.65	1.67	1.58
	12	12	12.65	1.00	0.95
High K	60	18	18.65	3.33	3.22
	40	18	18.65	2.22	2.14
	20	18	18.65	1.11	1.07
	12	18	18.65	0.67	0.64

4. Discussion

Inductively coupled plasma optical emission spectrometry is regarded as one of the "gold standard" techniques for trace element analysis. It utilizes specific wavelengths to detect and measure Na (568.263 nm and 568.821 nm) and K (766.491 nm and 769.897 nm) in the acid digested fluid, in this case HM, during the process. We found no statistically significant differences between Na concentrations as measured by the Na specific electrode and the ICP-OES in 65 whole HM samples (Figure 1C, Table 3).

Table 3. Human milk (HM) sodium and potassium concentrations measured using ion selective electrode (ISE) and inductively coupled plasma optical emission spectrometry (ICP-OES).

n = 65	Sodium (mM)			Potassium (mM)		
	ISE	ICP-OES	p value	ISE	ICP-OES	p value
Mean SD	6.18 2.47	5.91 3.37	0.20	11.70 2.21	11.10 1.55	0.01
Range	3.59–19.80	2.59–21.50		7.69–18.10	7.91–15.20	

For K, measurements were significantly higher on average with the ion specific electrode (ISE) compared to the ICP-OES measurements (Figure 2C, Table 3). Whilst the ISE and ICP-OES were significantly correlated (Figure 2A) and the values fell within 2 SD of the mean (Figure 2B) the confidence intervals of the mean difference also suggest a significant difference between the two methods. The design of the ISE for Na and K is based on a polymeric membrane such that the size of the molecular cavity on the membrane matches the size of the targeted ion for the measurement [15]. The only difference between Na and K ion selective electrodes is the type of polymeric membrane used. The Na ion selective electrode membrane is sodium ionophore II, while valinomycin is the polymeric membrane for the K ion selective electrode. The mean difference of 0.65 mM in the measurement of K between the two methods may be related the effect of the milk matrix [16,17]. Components in milk, such as proteins and other ions, could interfere with the interaction of K and the membrane of the ISE by partially blocking some of the molecular pores in the membrane. The matrix effect of milk may be more prominent on the ISE of K as the molecular cavity of the membrane of the K ISE is greater than that of the Na ISE.

Nevertheless, the measurement of Na and K with both methods was comparable and the mean differences of Na and K with both methods were within the limits of agreement (Table 4). Furthermore, within the first year of lactation, the mean concentrations of Na and K in milk ranged between 11 to 60 mM and 4 to 18.2 mM, respectively [18]. We calculated Na:K ratios using all permeations of high, medium, and low levels of Na and K to determine if the ratio would shift dramatically to alter diagnosis particularly in the case of identifying secretory activation. Indeed, we found the ratio not to be altered enough to change a clinical diagnosis. (Table 2).

Table 4. Limits of agreement for the measurement of Na and K concentrations using ICP-OES and the ion selective electrode.

Element	Mean Difference	CI mean Difference	Limits of Agreement		CI of Limits of Agreement	
			Lower	Upper	Lower	Upper
Na (mM)	0.26	−0.15, 0.68	−3.08	3.61	−3.81, −2.37	2.90, 4.34
K (mM)	0.65	0.17, 1.13	−3.19	4.49	−4.01, −2.37	3.67, 5.31

CI—95% confidence interval.

The accuracy of the ISE was comparable to ICP-OES with a significant correlation (Figures 1A and 2A) and good limits of agreement (Figures 1B and 2B). The ISE could therefore be used to measure the high sodium concentrations found in antepartum secretions, colostrum, and the milk from mastitic breast or milk during the involution phase [6,19]. Under all these conditions the integrity of the tight junctions is compromised resulting in widening of the paracellular pathway between the mammary epithelial cells allowing transfer of components between the circulation and milk [19].

Human milk sodium concentrations decrease rapidly in the first three days post-partum as secretory activation occurs in response to the withdrawal of progesterone. However, milk sodium levels have a nonlinear relationship with milk volume, suggesting changes are not due to dilution as milk volume increases [1]. Delayed secretory activation is a risk factor for reduced breastfeeding success [1]. HM sodium drops from 60 mM to 10 mM between days 1 and 5 postpartum [2]. As such, the ion selective probe is accurate enough to monitor HM sodium levels postpartum to confirm secretory activation particularly in high risk mothers such as primiparous mothers, those with maternal obesity, preterm birth, caesarean deliveries, and those who have had long and complicated deliveries [20–24].

Low milk supply is also a frequent concern for mothers, particularly primiparous mothers [3,25]. This concern may be either perceived or actual milk supply insufficiency. It is known that milk production at week 2 is predictive of milk production at week 6; therefore, the first 14 days are critical to the establishment of a good milk supply. Na:K ratios during the first week postpartum have been shown to be useful biochemical indicators of suboptimal milk production, and as a result, are predictors of shorter breastfeeding duration [4,9,26]. High Na:K ratios are indicative of incomplete tight junction closure. This may impact the volume of milk produced and thus the transition to full lactation [9]. Higher breastfeeding frequency is associated with lower sodium levels, and increased production. Dewey et al. [20] recommend that all mother and infant dyads be followed up at 72–96 h postpartum to ensure that secretory activation has occurred and a biochemical indicator such as ion selective probes that measure Na and K may provide rapid results to ensure early intervention to improve milk production.

The ISE may also be useful in immediate detection of mastitis particularly subclinical mastitis [27] via increases in Na:K (>1.0). Mastitis is a debilitating inflammatory breast disease, reported to result in cessation of breastfeeding in as many as 20% of cases; therefore, rapid detection would allow early treatment and resolution resulting in better breastfeeding outcomes. HM sodium levels decrease over time with mature milk to 4–5 mM, whereas HM Na levels of 12 mM and upwards are indicative of subclinical mastitis and mastitis. The Na:K ratio has been categorized as <0.6 normal, $\geq$0.6 and $\leq$1 slightly elevated, >1 very high [7]. Na:K above 1.0 is commonly used in the diagnosis of subclinical or clinical mastitis [7,27,28].

In conclusion, ion selective probes are sufficiently accurate to determine secretory activation by measurement of Na and K in the milk of lactating women. The use of ion selective probes may provide a useful point of care instrument to diagnose low milk supply and/or mammary infection. Early detection of these issues would allow timely intervention to ensure a successful lactation.

Author Contributions: Conceptualization, C.T.L. and D.G.; Methodology, C.T.L. and D.G.; Formal Analysis, C.T.L. and H.G.; Investigation, C.T.L.; Resources, D.G.; Data Curation, C.T.L. & H.G.; Writing-Review & Editing: C.T.L., H.G., D.G.; Visualization, C.T.L.; Supervision, D.G.; Project Administration, D.G.; Funding Acquisition, D.G.

Acknowledgments: We thank the participated mothers who donated their milk for this study. We thank Oscar Del Borrello for his technical support on the ICP-OES instrument.

References

1. Neville, M.C.; Allen, J.C.; Archer, P.C.; Casey, C.E.; Seacat, J.; Keller, R.P.; Lutes, V.; Rasbach, J.; Neifert, M. Studies in human lactation: milk volume and nutrient composition during weaning and lactogenesis. *Am. J. Clin. Nutr.* **1991**, *54*, 81–92. [CrossRef] [PubMed]
2. Cregan, M.D.; De Mello, T.R.; Kershaw, D.; McDougall, K.; Hartmann, P.E. Initiation of lactation in women after preterm delivery. *Acta. Obstet. Gynecol. Scand.* **2002**, *81*, 870–877. [CrossRef] [PubMed]
3. Wagner, E.A.; Chantry, C.J.; Dewey, K.G.; Nommsen-Rivers, L.A. Breastfeeding concerns at 3 and 7 days postpartum and feeding status at 2 months. *Pediatrics* **2013**, *132*, e865–e875. [CrossRef] [PubMed]

4. Murase, M.; Wagner, E.A.; Chantry, C.J.; Dewey, K.G.; Nommsen-Rivers, L.A. The relation between breast milk sodium to potassium ratio and maternal report of a milk supply concern. *J. Pediatr.* **2017**, *181*, 294–297.e3. [CrossRef] [PubMed]
5. Lemay, D.G.; Ballard, O.A.; Hughes, M.A.; Morrow, A.L.; Horseman, N.D.; Nommsen-Rivers, L.A. RNA sequencing of the human milk fat layer transcriptome reveals distinct gene expression profiles at three stages of lactation. *PLoS ONE* **2013**, *8*, e67531. [CrossRef] [PubMed]
6. Fetherston, C.M.; Lai, C.; Hartmann, P.E. Relationships between symptoms and changes in breast physiology during lactation mastitis. *Breastfeed. Med.* **2006**, *1*, 136–145. [CrossRef] [PubMed]
7. Filteau, S.M.; Rice, A.L.; Ball, J.J.; Chakraborty, J.; Stoltzfus, R.; de Francisco, A.; Willumsen, J.F. Breast milk immune factors in Bangladeshi women supplemented postpartum with retinol or beta-carotene. *Am. J. Clin. Nutr.* **1999**, *69*, 953–958. [CrossRef] [PubMed]
8. Prentice, A.; Prentice, A. Unilateral breast dysfunction in lactating Gambian women. *Ann. Trop. Paediatr.* **1984**, *4*, 19–23. [CrossRef] [PubMed]
9. Humenick, S.; Hill, P.; Thompson, J.; Hart, A. Breast-milk sodium as a predictor of breastfeeding patterns. *Can. J. Nurs. Res.* **1997**, *30*, 67–81.
10. Arthur, P.; Hartmann, P.; Smith, M. Measurement of the milk intake of breast-fed infants. *J. Pediatr. Gastroenterol. Nutr.* **1987**, *6*, 758–763. [CrossRef] [PubMed]
11. R Core Team. R: A Language and Environment for Statistical Computing. Available online: ftp://ftp.uvigo.es/CRAN/web/packages/dplR/vignettes/intro-dplR.pdf (accessed on 1 August 2018).
12. R Studio Team. R Studio: Integrated Development for R. Available online: https://www.rstudio.com/ (accessed on 1 August 2018).
13. Sarkar, D. Lattice: Trellis Graphics for R. Available online: https://cran.r-project.org/web/packages/lattice/index.html (accessed on 1 August 2018).
14. Bland, J.M.; Altman, D.G. Statistical methods for assessing agreement between two methods of clinical measurement. *Lancet* **1986**, *1*, 307–310. [CrossRef]
15. Hauser, P.C. Determination of alkali ions in biological and environmental samples. In *The Alkali Metal Ions: Their Role for Life*; Sigel, A., Sigel, H., Sigel, R.K.O., Eds.; Springer: Cham, Germany, 2016; pp. 11–25.
16. Payne, R.; Buckley, B.; Rawson, K. Protein interference with ion-selective electrode measurement depends on reference electrode composition and design. *Ann. Clin. Biochem.* **1991**, *28*, 68–72. [CrossRef] [PubMed]
17. Dimeski, G.; Badrick, T.; St John, A. Ion selective electrodes (ISEs) and interferences—A review. *Clin. Chim. Acta* **2010**, *411*, 309–317. [CrossRef] [PubMed]
18. Atkinson, S.; Alston-Mills, B.; Lönnerdal, B.; Neville, M.C. Major minerals and ionic constituents of human and bovine milks. In *Handbook of Milk Composition*; Elsevier: Newyork, NY, USA, 1995; pp. 593–622.
19. Neville, M.C.; Keller, R.P.; Seacat, J.; Casey, C.E.; Allen, J.C.; Archer, P. Studies on human lactation. I. Within-feed and between-breast variation in selected components of human milk. *Am. J. Clin. Nutr.* **1984**, *40*, 635–646. [CrossRef] [PubMed]
20. Dewey, K.G.; Nommsen-Rivers, L.A.; Heinig, M.J.; Cohen, R.J. Risk factors for suboptimal infant breastfeeding behavior, delayed onset of lactation, and excess neonatal weight loss. *Pediatrics* **2003**, *112*, 607–619. [CrossRef] [PubMed]
21. Chapman, D.J.; Perez-Escamilla, R. Identification of risk factors for delayed onset of lactation. *J. Am. Diet. Assoc.* **1999**, *99*, 450–454. [CrossRef]
22. Hildebrandt, H. Maternal perception of lactogenesis time: A clinical report. *J. Hum. Lact.* **1999**, *15*, 317–323. [CrossRef] [PubMed]
23. Hall, R.T.; Mercer, A.M.; Teasley, S.L.; McPherson, D.M.; Simon, S.D.; Santos, S.R.; Meyers, B.M.; Hipsh, N.E. A breast-feeding assessment score to evaluate the risk for cessation of breast-feeding by 7 to 10 days of age. *J. Pediatr.* **2002**, *141*, 659–664. [CrossRef] [PubMed]
24. Meier, P.P.; Engstrom, J.L.; Mingolelli, S.S.; Miracle, D.J.; Kiesling, S. The rush mothers' milk club: Breastfeeding interventions for mothers with very-low-birth-weight Infants. *J. Obstet. Gynecol. Neonatal Nurs.* **2004**, *33*, 164–174. [CrossRef] [PubMed]
25. Li, R.; Fein, S.B.; Chen, J.; Grummer-Strawn, L.M. Why mothers stop breastfeeding: Mothers' self-reported reasons for stopping during the first year. *Pediatrics* **2008**, *122* (Suppl. 2), S69–S76. [CrossRef]

26. Morton, J.A. The clinical usefulness of breast milk sodium in the assessment of lactogenesis. *Pediatrics* **1994**, *93*, 802–806. [PubMed]
27. Aryeetey, R.N.; Marquis, G.S.; Timms, L.; Lartey, A.; Brakohiapa, L. Subclinical mastitis is common among Ghanaian women lactating 3 to 4 months postpartum. *J. Hum. Lact.* **2008**, *24*, 263–267. [CrossRef] [PubMed]
28. Buescher, E.S.; Hair, P.S. Human milk anti-inflammatory component contents during acute mastitis. *Cell. Immunol.* **2001**, *210*, 87–95. [CrossRef] [PubMed]

14

Mother–Infant Physical Contact Predicts Responsive Feeding among U.S. Breastfeeding Mothers

Emily E. Little [1,*], Cristine H. Legare [2] and Leslie J. Carver [1]

[1] Department of Psychology, University of California, San Diego, CA 92093, USA; ljcarver@ucsd.edu
[2] Department of Psychology, The University of Texas at Austin, TX 78712, USA; legare@austin.utexas.edu
* Correspondence: emelysialittle@gmail.com

Abstract: Responsive feeding—initiating feeding in response to early hunger cues—supports the physiology of lactation and the development of infant feeding abilities, yet there is a dearth of research examining what predicts responsive feeding. In non-Western proximal care cultures, there is an association between responsive feeding and mother–infant physical contact, but this has not been investigated within Western populations. In two studies, we tested whether mother–infant physical contact predicted feeding in response to early hunger cues versus feeding on a schedule or after signs of distress among U.S. breastfeeding mothers. With an online questionnaire in Study 1 (n = 626), physical contact with infants (via co-sleeping and babywearing) predicted increased likelihood of self-reported responsive feeding. Mothers who reported responsive feeding were more likely to exclusively breastfeed for the first six months, breastfeed more frequently throughout the day, and had a longer planned breastfeeding duration than mothers who reported feeding on a schedule or after signs of infant distress. In Study 2 (n = 96), a three-day feeding log showed that mother–infant physical contact predicted feeding in response to early hunger cues but mother–infant proximity (without physical contact) did not. In sum, our results demonstrate that physical contact with infants may shape breastfeeding behavior among U.S. mothers, highlighting a connection between social interaction and infant nutrition that warrants further investigation.

Keywords: responsive feeding; breastfeeding; breastmilk; babywearing; co-sleeping; mother–infant interaction; feeding cues; maternal responsiveness; mother–infant physical contact; proximal care

---

1. Introduction

Breastfeeding is internationally recognized as the optimal nutrition for infant health and development [1,2], yet most U.S. mothers do not meet the World Health Organization's recommendation of exclusive breastfeeding for six months and continued breastfeeding for 24 months and beyond [3–5]. Responsive feeding—initiating feeding in response to early hunger cues such as lip smacking and bringing hands to mouth—decreases breastfeeding challenges by supporting the physiology of lactation and the development of infant feeding abilities [6–8]. Most mothers in the U.S. report crying as the primary reason for initiating feeding, which is an indication of infant distress rather than an early cue for hunger [9]. Ethnographic accounts of infant care report high levels of responsive feeding among mothers in proximal care cultures in which infants are in near-constant physical contact with mothers [10,11]. No research to date has systematically documented the association between mother–infant physical contact and responsive feeding among U.S. mothers. Here, we use convergent methods—an online questionnaire and an at-home feeding log—to examine whether mother–infant physical contact facilitates increased responsive feeding among U.S. breastfeeding mothers.

Ethnographic accounts of infant care in non-Western cultures show that responsive feeding is associated with proximal caretaking practices, a style of parenting characterized by mother–infant physical contact through the day and night. For example, Konner and colleagues note that !Kung San caregivers of Northwestern Botswana are in near-constant physical contact with infants and respond to their needs quickly [12]. Hewlett and colleagues have noted similar practices among the Aka foragers of Central Africa, who also keep infants close throughout the majority of the day and respond promptly to signs of distress [13]. Responsiveness in this context of physical closeness often manifests in the form of offering the breast for nursing [14–16]. Breastfeeding promptly in response to early hunger cues may preclude the need for infants to display overt signs of distress [17,18]. When in sustained body contact, mothers can sense infants' needs via subtle physical movements and do not wait to see or hear overt signs of discomfort [19,20]. This leads to high frequency of breastfeeding in proximal care cultures, up to several times per hour [21,22]. Mothers also show acute awareness of subtle elimination signals, demonstrated by moving infants into an appropriate position immediately before infants empty their bowels [23].

A limitation of the ethnographic literature is that the connection between high levels of physical contact and increased maternal responsiveness is embedded within the broader parenting profile of proximal care, comprising a distinct set of parenting beliefs that may also be driving increased responsiveness. These beliefs are referred to as parental ethnotheories, or cultural parenting models used to define parental roles and goals for children [24]. It is an open question whether the mother–infant physical contact characteristic of proximal care facilitates increased responsiveness or whether the increased responsiveness is simply part of the psychological model of socialization goals and parenting beliefs.

The connection between mother–infant physical contact and maternal responsiveness has not been investigated outside of the proximal care context of small-scale, indigenous communities. Infant care among middle-class Euro-American parents in the U.S. is described as distal care, which is characterized by face-to-face interaction and object stimulation [25]. Yet a movement within many Western countries to adopt philosophies of "natural parenting" and "attachment parenting" has motivated some parents to adopt a parenting style that resembles proximal care, emphasizing high levels of physical contact and extended breastfeeding. There is a dearth of information about these practices in Western culture. One study reported that parents in London who identify with proximal care parenting philosophies had over 50% more physical contact with their infant than parents practicing distal care, which resulted in the proximal care infants crying 50% less and breastfeeding for longer [26]. The extent to which the practices of proximal care—including babywearing (carrying infants for extended periods on the body using a sling or wrap) and co-sleeping (bed-sharing with infants to maintain physical contact throughout the night)—predict increased maternal responsiveness during feeding among U.S. mothers is currently unknown.

Our objective in the current investigation was to test whether mother–infant physical contact predicts variation in responsive feeding among U.S. breastfeeding mothers. Though very little is known about the predictors of responsive feeding among U.S. mothers, mothers who breastfeed directly from the breast—in comparison with bottle-feeding—are more likely to be responsive to early hunger cues [27] and are also more likely to breastfeed for a longer duration [28,29]. This disparity in responsive feeding between direct breast- versus bottle-feeding has been explained by several different factors, including the salient visual cue of the emptying bottle, prompting mothers to use quantity consumed to guide feeding rather than infant hunger and fullness cues [30]. Another potential explanation is the increased maternal sensitivity promoted by the oxytocin release during skin-to-skin contact [31]. We examined predictors of responsive feeding solely among mothers feeding directly from the breast.

In two studies, we used convergent evidence—a self-report questionnaire (Study 1) and an at-home feeding log (Study 2)—to test the hypothesis that mother–infant physical contact predicts responsiveness to infant hunger cues among U.S. breastfeeding mothers. Whereas questionnaires can assess overall reported responsiveness or philosophies about feeding, evidence can be strengthened if it is combined with live documentation of each feeding session, allowing us to capture not only variation between individuals in feeding strategies but also variation within individuals in their likelihood of responding to early hunger cues. Cross-cultural variation in mother–infant physical contact is associated with a set of socialization goals characteristic of proximal care culture, and even subtle differences in beliefs and intentions regarding breastfeeding can affect breastfeeding behavior [32]. We therefore used Keller's [33] parental ethnotheories questionnaire to assess maternal beliefs about breastfeeding and responsiveness in Studies 1 and 2. We hypothesized that mother–infant physical contact would be associated with increased maternal responsiveness to infant hunger cues in the context of breastfeeding.

2. Study 1

Responsive feeding supports the supply and demand physiology of lactation and works in accordance with the range of individual variation in infant feeding needs [34]. It may also help protect against perceived insufficient milk syndrome, one of the primary reasons mothers end breastfeeding earlier than planned [35]. Though many lactation education programs now recommend responsive feeding as best practice for successful breastfeeding [36], alternate recommendations also exist. For example, starting in the 18th century, European male pediatricians recommended that infants be fed on a strictly regulated schedule [37], a practice which is still promoted today, both informally by parenting blogs and in certain health care settings. Waiting for crying and feeding on a set schedule are both problematic, because they neglect the ability of infants to communicate their hunger, creating a mismatch between infant hunger and feeding time. This mismatch has been linked to problems with early self-regulation and childhood obesity [38–40], in addition to breastfeeding-specific problems of latching difficulties and perceived insufficient milk supply, all of which may contribute to ending breastfeeding earlier than recommended.

Despite the known consequences of not practicing responsive feeding, there is a dearth of information regarding what individual level factors predict responsive feeding, especially among middle-class Euro-American mothers. Study 1 addressed two research question. First, do behaviors consistent with proximal care (i.e., babywearing, co-sleeping) predict a responsive breastfeeding philosophy? We hypothesized that mothers who practiced high level of physical contact through the day (via babywearing) and through the night (via co-sleeping) would be more likely to report a responsive feeding philosophy. Second, does having a responsive feeding philosophy predict improved breastfeeding outcomes? We predicted that self-reported responsive feeding would be associated with an increased likelihood of exclusive breastfeeding for the first six months, increased feeding frequency, and longer planned breastfeeding duration.

2.1. Materials and Methods

This study was conducted in accordance with the Declaration of Helsinki, and the protocol was approved by the Institutional Review Board of University of California, San Diego (protocol number 130567 "Culture and Infant-Caregiver Interactions"). We recruited mothers ($n = 626$) of newborn to 24-month-old infants to fill out an online questionnaire. These dyads were recruited from social media postings within U.S.-based parenting groups. After mothers expressed interest in participating in the study, they were contacted electronically by a research assistant who explained the protocol and obtained consent. Participants filled out the anonymous online questionnaire from their home.

Demographic information for the sample is included in Table 1.

Table 1. Demographic information for the participants in Study 1.

Maternal and Infant Characteristics	Range	*M*	*SD*
Infant Age	0.23–24.91	9.36	5.92
Maternal Age	20–44	30.71	(4.29)
Daycare	0–60	9.70	(15.59)
		n	%
Maternal Education			
High School		174	30.16%
College Degree		204	35.36%
Graduate Degree		199	34.49%
Maternal Employment			
Home		345	55.11%
Working		281	44.89%

M is the mean response of each category; *SD* is the standard deviation of each category; *n* is number of caregivers in the sample who fit into each category; percentages provided are based on the total sample. Infant age was measured in months, maternal age was measured in years, and daycare was measured as hours per week that the child spends in daycare.

The online questionnaire (administered through Google Forms) assessed demographic factors; parenting practices that facilitate mother–infant physical contact (babywearing, co-sleeping); maternal beliefs; and infant feeding philosophies, practices, and outcomes. We collected basic sociodemographic information from all mothers and controlled for these factors in each statistical model, including infant age (in months), maternal education level (high school, college, or graduate degree), current employment status (at home not working, working outside of the home), and hours per week that the child spends in daycare. These factors were chosen because past research has indicated these variables may be important for predicting breastfeeding behavior [41], and they play a role in how much time the mother spends with her child, potentially impacting ability to recognize or respond to feeding cues.

To assess mother–infant physical contact during the day, mothers were asked about infant carrying practices: "What is the primary method you use to transport your baby?" with the following response options: babywearing or other (i.e., "arms", "stroller/seat"). To assess nighttime physical contact, mothers were asked "Where does your baby currently sleep?" with the following response categories: co-sleeping ("In the same bed as me") or mixed/other ("in the same room, but a separate bed", "in a separate room", or "mixed").

Maternal beliefs about responsiveness were assessed with Keller's 10-question parental ethnotheory questionnaire that solicits degree of agreement with parenting statements regarding the care of a three-month-old infant. Responses to each item were on a scale from one (completely disagree) to five (completely agree). Responses from each participant were compiled to form a proximal care belief score, calculated by summing responses from all questions aimed at measuring alignment with goals of proximal care parenting culture then subtracting the sum of responses to all questions designed to test alignment with goals of distal care parenting culture. The range of possible scores was negative 20 to positive 20. Positive scores indicated that mothers were more aligned with the values of proximal care culture than distal care culture, and a higher score indicated a greater agreement with the parenting goals characteristic of proximal care culture.

To assess feeding philosophy, each mother was asked to choose the option that best described her feeding strategy with the options: responsive ("on demand") or schedule/mixed ("feeding schedule", "mix of both"). To assess breastfeeding outcomes, mothers of infants six months of age and younger were asked about exclusive breastfeeding (only breastmilk, as recommended by the World Health Organization and other international health organizations for the first six months of life) versus non-exclusive breastfeeding (supplementing breastmilk with formula, solids, or other liquids). Breastfeeding frequency throughout the day was assessed by asking mothers how many times per day they usually breastfeed their child (number). We assessed planned breastfeeding duration by asking mothers how many months they planned to breastfeed their child for (number in months).

In our analyses, we first sought to describe the beliefs and practices of U.S. breastfeeding mothers. We then examined the degree to which engagement in the beliefs and practices of proximal care predicted responsive feeding and whether responsive feeding predicted breastfeeding behavior. To examine whether proximal care beliefs (proximal care belief score) and practices (babywearing, co-sleeping) predicted self-reported responsive breastfeeding, we conducted multistep logistic regressions with feeding philosophy (responsive, scheduled/mixed) as the outcome measures and proximal care beliefs (proximal care beliefs score) and practices (babywearing, co-sleeping, or both) as the predictor measures, controlling for infant age, maternal education and employment, and hours per week that the child spends in daycare.

To examine whether reporting a responsive feeding philosophy predicted improved breastfeeding outcomes, we conducted separate logistic regressions with feeding strategy (responsive, scheduled/mixed) as the predictor measure—controlling for infant age, maternal education, maternal employment, and hours per week that the child spent in daycare—and exclusive breastfeeding (yes versus no) as the outcome measure (for mothers of infants six months of age and younger, $n = 217$). Controlling for the same demographic variables, we conducted linear regressions with breastfeeding frequency (number of times per day) and planned duration of breastfeeding (in months) as continuous outcome measures.

2.2. Results

All descriptive statistics for Study 1 are included in Table 2.

Table 2. Descriptive statistics for the participants in Study 1.

Maternal Characteristics	*n*	%
Feeding Philosophy		
Responsive Feeding	441	71.13%
Other (Schedule/Mixed)	179	28.87%
Co-sleeping		
Yes	266	42.42%
No	361	57.58%
Babywearing		
Yes	439	73.41%
No	159	26.59%
Exclusive Breastfeeding (for infants 6 months and younger, $n = 217$)		
Yes	177	81.94%
No	39	18.06%
	M	***SD***
Maternal Beliefs		
Proximal Care Belief Score	6.85	5.73
Breastfeeding Duration	21.55	11.76
Breastfeeding Frequency	6.92	4.33

M is the mean response of each category; *SD* is the standard deviation of each category; *n* is number of participants in the sample.

We first tested proximal care predictors of responsive breastfeeding. In Step 1 of the model, controlling for infant age, maternal education, maternal employment, and hours per week in daycare, proximal care belief score predicted a self-reported responsive feeding style, $\beta = 0.10$, $SE = 0.02$, $\chi^2 = 24.37$, $p < 0.0001$ (β is the effect estimate, SE is the standard error, χ^2 is the chi-squared statistic, and p is the calculated probability). In Step 2, physical contact throughout the day and night (via babywearing and co-sleeping) predicted reporting an on-demand feeding philosophy, $\beta = 0.62$, $SE = 0.21$, $\chi^2 = 9.13$, $p < 0.001$; see Table 3.

Table 3. Results of the logistic regression predicting responsive breastfeeding philosophy from proximal care practices and beliefs in Study 1.

	Step 1						Step 2					
Multivariate Analyses	β	*SE*	χ^2	*p*	*Lower 95%*	*Upper 95%*	β	*SE*	χ^2	*p*	*Lower 95%*	*Upper 95%*
Intercept	1.32	0.24	30.37	<0.0001	0.86	1.80	1.38	0.27	26.94	<0.0001	0.87	1.92
Infant Age	−0.07	0.02	15.18	<0.0001	−0.11	−0.04	−0.07	0.02	15.20	<0.0001	−0.11	−0.04
Maternal Education												
High School (ref)												
College	−0.03	0.15	0.04	0.85	−0.32	0.27	−0.07	0.15	0.20	0.65	−0.37	0.23
Graduate	−0.17	0.15	1.32	0.25	−0.47	0.12	−0.10	0.15	0.41	0.52	−0.40	0.20
Maternal Employment												
Home (ref)												
Working	0.33	0.14	5.68	0.02	0.06	0.60	0.34	0.14	5.84	0.02	0.07	0.61
Daycare	−0.02	0.01	7.52	0.01	−0.04	−0.01	−0.02	0.01	6.50	0.01	−0.04	−0.01
Maternal Beliefs												
Proximal Care Belief Score	0.10	0.02	24.37	<0.0001	0.06	0.14	0.08	0.02	12.06	<0.001	0.03	0.12
Mother-Infant Physical Contact												
Neither (ref)												
Babywearing Only							0.01	0.18	0.00	0.97	−0.34	0.35
Co-sleeping Only							−0.16	0.30	0.27	0.60	−0.73	0.46
Babywearing and Co-sleeping							0.62	0.21	9.13	<0.001	0.22	1.03

β is the effect estimate; *SE* is the standard error; χ^2 is the chi-squared statistic; *p* is the calculated probability; *lower 95%* is the lower bounds of the 95% confidence interval; *upper 95%* is the upper bounds of the 95% confidence interval.

We next tested breastfeeding outcomes associated with responsive breastfeeding philosophy with three separate models. Controlling for infant age, maternal education, maternal employment, and hours per week in daycare, responsive feeding philosophy predicted increased likelihood of exclusive breastfeeding (for infants under six months), $\beta = 0.50$, $SE = 0.24$, $\chi^2 = 4.33$, $p = 0.04$ (Model 1, see Table 4); increased frequency of breastfeeding times per day $\beta = 0.84$, $SE = 0.23$, $\chi^2 = 3.64$, $p < 0.001$ (Model 2, see Table 4); and longer planned breastfeeding duration, $\beta = 2.40$, $SE = 0.70$, $\chi^2 = 3.44$, $p < 0.001$ (Model 3, see Table 4).

Table 4. Results of the logistic regression predicting exclusive breastfeeding (feeding only breastmilk to infants under six months) from self-reported responsive feeding (Model 1), results of the linear regression predicting feeding frequency (average number of breastfeeding sessions per day) from self-reported responsive feeding (Model 2), and results of the linear regression predicting planned breastfeeding duration (in months) from self-reported responsive feeding (Model 3) in Study 1.

Model 1: Exclusive Breastfeeding	β	*SE*	χ^2	*p*	*Lower 95%*	*Upper 95%*
Intercept	2.19	0.54	16.41	<0.0001	1.18	3.32
Infant Age	−0.27	0.12	4.78	0.03	−0.53	−0.03
Maternal Education						
High School (ref)						
College	0.10	0.32	0.10	0.75	−0.50	0.75
Graduate	−0.30	0.30	1.00	0.32	−0.89	0.30
Maternal Employment						
Home (ref)						
Working	0.11	0.25	0.20	0.65	−0.37	0.63
Daycare	0.01	0.02	0.37	0.54	−0.02	0.05
Feeding Philosophy						
Schedule/Other (ref)						
Responsive Feeding	0.50	0.24	4.33	0.04	0.02	0.97
Model 2: Breastfeeding Frequency	β	*SE*	χ^2	*p*	*Lower 95%*	*Upper 95%*
Intercept	8.58	0.43	19.72	<0.0001	7.73	9.43
Infant Age	−0.18	0.03	−5.36	<0.0001	−0.25	−0.12
Maternal Education						
High School (ref)						
College	0.24	0.30	0.80	0.42	−0.34	0.82
Graduate	−0.26	0.29	−0.91	0.36	−0.82	0.30
Maternal Employment						
Home (ref)						
Working	−0.29	0.25	−1.15	0.25	−0.77	0.20
Daycare	−0.03	0.02	−1.85	0.07	−0.06	0.00
Feeding Philosophy						
Schedule/Other (ref)						
Responsive Feeding	0.84	0.23	3.64	<0.001	0.39	1.29
Model 3: Breastfeeding Duration	β	*SE*	χ^2	*p*	*Lower 95%*	*Upper 95%*
Intercept	15.75	1.41	11.17	<0.0001	12.98	18.52
Infant Age	0.45	0.11	4.15	<0.0001	0.24	0.67
Maternal Education						
High School (ref)						
College	−1.80	0.94	−1.92	0.06	−3.64	0.05
Graduate	1.11	0.86	1.28	0.20	−0.59	2.81
Maternal Employment						
Home (ref)						
Working	−2.60	0.82	−3.19	<0.001	−4.21	−0.99
Daycare	0.00	0.05	0.04	0.97	−0.10	0.10
Feeding Philosophy						
Schedule/Other (ref)						
Responsive Feeding	2.40	0.70	3.44	<0.001	1.03	3.77

Exclusive breastfeeding was defined as feeding only breastmilk to infants and this model only included a sub-sample of infants under six months of age ($n = 217$); breastfeeding frequency was defined as the average number of breastfeeding sessions per day; breastfeeding duration was the planned number of months of breastfeeding.

2.3. Discussion

We documented beliefs and practices consistent with proximal care and their relation to self-reported breastfeeding behavior among U.S. mothers. Our first research aim was to assess whether behaviors consistent with proximal care (i.e., mother–infant physical contact throughout the day and night via babywearing and co-sleeping) predicted increased likelihood of reporting a responsive breastfeeding philosophy. Consistent with our predictions, mothers who reported both babywearing and co-sleeping (but not babywearing or co-sleeping only) had an increased likelihood of reporting a responsive feeding philosophy. This finding aligns with ethnographic work showing high levels of breastfeeding responsiveness among populations that practice physical contact throughout the day and night. It is possible that mothers who only practice babywearing or only practice co-sleeping may engage in these practices for convenience, rather than for the desire to have constant physical closeness to infants. This distinction between constant day and night physical contact versus just babywearing or just co-sleeping warrants further investigation.

Our second research aim was to examine whether having a responsive feeding philosophy predicted improved breastfeeding outcomes. Reporting a responsive feeding philosophy predicted increased likelihood of exclusive breastfeeding during the first six months of life, increased feeding frequency, and longer planned breastfeeding duration. The finding regarding planned breastfeeding duration was limited by the fact that this was only in relation to the planned—rather than actual—breastfeeding duration. Future work should employ a longitudinal design to see if responsive feeding does in fact predict actual breastfeeding duration.

One general limitation of this study is that it only reports whether the mother would describe herself as a responsive feeder, which may be closer to her ideal behavior rather than reflecting the mother's actual behavior at time of feeding. To address this in Study 2, we had mothers fill out a three-day at-home feeding log. At the time of each feeding, mothers documented the reason for feeding their child, as well as their distance from their child (i.e., in physical contact versus not in physical contact) preceding feeding onset, with the aim of capturing a more accurate depiction of the mother's feeding behavior and how it relates to mother–infant physical contact.

3. Study 2

The primary objective of Study 2 was to examine whether individual variation in mother–infant physical contact predicted increased likelihood of feeding in response to early hunger cues (e.g., rooting, lip smacking) rather than waiting for the onset of distress (i.e., crying) or feeding for other reasons (comfort, schedules). Mothers filled out an at-home feeding log for three days. For each feeding, mothers documented the location of the infant (i.e., mother–infant contact) preceding feed onset and the reason for initiating feeding. In line with past ethnographic work citing an association between mother–infant physical contact and increased breastfeeding frequency [42], we predicted increased responsiveness to infant hunger cues when a feeding was preceded by mother–infant physical contact in comparison with mother–infant proximity (without direct physical contact).

Hunger is not the only reason a mother might breastfeed her baby, as feeding may be motivated by mother-led contextual reasons (e.g., work constraints, doctor-recommended schedules, or concerns about breastfeeding in public). Mothers may also feed for infant-led contextual reasons (e.g., use nursing as a strategy for comforting infants, as well as decreasing crying and helping infants get to sleep) [43]. Our second objective was to examine whether increased physical contact predicted increased likelihood of feeding to comfort the infant (as reported by the mother) rather than for adult-led contextual reasons. Based on the proposal that physical contact facilitates mother–infant bonding [44], we predicted that when mothers report feeding for non-hunger reasons, the feeding session would be more likely to be preceded by physical contact when feeding in response to infant-led (i.e., comfort) reasons versus adult-led contextual reasons.

As in Study 1, we tested mothers' degree of alignment with the beliefs of proximal care culture with Keller's parental ethnotheory questionnaire. We controlled for these beliefs in all analyses to test whether feeding responsiveness could be attributed to increased mother–infant physical contact, beyond the variation attributed to maternal beliefs. We also tested—and controlled for—the same demographic factors that were included as controls in Study 1 (infant age, maternal education, maternal employment, and hours per week in daycare). These societal factors are some of the primary differences between proximal care and distal care cultures, have been identified as shaping breastfeeding outcomes in the breastfeeding literature, and also may be important because they affect the amount of time a mother spends with her infant.

3.1. Materials and Methods

This study was conducted in accordance with the Declaration of Helsinki, and the protocol was approved by the Institutional Review Board of University of California, San Diego (protocol number 130567 "Culture and Infant-Caregiver Interactions"). Study 2 comprised a subset of the participants from Study 1 (recruitment methods and eligibility were identical to Study 1). Only mothers who logged at least 12 breastfeeding sessions over a period of three consecutive days were included in the sample. Because we were only sampling from populations of breastfeeding mothers, the participants in this study are a unique sample and are not representative of U.S. mothers at large.

We used an online questionnaire (Google Forms) to solicit demographic information from each mother, including infant age, maternal age, maternal education, maternal employment (currently working outside of the home versus not), and average hours per week that the infant spends in daycare. Maternal beliefs about responsiveness were assessed with the same questions from Keller's parental ethnotheory questionnaire that was used in Study 1.

The feeding log consisted of three questions: (1) feed method (breastmilk from breast, breastmilk from bottle, formula in bottle, other liquids, other solids, and other), (2) location of the infant before feeding onset (in physical contact, in visual proximity, and no contact), and (3) reason for feeding (hunger: early cues, hunger: distress, non-hunger: infant-led, and non-hunger: mother-led). The date and time of the feeding session was automatically recorded by the online form. For each of these questions, a list of options was provided and only one response could be chosen for each question. For the question: "Where was your baby when you decided to feed him/her?", there were three pre-determined mutually exclusive categories of responses with regard to mother–infant contact: (1) physical contact (mother was in direct physical contact with the infant), (2) visual proximity (the mother was near enough to see the infant, but not in physical contact), and (3) no contact (the infant was out of sight or with another caregiver). For the question: "Why did you decide to start feeding your baby?", there were four pre-determined mutually exclusive categories of responses: (1) hunger: early cues, (2) hunger: distress, (3) non-hunger: infant-led, and (4) non-hunger: mother-led.

Feedings were coded as being in response to cues if the mother indicated that the feeding was initiated because the infant had shown either visual communication (e.g., facial expression), vocal communication (e.g., lip smacking), or physical communication (e.g., breast nuzzling, squirming) that indicated hunger (but not to the point of distress or crying). Feedings were coded as being in response to distress if the mother indicated she had decided to feed because the infant was crying or showing clear distress. Non-hunger feedings were coded as infant-led if the mother initiated feeding for a reason other than hunger that was centered around the well-being of the baby (e.g., wanted to comfort the baby, wanted to calm the baby before getting shots). Non-hunger feedings were coded as mother-led if the mother initiated feeding for a reason other than hunger that was centered around adult-dictated logistical reasons such as schedules (e.g., needing to leave for work) or other maternally-motivated reasons (e.g., breasts feeling engorged).

After indicating interest in the study, mothers were contacted electronically by a research assistant to give details about the feeding log procedure and obtain informed consent. Mothers were instructed to fill out the maternal questionnaire first, then fill out the feeding log during a consecutive three-day period of their choice. Both the questionnaire and the feeding log were administered online via a web browser or smartphone app.

We used generalized mixed-effects logistic regression models to test whether maternal beliefs (proximal care belief score) and immediate physical contact (versus visual contact or no contact) predicted reason for feeding. We analyzed hunger-related reasons for feeding (early cues versus distress) separately from non-hunger reasons for feeding (infant-led versus mother-led). In these models, we controlled for infant age, maternal education, maternal employment, and infant hours in daycare by including these as fixed effects. We included random intercepts for subject, as well as random slopes to account for the multiple responses for each participant [45]. These analyses were conducted using the lme4 package within R Studio software, Version 1.0.44 (RStudio, Inc., Boston, MA, USA) [46].

3.2. Results

Ninety-nine breastfeeding mothers completed the feeding log and were included in the final analyses. Infants were 0- to 12-month-olds (51 female, 5.66 months, standard deviation (*SD*) = 3.25). Mothers were 21 to 42 years old (*M* = 30.97 years, *SD* = 4.64) and had completed high school (30.61%), college (38.78%) or a graduate program (30.61%). The average household income of the sample was $78,703 (*SD* = $50,064). Mothers were multiparous (had more than one child, 75.26%) and were exclusively breastfeeding (65.66%). Many of the mothers were not currently working (60.20%), and infant hours in daycare ranged from zero to 55 h per week (*M* = 4.41 h, *SD* = 11.52).

Mothers logged from 12–47 breastfeeding sessions over the course of three days (*M* = 25.86, *SD* = 8.34); see Table 5. An average of 14.15 of the feedings were initiated when the infant was in physical contact with the mother (*SD* = 7.37, 3–39 feeds). The most common reason for feeding was early hunger cues (*M* = 30.52%, *SD* = 16.91%), followed by late cues (*M* = 34.59%, *SD* = 21.53%), infant-led non-hunger reasons (*M* = 17.42%, *SD* = 15.34%), and mother-led non-hunger reasons (*M* = 17.26%, *SD* = 14.33%). Proximal care belief scores ranged from −8 to +17 (*M* = 5.84, *SD* = 5.88) out of a possible range of −20 to +20.

Table 5. Descriptive statistics for Study 2.

Feeding and Infant Care Characteristics	Range	*M*	*SD*
Total Breastfeeding Sessions	12–47	23.63	7.77
Initiated in Physical Contact	3–39	13.07	6.74
Initiated in Visual Contact	0–24	7.85	4.54
Hunger—Early Cues	0–23	6.06	4.19
Hunger—Distress	2–22	10.85	5.45
Non-Hunger—Infant-Led	0–9	3.02	2.79
Non-Hunger—Mother-Led	0–9	3.05	2.62
		n	%
Exclusive Breastfeeding for 6 Months			
Yes		35	85.37%
No		6	14.63%
Babywearing			
Yes		29	70.73%
No		12	29.27%
Co-sleeping			
Yes		17	41.46%
No		24	58.54%

M is the mean response of each category; *SD* is the standard deviation of each category; *n* is number of participants in the sample.

Mother–infant physical contact predicted feeding in response to early hunger cues in comparison with distress, $\beta = 0.991$, $SE = 0.315$, $z = 3.149$, $p = 0.002$; see Table 6. Mothers who initiated more feedings while in physical contact (i.e., the median 53% or more) had a higher percentage of feeds initiated in response to early cues (*M* = 33.24%, *SE* = 2.41) than mothers who initiated fewer feedings (less than 53%) while in physical contact (*M* = 25.67%, *SE* = 2.59). Visual contact did not predict feeding in response to early cues versus distress, $\beta = 0.002$, $SE = 0.200$, $z = 0.007$, $p = 0.994$.

Table 6. Model Predicting Responsiveness to Cues. Fixed effects for the mixed-effects model predicting initiating hunger-related feedings in response to early cues (in comparison with crying) in Study 2.

Multivariate Analyses	β	SE	z	p
Infant Age	−0.030	0.044	−0.665	0.506
Maternal Education				
High School (ref)				
College	−0.081	0.343	−0.235	0.814
Graduate	0.740	0.390	1.898	0.058
Maternal Employment				
Home (ref)				
Working	−0.604	0.326	−1.853	0.064
Daycare	0.044	0.016	2.844	0.004
Maternal Beliefs				
Proximal Care Belief Score	0.030	0.027	1.106	0.269
Mother–Infant Physical Contact				
No Contact (ref)				
Visual Contact	0.002	0.300	0.007	0.994
Physical Contact	0.991	0.315	3.149	0.002

β is the effect estimate; *SE* is the standard error; *z* is the z-score; *p* is the calculated probability.

For non-hunger feedings, the bivariate regression analysis revealed that physical contact predicted feeding for infant-led versus mother-led reasons, $\beta = 1.271$, $SE = 0.261$, $z = 4.868$, $p < 0.0001$. Controlling for demographic factors and multiple responses (i.e., feeding log entries), we found that physical contact predicted feeding for infant-led versus mother-led reasons, $\beta = 1.246$, $SE = 0.304$, $z = 4.095$, $p < 0.0001$; see Table 7. Mothers with more feedings initiated in physical contact had a lower percentage of feeds initiated for mother-led reasons ($M = 14.54\%$, $SE = 1.94$) than mothers with fewer feedings initiated in physical contact ($M = 22.22\%$, $SE = 2.08$). In contrast, visual contact did not predict feeding for infant-led versus mother-led reasons, $\beta = 0.397$, $SE = 0.288$, $z = 1.379$, $p = 0.168$.

Table 7. Model Predicting Responsiveness to Cues. Fixed effects for the mixed-effects model predicting initiating non-hunger feedings in response to infant comfort (in comparison with adult-determined reasons) in Study 2.

Multivariate Analyses	β	SE	z	p
Infant Age	0.067	0.044	1.514	0.130
Maternal Education				
High School (ref)				
College	0.027	0.345	0.079	0.937
Graduate	0.085	0.403	0.210	0.833
Maternal Employment				
Home (ref)				
Working	−0.446	0.319	−1.397	0.162
Daycare	−0.013	0.015	−0.897	0.369
Maternal Beliefs				
Proximal Care Belief Score	0.057	0.022	2.665	0.008
Mother–Infant Physical Contact				
No Contact (ref)				
Visual Contact	0.397	0.288	1.379	0.168
Physical Contact	1.246	0.304	4.095	<0.0001

3.3. Discussion

These data provide support for the proposal that mother–infant physical contact influences maternal responsiveness to early hunger cues during breastfeeding. Consistent with our predictions, mothers were more likely to respond to early hunger cues when in physical contact with their infant. Visual contact did not predict reason for feeding, suggesting that it is something unique about physical contact that facilitates increased maternal responsiveness. In addition, increased responsiveness to hunger cues was not simply attributed to increased feeding frequency overall.

We tested whether physical contact predicted infant-led non-hunger reasons for feeding. When feeding for non-hunger contextual reasons, mothers were more likely to feed for infant-led reasons (e.g., to comfort the infant) rather than adult-led reasons (e.g., schedules) if the feeding was preceded by mother–infant physical contact. Visual contact was not associated with feeding for non-hunger reasons, suggesting that there is something special about direct physical contact that facilitates infant-led motivations for feeding above and beyond just having the infant in proximity.

In addition to testing specific research questions, we also sought to document proximal care parenting practices among Euro-American middle class parents. Though caregiving in U.S. culture is typically characterized as distal care; the mothers in our sample participated in many parenting practices typical of proximal care culture, including babywearing and co-sleeping. This study provides insight into how proximal care practices might shape other components of infant-caregiver interaction during feeding. More research is needed to examine the implications of these practices for infant health and nutrition.

4. General Discussion

Convergent methods were used to test whether mother–infant physical contact predicts increased responsiveness to early hunger cues during breastfeeding. Both the self-report questionnaire and the at-home feeding log showed that maternal beliefs and practices characteristic of proximal care culture predicted increased maternal responsiveness to infant hunger cues during breastfeeding. We discuss potential mechanisms underlying the connection between physical contact and maternal responsiveness, present potential directions for future research, and discuss broader implications of this work for protecting and promoting breastfeeding.

4.1. Mechanisms Underlying the Effect of Physical Contact

Our data show that mother–infant physical contact predicts increased responsiveness to infant hunger cues during breastfeeding, beyond any variation explained by underlying beliefs about responsiveness. Thus, mother-infant physical contact may facilitate increased maternal awareness of her infant's emotional state and communicative intentions, allowing her to increase her responsiveness to subtle movements or physiological changes in the infant that cannot be observed but can be felt. The release of oxytocin—a neuropeptide involved in mammalian social bonds—during mother–infant physical contact may also underlie the effect of physical contact on maternal responsiveness. Oxytocin is associated with some aspects of responsiveness, including responding to infant crying [47] and infant laughing [48]. Because oxytocin is released during skin-to-skin contact [49], infant holding without direct skin-to-skin [50], and even in response to infant vocalizations [51], oxytocin release likely plays a role in the relationship between mother–infant physical contact and maternal responsiveness demonstrated in these studies. Though measuring oxytocin was outside of the scope of the current project, future research should measure the effect of mother–infant contact on maternal responsiveness while accounting for potential changes in oxytocin levels.

4.2. Limitations and Broader Implications

Because we did not directly manipulate mother–infant physical contact in these studies, we cannot determine the causal relationship between mother–infant physical contact and responsive feeding. We hope these studies motivate controlled experimental studies to continue investigating our hypothesis that mother–infant physical contact facilitates increased responsiveness to infant hunger cues during breastfeeding. Because we specifically sampled from the population of breastfeeding mothers, mothers in our study were more likely to be older, more educated, and have a higher income than the general population. We therefore cannot determine whether these findings generalize to the population of U.S. mothers at large. Many studies have reported that crying is the most commonly reported indication of hunger used by U.S. mothers to initiate feeding [52]. The fact that mothers in this sample initiated feeding more often due to early hunger cues rather than distress in Study 2 demonstrates higher levels of responsiveness than the average population. Past research shows that breastfeeding mothers show different patterns of interaction and responsiveness than bottle-feeding mothers. Breastfeeding mothers—in comparison with bottle-feeding mothers—are more likely to show an increase in oxytocin levels after holding their infant [53] and are more likely to show neural activation in response to their infant's cry [54], suggesting that the variation in responsiveness found in these studies may be specific to breastfeeding mothers.

Populations show substantial variation in the modality of infant-caregiver interaction, especially with regard to physical contact [55]. The amount of physical contact with infants in Western, educated, industrialized, rich, and democratic—"WEIRD" societies, which comprise the majority of research on infant nutrition and development [56,57]—is substantially lower than in many other human populations [58,59]. Infant care in WEIRD societies is increasingly dominated by products that limit physical contact between infants and caregivers (e.g., cribs, strollers, playpens, and bouncers). Because human infants are like all other primates in their need to maintain close contact with mothers, this lack of physical contact represents a caregiving method that is unique from a cultural and historical perspective [60]. Though past research has identified the importance of cultural ecologies on breastfeeding behavior—including both cultural beliefs and behaviors [61]—our data suggest that amount of physical contact with infants may shape breastfeeding behavior, presenting a new avenue for exploring the intersection between social interaction and early nutrition.

Skin-to-skin contact is beneficial for physiological stability, physical growth, and breastfeeding initiation for both preterm and full-term infants, yet investigating the implications of mother–infant physical contact for responsiveness to hunger cues during breastfeeding is surprisingly understudied. Randomized controlled trials with preterm infants show that skin-to-skin contact immediately after birth increases the likelihood of breastfeeding in the hospital and throughout the first postpartum months [62], while also leading to a more stable heartbeat, respiratory rate, body temperature, and other benefits [63]. Intervention studies with full-term infants show that increased physical contact through carrying facilitates more secure attachment [64] and increased frequency of breastfeeding [65]. There are still substantial gaps in our knowledge of the processes underlying the effects of skin-to-skin and physical contact, leaving many questions unanswered about how and why physical contact can be used to improve breastfeeding outcomes for infants. Because increasing mother–infant physical contact is both a viable and inexpensive potential intervention, this area warrants further research.

4.3. Conclusions

Breastmilk is internationally recognized as the optimal nutrition for infant health and development. Neglecting to recognize and respond to subtle feeding cues exacerbates both physiological and psychological breastfeeding challenges, yet many mothers feed on a schedule or report crying rather than early hunger cues as the primary motivation for initiating feeding. Our data suggest that culturally-mediated parenting practices like mother–infant physical contact may shape maternal responsiveness to early hunger cues, providing a new potential opportunity for intervention to support breastfeeding mothers in meeting their goals.

Author Contributions: Conceptualization, E.E.L.; Methodology, E.E.L.; Formal Analysis, E.E.L.; Investigation, E.E.L.; Writing-Original Draft Preparation, E.E.L.; Writing—Review & Editing, C.H.L. and L.J.C.; Supervision, C.H.L. and L.J.C.

References and Note

1. Victora, C.G.; Bahl, R.; Barros, A.J.; França, G.V.; Horton, S.; Krasevec, J. Breastfeeding in the 21st century: Epidemiology, mechanisms, and lifelong effect. *Lancet* **2016**, *387*, 475–490. [PubMed]
2. Bode, L.; McGuire, M.; Rodriguez, J.M.; Geddes, D.T.; Hassiotou, F.; Hartmann, P.E.; McGuire, M.K. It's alive: Microbes and cells in human milk and their potential benefits to mother and infant. *Adv. Nutr.* **2014**, *5*, 571–573. [CrossRef] [PubMed]
3. World Health Organization. Health Topics—Breastfeeding. Available online: http://www.who.int/topics/breastfeeding/en/ (accessed on 16 August 2018).
4. Bartick, M.C.; Schwarz, E.B.; Green, B.D.; Jegier, B.J.; Reinhold, A.G.; Colaizy, T.T.; Bogen, D.L.; Schaefer, A.J.; Stuebe, A.M. Suboptimal breastfeeding in the United States: Maternal and pediatric health outcomes and costs. *Matern. Child Nutr.* **2017**, *13*, e12366. [CrossRef]
5. Centers for Disease Control and Prevention. Breastfeeding Report Card—United States. 2018. Available online: https://www.cdc.gov/breastfeeding/pdf/2018breastfeedingreportcard.pdf (accessed on 16 August 2018).
6. Shloim, N.; Vereijken, C.M.; Blundell, P.; Hetherington, M.M. Looking for cues-infant communication of hunger and satiation during milk feeding. *Appetite* **2017**, *108*, 74–82. [PubMed]
7. Woolridge, M.W. Baby-controlled breastfeeding: Biocultural implications. In *Breastfeeding: Biocultural Perspectives*; Stuart-Macadam, P., Dettwyler, K.A., Eds.; Walter de Gruyter: Hawthorne, NY, USA, 1995; pp. 217–242.
8. Kent, J.C. How breastfeeding works. *J. Midwifery Women's Health* **2007**, *52*, 564–570. [CrossRef]
9. Kirk, A.T.; Alder, S.C.; King, J.D. Cue-based oral feeding clinical pathway results in earlier attainment of full oral feeding in premature infants. *J. Perinatol.* **2007**, *27*, 572–578. [PubMed]
10. Hodges, E.A.; Hughes, S.O.; Hopkinson, J.; Fisher, J.O. Maternal decisions about the initiation and termination of infant feeding. *Appetite* **2008**, *50*, 333–339. [CrossRef] [PubMed]
11. Konner, M. Hunter-gatherer infancy and childhood. In *Hunter-Gatherer Childhoods: Evolutionary, Developmental, & Cultural Perspectives*; Hewlett, B.S., Lamb, M.E., Eds.; Aldine Transaction: New Brunswick, NJ, USA, 2005; pp. 19–64.
12. Hewlett, B.S.; Lamb, M.E. Integrating evolution, culture and developmental psychology: Explaining caregiver-infant proximity and responsiveness in central Africa and the USA. In *Between Culture and Biology: Perspectives on Ontogenetic Development*; Cambridge University Press: Cambridge, UK, 2002; Volume 8, pp. 241–269.
13. Konner, M. Hunter-gatherer infancy and childhood: The! Kung and others. In *Hunter-Gatherer Childhoods*; Routledge: Oxford, UK, 2017; pp. 19–64.
14. Hewlett, B.S.; Lamb, M.E.; Shannon, D.; Leyendecker, B.; Schölmerich, A. Culture and early infancy among central African foragers and farmers. *Dev. Psychol.* **1998**, *34*, 653–661. [CrossRef] [PubMed]
15. Richman, A.L.; Miller, P.M.; LeVine, R.A. Cultural and educational variations in maternal responsiveness. *Dev. Psychol.* **1992**, *28*, 614–621.
16. Morelli, G.A.; Rogoff, B.; Oppenheim, D.; Goldsmith, D. Cultural variation in infants' sleeping arrangements: Questions of independence. *Dev. Psychol.* **1992**, *28*, 604–613. [CrossRef]
17. Kärtner, J.; Keller, H.; Yovsi, R.D. Mother–infant interaction during the first 3 months: The emergence of culture-specific contingency patterns. *Child Dev.* **2010**, *81*, 540–554. [CrossRef] [PubMed]
18. LeVine, R.A.; Miller, P.M.; Richman, A.L.; LeVine, S. Education and mother-infant interaction: A Mexican case study. In *Parents' Cultural Belief Systems: Their Origins, Expressions, and Consequences*; Harkness, S., Super, M.K., Eds.; The Guilford Press: San Antonio, TX, USA, 1996; pp. 254–269.
19. Caudill, W.A.; Schooler, C. Child behavior and child rearing in Japan and the United States: An interim report. *J. Nerv. Ment. Dis.* **1973**, *157*, 323–338. [CrossRef]
20. Kärtner, J.; Keller, H.; Lamm, B.; Abels, M.; Yovsi, R.D.; Chaudhary, N.; Su, Y. Similarities and differences in contingency experiences of 3-month-olds across sociocultural contexts. *Infant Behav. Dev.* **2008**, *31*, 488–500. [CrossRef] [PubMed]
21. Barr, R.G.; Konner, M.; Bakeman, R.; Adamson, L. Crying in! Kung San infants: A test of the cultural specificity hypothesis. *Dev. Med. Child Neurol.* **1991**, *33*, 601–610. [CrossRef] [PubMed]
22. Dettwyler, K.A. More than nutrition: Breastfeeding in urban Mali. *Med. Anthropol. Q.* **1988**, *2*, 172–183. [CrossRef]

23. Chapin, B.L. Attachment in rural Sri Lanka: The shape of caregiver sensitivity, communication, and autonomy. In *Attachment Reconsidered*; Palgrave Macmillan: New York, NY, USA, 2013; pp. 143–163.
24. Harkness, S.; Super, C.M. Themes and variations: Parental ethnotheories in Western cultures. In *Parenting Beliefs, Behaviors, and Parent-Child Relations: A Cross-Cultural Perspective*; Rubin, K.H., Chung, O.B., Eds.; Psychology Press: Florence, KY, USA, 2006; pp. 61–79.
25. Keller, H.; Borke, J.; Staufenbiel, T.; Yovsi, R.D.; Abels, M.; Papaligoura, Z.; Jensen, H.; Lohaus, A.; Chaudhary, N.; Lo, W.; et al. Distal and proximal parenting as alternative parenting strategies during infants' early months of life: A cross-cultural study. *Int. J. Behav. Dev.* **2009**, *33*, 412–420. [CrossRef]
26. St James-Roberts, I.; Alvarez, M.; Csipke, E.; Abramsky, T.; Goodwin, J.; Sorgenfrei, E. Infant crying and sleeping in London, Copenhagen and when parents adopt a "proximal" form of care. *Pediatrics* **2006**, *117*, e1146–e1155. [CrossRef] [PubMed]
27. Hodges, E.A.; Johnson, S.L.; Hughes, S.O.; Hopkinson, J.M.; Butte, N.F.; Fisher, J.O. Development of the responsiveness to child feeding cues scale. *Appetite* **2013**, *65*, 210–219. [CrossRef] [PubMed]
28. Pinchevski-Kadir, S.; Shust-Barequet, S.; Zajicek, M.; Leibovich, M.; Strauss, T.; Leibovitch, L.; Morag, I. Direct feeding at the breast is associated with breast milk feeding duration among preterm infants. *Nutrients* **2017**, *9*, 1202. [CrossRef] [PubMed]
29. Pang, W.W.; Bernard, J.Y.; Thavamani, G.; Chan, Y.H.; Fok, D.; Soh, S.E.; Chua, M.C.; Lim, S.B.; Shek, L.P.; Yap, F.; et al. Direct vs. expressed breast milk feeding: Relation to duration of breastfeeding. *Nutrients* **2017**, *9*, 547. [CrossRef] [PubMed]
30. Dewey, K.G.; Lonnerdal, B. Infant self-regulation of breast milk intake. *Acta Paediatr.* **1986**, *75*, 893–898. [CrossRef]
31. Uvnäs-Moberg, K. Oxytocin may mediate the benefits of positive social interaction and emotions. *Psychoneuroendocrinology* **1998**, *23*, 819–835. [CrossRef]
32. Perrella, S.L.; Williams, J.; Nathan, E.A.; Fenwick, J.; Hartmann, P.E.; Geddes, D.T. Influences on breastfeeding outcomes for healthy term and preterm/sick infants. *Breastfeed. Med.* **2012**, *7*, 255–261. [CrossRef]
33. Keller, H.; Poortinga, Y.H.; Scholmerich, A.; Butterworth, G.; Schölmerich, A. *Between Culture and Biology: Perspectives on Ontogenetic Development*; Cambridge University Press: Cambridge, UK, 2002; Volume 8.
34. Kent, J.C.; Mitoulas, L.R.; Cregan, M.D.; Ramsay, D.T.; Doherty, D.A.; Hartmann, P.E. Volume and frequency of breastfeedings and fat content of breast milk throughout the day. *Pediatrics* **2006**, *117*, e387–e395. [CrossRef] [PubMed]
35. Colombo, L.; Crippa, B.L.; Consonni, D.; Bettinelli, M.E.; Agosti, V.; Mangino, G.; Bezze, E.N.; Mauri, P.A.; Zanotta, L.; Roggero, P.; et al. Breastfeeding determinants in healthy term newborns. *Nutrients* **2018**, *10*, 48. [CrossRef] [PubMed]
36. Ventura, A.K. Associations between breastfeeding and maternal responsiveness: A systematic review of the literature. *Adv. Nutr.* **2017**, *8*, 495–510. [CrossRef] [PubMed]
37. Manz, F.; Manz, I.; Lennert, T. Zur Geschichte der ärztlichen Stillempfehlungen in Deutschland. *Monatsschrift Kinderheilkunde* **1997**, *145*, 572–587. [CrossRef]
38. Iacovou, M.; Sevilla, A. Infant feeding: The effects of scheduled vs. on-demand feeding on mothers' wellbeing and children's cognitive development. *Eur. J. Public Health* **2012**, *23*, 13–19. [CrossRef] [PubMed]
39. Li, R.; Fein, S.B.; Grummer-Strawn, L.M. Do infants fed from bottles lack self-regulation of milk intake compared with directly breastfed infants? *Pediatrics* **2010**. [CrossRef] [PubMed]
40. Ventura, A.K.; Mennella, J.A. An experimental approach to study individual differences in infants' intake and satiation behaviors during bottle-feeding. *Child. Obes.* **2017**, *13*, 44–52. [CrossRef] [PubMed]
41. Piper, S.; Parks, P.L. Predicting the duration of lactation: Evidence from a national survey. *Birth* **1996**, *23*, 7–12. [CrossRef] [PubMed]
42. Fouts, H.N.; Hewlett, B.S.; Lamb, M.E. A biocultural approach to breastfeeding interactions in Central Africa. *Am. Anthropol.* **2012**, *114*, 123–136. [CrossRef] [PubMed]
43. True, M.; Pisani, L.; Oumar, F. Infant-mother attachment among the Dogon of Mali. *Child Dev.* **2001**, *72*, 1451–1466. [CrossRef] [PubMed]
44. Tessier, R.; Cristo, M.; Velez, S.; Girón, M.; de Calume, Z.F.; Ruiz-Paláez, J.G.; Charpak, Y.; Charpak, N. Kangaroo mother care and the bonding hypothesis. *Pediatrics* **1998**, *102*, e17. [CrossRef] [PubMed]
45. Pinheiro, J.; Bates, D.; DebRoy, S.; Sarkar, D. Linear and nonlinear mixed effects models. R package version 3. 2014. pp. 1–137.

46. Bates, D.; Maechler, M.; Bolker, B. *lme4: Linear Mixedeffects Models Using S4 Classes;* R Package Version 0.999375-42; R Foundation for Statistical Computing: Vienna, Austria, 2011.
47. Bakermans-Kranenburg, M.J.; van IJzendoorn, M.H.; Riem, M.M.; Tops, M.; Alink, L.R. Oxytocin decreases handgrip force in reaction to infant crying in females without harsh parenting experiences. *Soc. Cogn. Affect. Neurosci.* **2011**, *7*, 951–957. [CrossRef] [PubMed]
48. Riem, M.M.; Bakermans-Kranenburg, M.J.; van IJzendoorn, M.H.; Out, D.; Rombouts, S.A. Attachment in the brain: Adult attachment representations predict amygdala and behavioral responses to infant crying. *Attach. Hum. Dev.* **2012**, *14*, 533–551. [CrossRef] [PubMed]
49. Neumann, I.D. Brain oxytocin: A key regulator of emotional and social behaviours in both females and males. *J. Neuroendocrinol.* **2008**, *20*, 858–865. [CrossRef] [PubMed]
50. Light, K.C.; Smith, T.E.; Johns, J.M.; Brownley, K.A.; Hofheimer, J.A.; Amico, J.A. Oxytocin responsivity in mothers of infants: A preliminary study of relationships with blood pressure during laboratory stress and normal ambulatory activity. *Health Psychol.* **2000**, *19*, 560–567. [CrossRef] [PubMed]
51. Seltzer, L.J.; Ziegler, T.E.; Pollak, S.D. Social vocalizations can release oxytocin in humans. *Proc. R. Soc. Lond. B Biol. Sci.* **2010**, *277*, 2661–2666. [CrossRef] [PubMed]
52. Gross, R.S.; Fierman, A.H.; Mendelsohn, A.L.; Chiasson, M.A.; Rosenberg, T.J.; Scheinmann, R.; Messito, M.J. Maternal perceptions of infant hunger, satiety, and pressuring feeding styles in an urban Latina WIC population. *Acad. Pediatr.* **2010**, *10*, 29–35. [CrossRef] [PubMed]
53. Heinrichs, M.; Baumgartner, T.; Kirschbaum, C.; Ehlert, U. Social support and oxytocin interact to suppress cortisol and subjective responses to psychosocial stress. *Biol. Psychiatry* **2003**, *54*, 1389–1398. [CrossRef]
54. Kim, P.; Feldman, R.; Mayes, L.C.; Eicher, V.; Thompson, N.; Leckman, J.F.; Swain, J.E. Breastfeeding, brain activation to own infant cry, and maternal sensitivity. *J. Child Psychol. Psychiatry* **2011**, *52*, 907–915. [CrossRef] [PubMed]
55. Little, E.E.; Carver, L.J.; Legare, C.H. Cultural variation in triadic infant caregiver object exploration. *Child Dev.* **2016**, *87*, 1130–1145. [CrossRef] [PubMed]
56. Henrich, J.; Heine, S.J.; Norenzayan, A. Most people are not WEIRD. *Nature* **2010**, *466*, 29. [CrossRef] [PubMed]
57. Nielsen, M.; Haun, D.; Kärtner, J.; Legare, C.H. The persistent sampling bias in developmental psychology: A call to action. *J. Exp. Child Psychol.* **2017**, *162*, 31–38. [CrossRef] [PubMed]
58. Bartick, M.; Tomori, C.; Ball, H.L. Babies in boxes and the missing links on safe sleep: Human evolution and cultural revolution. *Matern. Child Nutr.* **2018**, *14*, e12544. [CrossRef] [PubMed]
59. Trevathan, W.R.; McKenna, J.J. Evolutionary environments of human birth and infancy: Insights to apply to contemporary life. *Children's Environ.* **1994**, *1*, 88–104.
60. Lozoff, B.; Brittenham, G. Infant care: Cache or carry. *J. Pediatr.* **1979**, *95*, 478–483. [CrossRef]
61. Bazzano, A.N.; Kaji, A.; Felker-Kantor, E.; Bazzano, L.A.; Potts, K.S. Qualitative studies of infant and young child feeding in lower-income countries: A systematic review and synthesis of dietary patterns. *Nutrients* **2017**, *9*, 1140. [CrossRef] [PubMed]
62. Moore, E.R.; Anderson, G.C.; Bergman, N.; Dowswell, T. Early skin-to-skin contact for mothers and their healthy newborn infants. *Cochrane Database Syst. Rev.* **2012**. [CrossRef]
63. Ludington-Hoe, S.M.; Morgan, K.; Abouelfettoh, A. A clinical guideline for implementation of kangaroo care with premature infants of 30 or more weeks' postmenstrual age. *Adv. Neonatal Care* **2008**, *8*, S3–S23. [CrossRef]
64. Anisfeld, E.; Casper, V.; Nozyce, M.; Cunningham, N. Does infant carrying promote attachment? An experimental study of the effects of increased physical contact on the development of attachment. *Child. Dev.* **1990**, *61*, 1617–1627. [CrossRef] [PubMed]
65. Pisacane, A.; Continisio, P.; Filosa, C.; Tagliamonte, V.; Continisio, G.I. Use of baby carriers to increase breastfeeding duration among term infants: The effects of an educational intervention in Italy. *Acta Paediatr.* **2012**, *101*, e434–e438. [CrossRef] [PubMed]

15

Variability of Water-Soluble Forms of Choline Concentrations in Human Milk during Storage, after Pasteurization and among Women

Sara Moukarzel [1,‡], Alejandra M. Wiedeman [2,3,‡], Lynda S. Soberanes [2,4], Roger A. Dyer [2,3], Sheila M. Innis [2,3,†] and Yvonne Lamers [2,4,*]

1 Larsson-Rosenquist Foundation Mother-Milk-Infant Center of Research Excellence, University of California, San Diego, CA 92093, USA; smoukarzel@ucsd.edu

2 British Columbia Children's Hospital Research Institute, Vancouver, BC V5Z 4H4, Canada; awiedeman@bcchr.ca (A.M.W.); lynda.soberanes@gmail.com (L.S.S.); radyer@mail.ubc.ca (R.A.D.); sheila.innis@ubc.ca (S.M.I.)

3 Department of Pediatrics, Faculty of Medicine, The University of British Columbia, Vancouver, BC V5Z 4H4, Canada

4 Food, Nutrition, and Health Program, Faculty of Land and Food Systems, The University of British Columbia, Vancouver, BC V6T 1Z4, Canada

* Correspondence: yvonne.lamers@ubc.ca

† Deceased.

‡ Shared first authorship.

Abstract: Choline is critical for infant development and mother's milk is the sole source of choline for fully breastfed infants until six months of age. Human milk choline consists to 85% of water-soluble forms of choline including free choline (FC), phosphocholine (PhosC), and glycerophosphocholine (GPC). Donor milk requires safe handling procedures such as cold storage and pasteurization. However, the stability of water-soluble forms of choline during these processes is not known. The objectives of this research were to determine the effect of storage and pasteurization on milk choline concentration, and the diurnal intra- and inter-individual variability of water-soluble choline forms. Milk samples were collected from healthy women who were fully breastfeeding a full-term, singleton infant <6 months. Milk total water-soluble forms of choline, PhosC, and GPC concentrations did not change during storage at room temperature for up to 4 h. Individual and total water-soluble forms of choline concentrations did not change after storage for 24 h in the refrigerator or for up to one week in the household freezer. Holder pasteurization decreased PhosC and GPC, and thereby total water-soluble choline form concentrations by <5%. We did not observe diurnal variations in PhosC and total water-soluble forms of choline concentrations, but significant differences in FC and GPC concentrations across five sampling time points throughout one day. In conclusion, these outcomes contribute new knowledge for the derivation of evidence-informed guidelines for the handling and storage of expressed human milk as well as the development of optimized milk collection and storage protocols for research studies.

Keywords: human milk; donor milk; choline; phosphocholine; storage; pasteurization; milk banking; pumping; breastfeeding; lactation

1. Introduction

Choline is an essential nutrient with crucial roles in brain function, neurodevelopment, and growth [1,2]. Biological roles of choline include neurogenesis and synapse formation in the form of acetylcholine, membrane biogenesis, cell division, lipid transports, and myelination in the form of choline phospholipids, and as a methyl donor in the form of its oxidation product betaine [3–6]. Betaine contributes to the generation of *S*-adenosylmethionine, which is the main methyl donor involved in creatine and phosphatidylcholine synthesis, and DNA methylation, among other biochemical reactions [7]. Choline adequacy in early infancy and rapid stages of growth is critical to support membrane formation, cell proliferation, and parenchymal growth [6].

Exclusive breastfeeding ad libitum is the recommended feeding practice for the first six months of life, with continued breastfeeding up to two years of age [8]. Human milk contains various forms of the essential nutrient choline. The three water-soluble forms of choline, i.e., free choline (FC), phosphocholine (PhosC), and glycerophosphocholine (GPC), contribute to approximately 85% of total choline in human milk; the lipid-soluble phosphatidylcholine and sphingomyelin account for the remaining 15% [9–13].

The practice of human milk pumping and storage for later use is on the rise both at home and in clinical settings to accommodate various situations when feeding human milk at the breast is not possible, e.g., mothers returning to work; insufficient volume of mother's own milk, and need for donor milk [14,15]. Current guidelines for the safe handling of expressed human milk focus largely on microbiological safety, whereby Holder pasteurization (at 62.5 °C for 30 min) of donor milk is mandatory in all North American hospitals [16]. Additionally, it is recommended that milk be stored in the refrigerator at ≤4 °C for no more than eight days, and in the freezer at −17 °C for up to 12 months [17]. Whilst evidence suggests that refrigeration, freezing and pasteurization impact human milk concentration of folate, vitamin B6, vitamin C, and other nutrients to various degrees [18–21], the effect of pasteurization and short- and long-term storage at different temperatures on water-soluble forms of choline in expressed human milk is not known.

Water-soluble forms of choline concentrations in human milk may vary within and between women. Higher maternal dietary choline intake increases milk concentrations of water-soluble, yet not fat-soluble, forms of choline, as shown in a 12-week dose-response feeding study and a supplementation trial from 18 gestational weeks to 90 days postpartum [11,13]. No consistent changes in total concentration of water-soluble forms of choline in human milk were observed in six women over a time period of 72 h [22]. The diurnal changes and variability of individual water-soluble choline forms among women have not been studied to date. Understanding these variabilities has important implications for designing study protocols (e.g., sampling techniques) that focus on identifying the determinants of choline in human milk and infant outcomes due to milk choline consumption.

The objectives of this research were to determine the effect of cold storage and pasteurization on the concentrations of water-soluble forms of choline in human milk, and to determine the intra- and inter-individual variability of water-soluble forms of choline concentrations in human milk within a day. Water-soluble forms of choline seem stable during short-term cold storage and most forms remained unchanged after four hours of storage at room temperature and six months of storage at ultra-low freezing temperatures, as employed in research settings. Holder pasteurization significantly impacted milk concentrations of water-soluble forms of choline, but to a small extent that is outweighed by the microbiological safety benefits of pasteurization. We observed intra-individual variability of individual but not total water-soluble forms of choline throughout one day, and recommend standardized sampling protocols for research studies.

2. Materials and Methods

2.1. Participants and Study Design

The research consisted of two cross-sectional studies, i.e., the stability and variability study, as well as the secondary analysis of bio-banked milk samples for the pasteurization study. For all studies, healthy women who were exclusively breastfeeding a healthy, full-term and singleton infant <6 months of age were eligible to participate. Exclusion criteria included: suffering from diabetes mellitus Type 1 or 2, or any chronic disease involving fat metabolism, taking routine medications known to influence fat metabolism, or consumption of more than 1 alcoholic drink per day.

2.1.1. Stability Study

A convenience sample of 6 mothers of 2- to 6- month old infants was included in this study. Women were recruited through active and passive recruitment methods in the Greater Vancouver area in 2014. Signed informed consent was obtained prior to enrolment. Information on maternal and infant age, sociodemographic status, supplement use, and general infant health, was collected using a self-administered questionnaire. Ethical approval was granted by the University of British Columbia and the British Columbia Children's and Women's (C&W) Hospital Research Ethics Board (H12-03191).

Women provided a fresh complete milk expression collected in the morning (between 9:00–10:00 a.m.) using a commercial pump (Medela); samples were immediately transferred on ice to the lab to be aliquoted and analyzed. One milk aliquot was analyzed immediately, with the rest of the samples being stored at different temperatures for different durations (see Supplemental Table S1), prior to analysis.

2.1.2. Pasteurization Study

Mid-feed human milk samples (milk collected after breastfeeding or pumping milk for approximately 3 min) from mothers of 1-month old infants were used in the pasteurization study; these bio-banked samples were derived from a completed, randomized controlled trial studying the effect of DHA supplementation during pregnancy on the cognitive and visual outcomes on infants [23]. The study was approved by C&W REB (H03-70242). A subset of milk samples was randomly selected from the bio-banked samples that had been stored for 5–9 years at −80 °C. In the original study, milk samples were immediately frozen at home for a maximum time of 3 days, and transferred on ice to the lab where they were frozen at −80 °C until analysis. Original milk samples obtained from the participants were thawed on ice, homogenized by gentle mixing, and divided in two aliquots. The first aliquot was stored at −20 °C for 1–2 h, and the second aliquot underwent Holder pasteurization in a water bath. Water-soluble forms of choline were quantified before and after pasteurization on the same day.

2.1.3. Variability Study

Twenty women were enrolled in this cross-sectional study. Recruitment and enrolment procedures were similar to those described for the stability study. Sociodemographic, health and supplement use data were collected using the same self-administered questionnaire as in the stability study. Ethical approval was granted by the University of British Columbia and the British Columbia Children's and Women's Hospital Research Ethics Board (H12-03191).

Each participant provided 5 mid-feed milk samples at different times throughout one day. For feasibility purposes, the five different time points were flexible as follows: before breakfast, before lunch, 45–60 min after lunch, 45–60 min after dinner, and before bedtime. Participants were instructed to place the vials in their home freezers immediately after pumping. Frozen samples were transferred to the lab on ice the day after collection and stored at −80 °C for 2 weeks, when choline analysis was completed.

2.2. Human Milk Choline Quantitation

Concentrations of water-soluble forms of choline in milk were determined using isotope dilution liquid chromatography tandem mass spectrometry as previously described [24]. In brief, aliquots of 20 μL of human milk were transferred to Eppendorf tubes containing 10 μL of deuterium-labeled internal standards (choline-d9, PhosC-d9, GPC-d9) and vortexed. Protein was precipitated with 30 μL of methanol with 0.1% formic acid. The supernatant was recovered after centrifugation at 18,000 × *g* at 4 °C for 10 min, transferred to an autosampler vial and mixed with acetonitrile with 0.1% formic acid in dilutions of 1:5. The inter-assay and intra-assay coefficient of variation (CV) based on 5 replicates were as follows: For FC, 5.5% and 4.1%; for PhosC, 6.4% and 5.2%; and for GPC 9.5% and 2.3%; respectively.

2.3. Statistical Analysis

Participant characteristics are presented using descriptive statistics. Normality of data distribution was assessed using Shapiro–Wilk test. Differences in milk concentrations of water-soluble forms of choline under different storage conditions were determined using the related-samples Friedman test, followed by Wilcoxon signed-ranks test as post-hoc analysis and adjusted using the Bonferroni correction. Differences in water-soluble forms of choline concentrations after pasteurization were determined using the Wilcoxon signed-ranks test. Intra-individual variability in water-soluble forms of choline concentrations was determined using the related-samples Friedman test, followed by Wilcoxon signed-ranks test as post-hoc analysis and adjusted using the Bonferroni correction. Analyses were performed using the IBM SPSS statistics software (IBM SPSS Statistics for Windows, Version 25.0. SPSS Inc., Chicago, IL, USA). Level of significance was set at p values < 0.05.

3. Results

3.1. Participant Characteristics

The characteristics of women included in each study are summarized in Table 1.

Table 1. Participant characteristics of each study.

Characteristics Total Sample Size	Stability Study (n = 6)	Pasteurization Study (n = 33)	Variability Study (n = 20)
Age, *y*	35 ± 2 [1]	34 ± 4	32 ± 4
Postpartum, *mo*	4.0 (3.0) [2]	1	4.5 (3.0)
First-time breastfeeding, *n* (%)	6 (100)	20 (61)	10 (50)
Ethnic background, *n* (%)			
European	2 (33)	26 (79)	11 (55)
Latin American	2 (33)	2 (6)	4 (20)
Middle Eastern	0	3 (9)	3 (15)
First Nation	1 (17)	0	1 (5)
Chinese Asian	1 (17)	2 (6)	1 (5)

[1] Mean ± SD; [2] median (IQR).

3.2. Stability of Water-Soluble Choline Forms at Different Storage Conditions

The concentration of total water-soluble forms of choline, PhosC, and GPC did not significantly change during storage at room temperature for up to 4 h (Figure 1, Supplemental Table S2). Compared to fresh milk samples, i.e., baseline values, only FC concentration significantly increased after 3 h and 4 h of storage at room temperature.

We observed no changes in total water-soluble forms of choline and PhosC concentrations independent of condition and duration of cold storage, including in the refrigerator at 4 °C for 24 h, in the freezer at −20 °C for up to 1 week, and in the ultra-low freezer at −80 °C for up to 6 months (Figure 1, Supplemental Table S2). The concentration of FC and GPC did not change after storage at 4 °C for 24 h or at −20 °C for up to 1 week, but significantly increased between baseline and 6 months of storage at −80 °C.

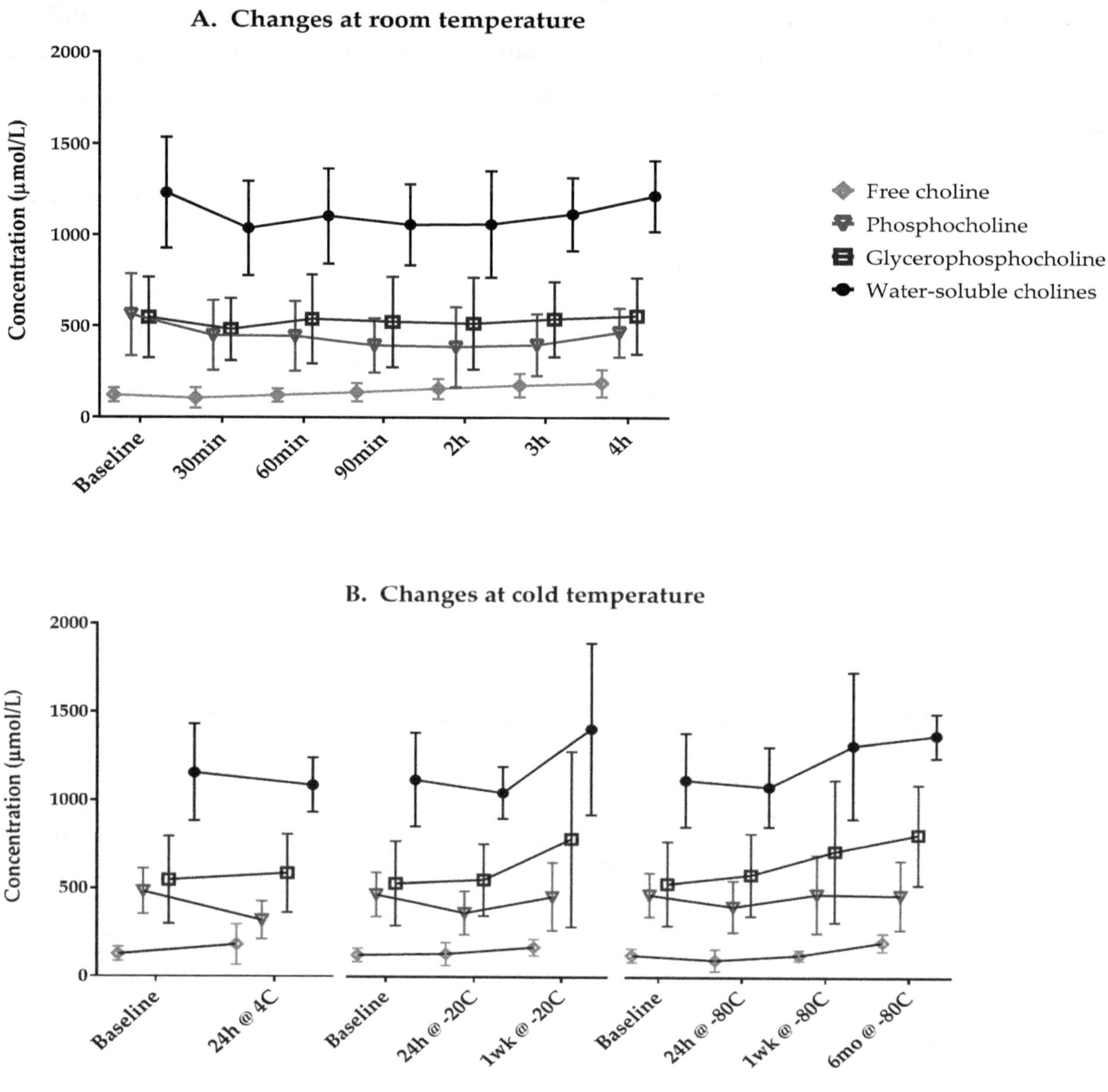

Figure 1. Changes in water-soluble forms of choline concentrations in human milk at (**A**) room temperature ($n = 6$) and (**B**) under different cold storage conditions ($n = 5$). Data presented as mean ± SD.

3.3. Stability of Water-Soluble Choline Forms during Pasteurization

Total water-soluble forms of choline concentrations significantly decreased by approximately 5% after Holder pasteurization in 33 milk samples (Table 2). This decrease seems to be largely driven by the decrease in the main water-soluble forms of choline in human milk, i.e., GPC and PhosC. The concentrations of GPC and PhosC showed a mean decrease of 4%–5%. Median FC concentration remained constant and did not seem to be impacted by exposure to pasteurization.

Table 2. Water-soluble forms of choline concentrations in human milk before and after Holder pasteurization [1].

Choline Form	Before, µmol/L	After, µmol/L	Difference, µmol/L	Difference, %	*p*-Value [2]
Free choline					
Mean ± SD	124 ± 60	124 ± 58	0.6 ± 14	1.3 ± 10	0.893
Median (min; max)	117 (47.9; 293)	120 (44.6; 275)	−1 (−29; 46)	−0.5 (−18; 33.0)	
Phosphocholine					
Mean ± SD	675 ± 220	632 ± 189	−43 ± 73	−4.7 ± 10	0.003
Median (min; max)	676 (230; 1131)	621 (261; 960)	−41 (−238; 111)	−6.5 (−21; 25)	
Glycerophosphocholine					
Mean ± SD	442 ± 181	425 ± 181	−17 ± 43	−3.6 ± 10	0.015
Median (min; max)	381 (243; 904)	387 (211; 994)	-20 (-122; 97)	-5.6 (-21; 26)	
Total water-soluble choline					
Mean ± SD	1241 ± 249	1186 ± 201	−56 ± 124	−3.4 ± 10	0.017
Median (min; max)	1229 (789; 1794)	1136 (792; 1566)	−63 (358; 231)	−4.8 (−20; 27)	

[1] $n = 33$ samples; [2] Wilcoxon signed-rank test to test for differences between before and after Holder pasteurization.

3.4. Intra- and Inter-Individual Variability of Water-Soluble Forms of Choline Concentrations

Total water-soluble forms of choline and PhosC concentrations did not vary significantly within a woman during the day based on analysis of five milk samples per mother (Table 3). However, significant changes in FC and GPC were found. Posthoc analysis showed a 22.7% increase in FC from T1 to T4 ($p = 0.027$) and a 12.2% decrease in GPC from T1 to T3 ($p = 0.027$).

Additionally, as shown in Figure 2, intra-individual variability in FC and GPC concentrations varied between women, whereby milk FC and GPC concentrations showed a large variability in some, i.e., 2 or 3 mothers, with milk samples of most other mothers reflecting minimal variability.

Table 3. Concentrations of water-soluble forms of choline in mid-feed milk samples collected at five different time points within one day [1].

Choline Form	T1	T2	T3	T4	T5	*p* [2]
Free choline						
Median (IQR)	119 (73.5)	125 (63.7)	131 (75.4)	146 (119)	132 (81.1)	0.029
Range	51.9–156	60.4–253	69.2–474	59.9–453	505–332	
Phosphocholine						
Median (IQR)	490 (328)	488 (270)	441 (359)	457 (330)	482 (335)	0.545
Range	138–906	82.1–1113	115–1120	78.9–1188	88.9–958	
Glycerophosphocholine						
Median (IQR)	625 (194)	559 (280)	549 (320)	533 (275)	682 (408)	0.008
Range	187–1363	107–1115	104–1188	99.1–1268	155–1445	
Total water-soluble choline						
Median (IQR)	1727 (366)	1219 (410)	1200 (308)	1289 (404)	1230 (344)	0.224
Range	955–2117	768–1817	809–1894	752–1896	652–2729	

[1] $n = 20$ mothers exclusively breastfeeding 2–6 months old infants. T1, milk collected before breakfast; T2, before lunch; T3, 45–60 min after lunch; T4, 45–60 min after dinner; T5, before bedtime. [2] p values for repeated-measures Friedman test for difference across time points within a woman.

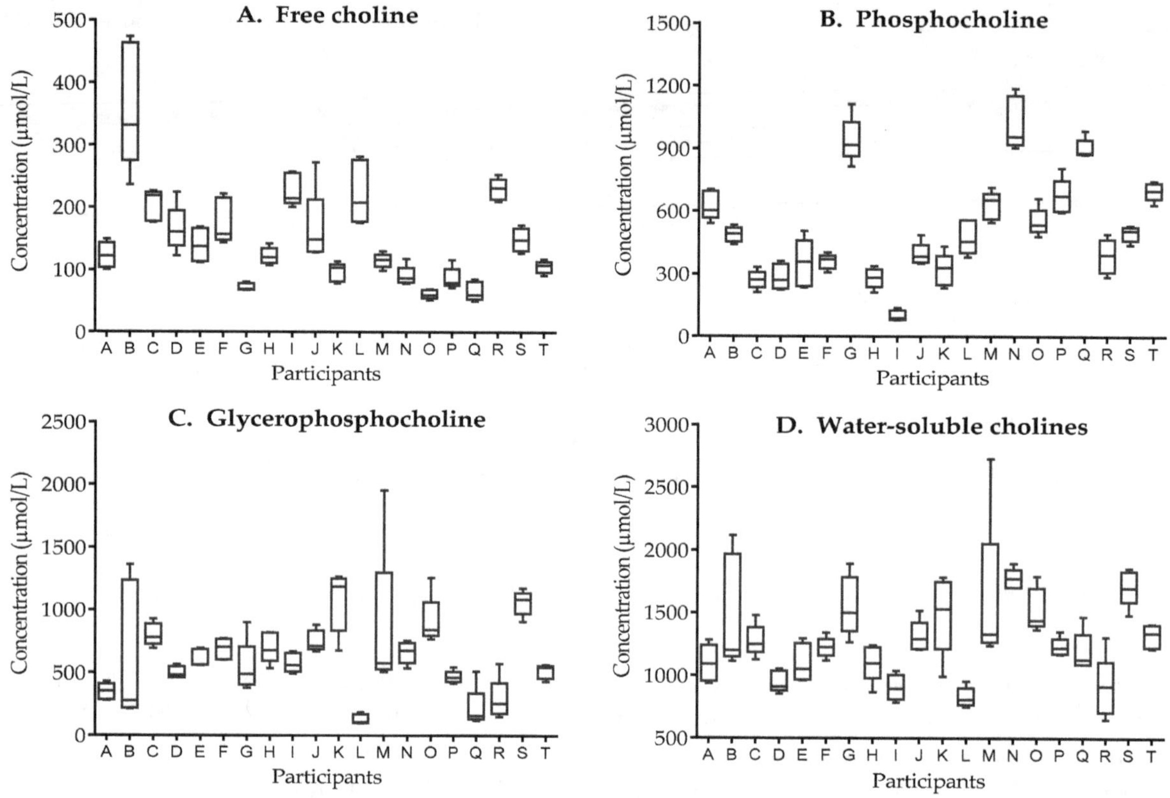

Figure 2. Intra-individual variability of human milk concentration of (**A**) free choline, (**B**) phosphocholine, (**C**) glycerophosphocholine, and (**D**) total water-soluble forms of choline. Boxes represent median and 25th–75th percentile; whiskers represent minimum and maximum values. Data for each participant (n = 20, represented on the x-axis) includes five mid-feed milk samples collected at separate feeds on a single day.

4. Discussion

In this study, we report three findings on the stability of water-soluble forms of choline in expressed human milk: First, storing human milk for 3 or 4 h at room temperature significantly increases milk FC concentration. Second, thawing human milk after 6 months of freezing at −80 °C significantly increases FC and GPC concentrations. Third, Holder pasteurization decreases PhosC and GPC concentrations, and thereby lowers total concentration of water-soluble forms of choline. Additionally, we report that total concentration of water-soluble forms of choline does not underlie diurnal variations within a woman; however, significant diurnal variations in FC and GPC concentrations may occur among some, but not all, women. These findings contribute to the literature being harnessed to develop evidence-informed guidelines for the handling and storage of expressed human milk as well as the development of optimized milk collection and storage protocols for research studies.

Milk expression for in-home use or human milk banking have become increasingly recognized as a first best alternative to direct breastfeeding. While ensuring microbiological safety of expressed milk remains a top priority, maintaining milk's bioactive and nutritional quality is an important weighing factor in developing milk handling and storage guidelines. The impact of storage and pasteurization on the immunological properties, digestive enzymes, antioxidant capacity, and macro- and micronutrient composition in human milk has been recently reviewed [19,25–29], with limited data on water-soluble forms of choline. In an older study, Zeisel et al. [22] compared fresh milk to either samples incubated for 15 min at 37 °C or to samples frozen for 72 h at −10 °C followed by incubation at 37 °C for 15 min. Using radioisotope labeled choline compounds, the authors showed that neither of the two milk handling and storage conditions resulted in significant changes in FC concentration. These findings combined with ours suggest that following current recommendation of keeping freshly expressed milk up to 4 h at room temperature should not significantly alter the composition of water-soluble forms of choline, except for minor possible increases in FC. The possible mechanism(s) underlying the increase in FC concentration cannot be determined in our study as designed.

The increase in FC concentration may be explained by the enzymatic breakdown of the lipid-soluble choline compounds phosphatidylcholine and sphingomyelin. The presence of these phospholipids within the milk fat globule membrane, a complex tri-layer of proteins and lipids, poses an analytical challenge for their accurate quantification [30]. In addition to identifying factors influencing the variability of choline forms in human milk in future studies, it is critical to also investigate whether changes in the composition of choline forms in milk, not total choline concentration per se, have functional implications for infant health and development. Choline has a wide array of functions that support infant growth and development. As an essential component of phosphatidylcholine and sphingomyelin, choline is involved in the maintenance of cell membrane structural integrity and signaling pathways, as well as in parenchymal growth, cell proliferation, and membrane formation [3–6]. Choline, via its oxidized form betaine, also functions as a methyl group donor in the generation of *S*-adenosylmethionine [7]. Additionally, choline is crucial for brain function as precursor of the neurotransmitter acetylcholine [4]. To date, the contribution of different choline forms in human milk to the variety in choline functions in the developing infant is largely unknown and merits further investigation.

The cold storage conditions we tested are relevant to home and clinical use (refrigeration temperature typically around 4 °C and freezing at −20 °C) and to storage conditions in research settings (ultra-low freeze storage at −80 °C). Our findings suggest that short-term storage of milk aliquots in the refrigerator (at 4 °C) for 1 day and in the home freezer (at −20 °C) for up to one week and long-term storage at −80 °C for up to 6 months does not alter the total concentration of water-soluble forms of choline in expressed human milk samples. However, milk FC and GPC concentrations increased in samples that were thawed after six months of ultra-low freeze storage (i.e., at −80 °C). The increase in FC and GPC concentrations after prolonged freezer storage may be explained by the breakdown of lipid-soluble forms of choline, similar to the increase in FC concentration in milk stored at room temperature for 4 h. Similar changes were observed in serum samples that were inappropriately processed and stored, with increasing concentration of total water-soluble choline concentration [31]. We were limited to six participants for the stability study as it was logistically challenging to recruit participants willing to commute to our research site, provide a fresh milk sample, and provide the sample as a complete milk expression. We however compensated in our statistical analysis for this limitation (i.e., possible high variability across samples due to small sample size) by using related-samples analyses rather than independent comparisons across conditions. Future research is warranted to enhance the stability data by testing more milk samples as well as more frequent and longer duration intervals to identify whether and when water-soluble forms of choline concentration or composition may change in different cold storage conditions.

To our knowledge, this study is the first to test the effect of pasteurization on water-soluble forms of choline concentrations in human milk. We showed that Holder pasteurization lowered milk PhosC and GPC concentrations by about 5%, and thereby total water-soluble forms of choline concentration by 3%. Limitation of our study was the use of previously frozen milk samples, for 5–9 years at −80 °C, which is not consistent with clinical practice of pooling human milk and it undergoing pasteurization. We used biobanked milk samples because of low milk volumes collected in the stability and variability study, as well as to reduce participant burden. Additionally, for this preliminary study, we were mainly focusing on the comparison of choline concentrations between before and after pasteurization. We acknowledge that the long-term storage at −80 °C may have affected the milk concentrations of the water-soluble forms of choline; however, the total water-soluble choline concentration in the pre-pasteurized samples was similar to that of the fresh milk samples in the stability study (1241 μmol/L versus 1231 μmol/L, respectively), as well as compared to those reported in the literature [11,24,32]. This seems to reflect that the total water-soluble choline concentration was not affected by the long-term storage at −80 °C and that our findings may contribute to the literature of how human milk is altered by pasteurization.

Considering the crucial benefits of pasteurization for microbiological safety, we evaluate the <5% decrease in milk concentration of water-soluble forms of choline as minor yet recommend the confirmation of our findings in a second and larger study. The impact of pasteurization on lipid-soluble choline compounds should also be investigated in future studies. If confirmed, our finding of a 5% decrease should reassure clinicians that the benefits of providing pasteurized human milk continue to outweigh the risk of nutrient losses. Indeed, despite previous reports of a decrease in several nutrients, including folate, vitamin C and B6, due to pasteurization [18,25,26], the use of pasteurization techniques continues to ensure the biologically-safe provision of human milk at hospital settings around the globe.

In regards to the variability of water-soluble forms of choline concentration in expressed human milk, we observed diurnal changes in milk FC and GPC concentrations, but not in PhosC and total water-soluble choline forms. The total concentration of water-soluble forms of choline in expressed human milk we found was similar to the concentrations previously reported by our team for Canadian lactating women [24,32] and by Fischer et al. for US women [11]. Because no substantial diurnal changes were observed and the total concentration of water-soluble forms of choline in human milk seems stable, we conclude that the time point of milk sample collection in studies on water-soluble forms of choline may not influence the study outcomes. However, because of the diverse intra-individual variability of FC and GPC concentration within a day, we recommend to standardize the time of milk sample collection across study participants. The influencing factors of the intra-individual variability for some of the water-soluble choline forms, when present, are not fully elucidated but may be related to dietary intake of choline and/or genetic variants related to choline absorption, distribution, and metabolism [11]. The effect of acute versus long-term dietary choline intake on milk composition of water-soluble forms of choline merits further investigation.

In conclusion, we provide new information on the stability of water-soluble forms of choline concentration that will help in the development of evidence-based guidelines for the safe handling and storage of expressed milk samples. Because breast milk is the recommended sole source of nutrients, including that of choline, for infants under the age of 6 months, the handling of expressed milk needs to address microbiological safety as well as nutrient-protective needs. Further research is warranted on the effect of acute versus long-term dietary choline intake on the composition of choline forms in human milk as well as the metabolic and functional significance of individual choline forms on infant growth and development.

Author Contributions: The authors' contributions were as follows: S.M.I., L.S.S., and A.M.W. designed the research; L.S.S., S.M., and A.M.W. coordinated and conducted the studies from which the milk samples were obtained; R.A.D. contributed to laboratory analysis; A.M.W. and Y.L. analyzed the data; L.S.S. prepared the initial draft of the manuscript; S.M., A.M.W., and Y.L. provided critical input into the writing and editing of the manuscript. All authors have read and approved the final version of the manuscript.

Acknowledgments: We thank all study participants for their time and efforts.

References

1. Zeisel, S.; Niculescu, M. Perinatal choline influences brain structure and function. *Nutr. Rev.* **2006**, *64*, 197–203. [CrossRef] [PubMed]
2. Zeisel, S.H. Nutritional Importance of Choline for Brain Development. *J. Am. Coll. Nutr.* **2004**, *23*, 621S–626S. [CrossRef] [PubMed]
3. Zeisel, S.H. Choline: Critical Role During Fetal Development and Dietary Requirements in Adults. *Annu. Rev. Nutr.* **2006**, *26*, 229–250. [CrossRef]
4. Zeisel, S.H.; Blusztajn, J.K. Choline and Human Nutrition. *Rev. Nutr* **1994**, *14*, 269–296. [CrossRef]

5. Zeisel, S.H. Biochemistry, physiology, and pharmacology. *Ann. Rev. Nutr.* **1981**, *1*, 121. [CrossRef]
6. Jiang, X.; West, A.A.; Caudill, M.A. Maternal choline supplementation: A nutritional approach for improving offspring health? *Trends Endocrinol. Metab.* **2014**, *25*, 263–273. [CrossRef]
7. Craig, S.A. Betaine in human nutrition. *Am. J. Clin. Nutr.* **2004**, *80*, 539–549. [CrossRef]
8. WHO Exclusive Breastfeeding for Six Months Best for Babies Everywhere. Available online: http://www.who.int/mediacentre/news/statements/2011/breastfeeding_20110115/en (accessed on 17 July 2019).
9. Holmes, H.C.; Snodgrass, G.J.A.I.; Iles, R.A. Changes in the choline content of human breast milk in the first 3 weeks after birth. *Eur. J. Pediatr.* **2000**, *159*, 198–204. [CrossRef]
10. Ilcol, Y.O.; Ozbek, R.; Hamurtekin, E.; Ulus, I.H. Choline status in newborns, infants, children, breast-feeding women, breast-fed infants and human breast milk. *J. Nutr. Biochem.* **2005**, *16*, 489–499. [CrossRef]
11. Fischer, L.M.; Da Costa, K.A.; Galanko, J.; Sha, W.; Stephenson, B.; Vick, J.; Zeisel, S.H. Choline intake and genetic polymorphisms influence choline metabolite concentrations in human breast milk and plasma. *Am. J. Clin. Nutr.* **2010**, *92*, 336–346. [CrossRef]
12. Holmes-McNary, M.Q.; Cheng, W.L.; Mar, M.H.; Fussell, S.; Zeisel, S.H. Choline and choline esters in human and rat milk and in infant formulas. *Am. J. Clin. Nutr.* **1996**, *64*, 572–576. [CrossRef] [PubMed]
13. Davenport, C.; Yan, J.; Taesuwan, S.; Shields, K.; West, A.A.; Jiang, X.; Perry, C.A.; Malysheva, O.V.; Stabler, S.P.; Allen, R.H.; et al. Choline intakes exceeding recommendations during human lactation improve breast milk choline content by increasing PEMT pathway metabolites. *J. Nutr. Biochem.* **2015**, *26*, 903–911. [CrossRef] [PubMed]
14. Jaeger, M.C.; Lawson, M.; Filteau, S. The impact of prematurity and neonatal illness on the decision to breast-feed. *J. Adv. Nurs.* **1997**, *25*, 729–737. [CrossRef] [PubMed]
15. Johns, H.M.; Forster, D.A.; Amir, L.H.; McLachlan, H.L. Prevalence and outcomes of breast milk expressing in women with healthy term infants: A systematic review. *BMC Pregnancy Childbirth* **2013**, *13*, 212. [CrossRef]
16. Jones, F. *Best Practice for Expressing, Storing and Handling Human Milk in Hospitals, Homes, and Child Care Settings*, 3rd ed.; Human Milk Banking Association of North America, Inc.: Fort Worth, TX, USA, 2011.
17. Eglash, A.; Simon, L.; Brodribb, W.; Reece-Stremtan, S.; Noble, L.; Brent, N.; Bunik, M.; Harrel, C.; Lawrence, R.A.; LeFort, Y.; et al. ABM Clinical Protocol #8: Human Milk Storage Information for Home Use for Full-Term Infants, Revised 2017. *Breastfeed. Med.* **2017**, *12*, 390–395.
18. Donnelly-Vanderloo, M.; O'Connor, D.L.; Shoukri, M. Impact of pasteurization and procedures commonly used to rethermalize stored human milk on folate content. *Nutr. Res.* **1994**, *14*, 1305–1316. [CrossRef]
19. Peila, C.; Moro, G.; Bertino, E.; Cavallarin, L.; Giribaldi, M.; Giuliani, F.; Cresi, F.; Coscia, A. The Effect of Holder Pasteurization on Nutrients and Biologically-Active Components in Donor Human Milk: A Review. *Nutrients* **2016**, *8*, 477. [CrossRef]
20. García-Lara, N.R.; Escuder-Vieco, D.; García-Algar, O.; De la Cruz, J.; Lora, D.; Pallás-Alonso, C. Effect of Freezing Time on Macronutrients and Energy Content of Breastmilk. *Breastfeed. Med.* **2012**, *7*, 295–301. [CrossRef]
21. Ahrabi, A.F.; Handa, D.; Codipilly, C.N.; Shah, S.; Williams, J.E.; McGuire, M.A.; Potak, D.; Aharon, G.G.; Schanler, R.J. Effects of Extended Freezer Storage on the Integrity of Human Milk. *J. Pediatr.* **2016**, *177*, 140–143. [CrossRef]
22. Zeisel, S.H.; Char, D.; Sheard, N.F. Choline, phosphatidylcholine and sphingomyelin in human and bovine milk and infant formulas. *J. Nutr.* **1986**, *116*, 50–58. [CrossRef]
23. Innis, S.M.; Friesen, R.W. Essential n-3 fatty acids in pregnant women and early visual acuity maturation in term infants. *Am. J. Clin. Nutr.* **2008**, *87*, 548–557. [CrossRef]
24. Moukarzel, S.; Soberanes, L.; Dyer, R.A.; Albersheim, S.; Elango, R.; Innis, S.M.; Moukarzel, S.; Soberanes, L.; Dyer, R.A.; Albersheim, S.; et al. Relationships among Different Water-Soluble Choline Compounds Differ between Human Preterm and Donor Milk. *Nutrients* **2017**, *9*, 369. [CrossRef]
25. Peters, M.D.J.; McArthur, A.; Munn, Z. Safe management of expressed breast milk: A systematic review. *Women Birth* **2016**, *29*, 473–481. [CrossRef]
26. Nessel, I.; Khashu, M.; Dyall, S.C. The effects of storage conditions on long-chain polyunsaturated fatty acids, lipid mediators, and antioxidants in donor human milk—A review. *Prostaglandins Leukot. Essent. Fat. Acids* **2019**, *149*, 8–17. [CrossRef]
27. Loikas, S.; Lopponen, M.; Suominen, P.; Moller, J.; Irjala, K.; Isoaho, R.; Kivela, S.L.; Koskinen, P.; Pelliniemi, T.T.

RIA for serum holo-transcobalamin: Method evaluation in the clinical laboratory and reference interval. *Clin. Chem.* **2003**, *49*, 455–462. [CrossRef]
28. O'Connor, D.L.; Ewaschuk, J.B.; Unger, S. Human milk pasteurization: Benefits and risks. *Curr. Opin. Clin. Nutr. Metab. Care* **2015**, *18*, 269–275. [CrossRef]
29. Gao, C.; Miller, J.; Middleton, P.F.; Huang, Y.C.; McPhee, A.J.; Gibson, R.A. Changes to breast milk fatty acid composition during storage, handling and processing: A systematic review. *Prostaglandins Leukot. Essent. Fat. Acids* **2019**, *146*, 1–10. [CrossRef]
30. Moukarzel, S.; Dyer, R.A.; Keller, B.O.; Elango, R.; Innis, S.M. Human milk plasmalogens are highly enriched in long-chain PUFAs. *J. Nutr.* **2016**, *146*, 2412–2417. [CrossRef]
31. Holm, P.I.; Ueland, P.M.; Kvalheim, G.; Lien, E.A. Determination of choline, betaine, and dimethylglycine in plasma by a high-throughput method based on normal-phase chromatography-tandem mass spectrometry. *Clin. Chem.* **2003**, *49*, 286–294. [CrossRef]
32. Wiedeman, A.M.; Whitfield, K.C.; March, K.M.; Chen, N.N.; Kroeun, H.; Sokhoing, L.; Sophonneary, P.; Dyer, R.A.; Xu, Z.; Kitts, D.D.; et al. Concentrations of Water-Soluble Forms of Choline in Human Milk from Lactating Women in Canada and Cambodia. *Nutrients* **2018**, *10*, 381. [CrossRef]

Permissions

All chapters in this book were first published by MDPI; hereby published with permission under the Creative Commons Attribution License or equivalent. Every chapter published in this book has been scrutinized by our experts. Their significance has been extensively debated. The topics covered herein carry significant findings which will fuel the growth of the discipline. They may even be implemented as practical applications or may be referred to as a beginning point for another development.

The contributors of this book come from diverse backgrounds, making this book a truly international effort. This book will bring forth new frontiers with its revolutionizing research information and detailed analysis of the nascent developments around the world.

We would like to thank all the contributing authors for lending their expertise to make the book truly unique. They have played a crucial role in the development of this book. Without their invaluable contributions this book wouldn't have been possible. They have made vital efforts to compile up to date information on the varied aspects of this subject to make this book a valuable addition to the collection of many professionals and students.

This book was conceptualized with the vision of imparting up-to-date information and advanced data in this field. To ensure the same, a matchless editorial board was set up. Every individual on the board went through rigorous rounds of assessment to prove their worth. After which they invested a large part of their time researching and compiling the most relevant data for our readers.

The editorial board has been involved in producing this book since its inception. They have spent rigorous hours researching and exploring the diverse topics which have resulted in the successful publishing of this book. They have passed on their knowledge of decades through this book. To expedite this challenging task, the publisher supported the team at every step. A small team of assistant editors was also appointed to further simplify the editing procedure and attain best results for the readers.

Apart from the editorial board, the designing team has also invested a significant amount of their time in understanding the subject and creating the most relevant covers. They scrutinized every image to scout for the most suitable representation of the subject and create an appropriate cover for the book.

The publishing team has been an ardent support to the editorial, designing and production team. Their endless efforts to recruit the best for this project, has resulted in the accomplishment of this book. They are a veteran in the field of academics and their pool of knowledge is as vast as their experience in printing. Their expertise and guidance has proved useful at every step. Their uncompromising quality standards have made this book an exceptional effort. Their encouragement from time to time has been an inspiration for everyone.

The publisher and the editorial board hope that this book will prove to be a valuable piece of knowledge for researchers, students, practitioners and scholars across the globe.

List of Contributors

Dandara G. Haag
Indigenous Oral Health Unit, Australian Research Centre for Population Oral Health, The University of Adelaide, Adelaide, SA 5005, Australia
School of Public Health, The University of Adelaide, Adelaide, SA 5005, Australia

Lisa M. Jamieson and Joanne Hedges
Indigenous Oral Health Unit, Australian Research Centre for Population Oral Health, The University of Adelaide, Adelaide, SA 5005, Australia

Lisa G. Smithers
School of Public Health, The University of Adelaide, Adelaide, SA 5005, Australia

Zoya Gridneva, Anna R. Hepworth and Ching T. Lai
School of Molecular Sciences, M310, The University of Western Australia, Crawley, Perth, WA 6009, Australia

Donna T. Geddes
School of Molecular Sciences, M310, The University of Western Australia, Crawley, Perth, WA 6009, Australia
School of Molecular Sciences, The University of Western Australia, 35 Stirling Hwy, Crawley, WA 6009, Australia

Leigh C. Ward
School of Chemistry and Molecular Biosciences, The University of Queensland, St. Lucia, Brisbane, QLD 4072, Australia

Céline J. Fischer Fumeaux, Lydie Beauport and Jean-François Tolsa
Clinic of Neonatology, Department Woman Mother Child, University Hospital of Lausanne, 1011 Lausanne, Switzerland

Marie-Claude Courtet-Compondu and Michael Affolter
Nestlé Institute of Food Safety & Analytical Science, Nestlé Research, 1000 Lausanne, Switzerland

Sagar K. Thakkar
Nestlé Research Asia, Singapore 138567, Singapore
Nestle Research Singapore Hub, Société des Produits Nestlé SA, 29 Quality Road, Singapore 618802, Singapore

Jacqueline C. Kent, Hazel Gardner and Ching-Tat Lai
School of Molecular Sciences, The University of Western Australia, 35 Stirling Hwy, Crawley, WA 6009, Australia

Kevin Murray
School of Population and Global Health, The University of Western Australia, 35 Stirling Hwy, Crawley, WA 6009, Australia

Alethea Rea
Centre for Applied Statistics, The University of Western Australia, Crawley, Perth, WA 6009, Australia

Catharina E. M. van Beijsterveldt
Department of Biological Psychology, Vrije Universiteit Amsterdam, 1081 BT Amsterdam, The Netherlands

Fiona A. Hagenbeek, Meike Bartels, Dorret I. Boomsma and Jenny van Dongen
Department of Biological Psychology, Vrije Universiteit Amsterdam, 1081 BT Amsterdam, The Netherlands
Amsterdam Public Health Research Institute, 1081 BT Amsterdam, The Netherlands

Gennady T. Sukhikh
Kulakov National Medical Research Center for Obstetrics, Gynecology and Perinatology, Moscow 101000, Russia

Veronika V. Odintsova
Department of Biological Psychology, Vrije Universiteit Amsterdam, 1081 BT Amsterdam, The Netherlands
Amsterdam Public Health Research Institute, 1081 BT Amsterdam, The Netherlands
Kulakov National Medical Research Center for Obstetrics, Gynecology and Perinatology, Moscow 101000, Russia

Matthew Suderman, Doretta Caramaschi and Caroline Relton
MRC Integrative Epidemiology Unit, Bristol Medical School, Population Health Science, University of Bristol, Bristol BS8 1TH, UK

Noah A. Kallsen, Erik A. Ehli and Gareth E. Davies
Avera Institute for Human Genetics, Sioux Falls, SD 57101, USA

Vassilios Fanos
Neonatal Intensive Care Unit, Department of Surgical Sciences, AOU and University of Cagliari, 09121 Cagliari, Italy

Setareh Shahab-Ferdows
USDA/ARS Western Human Nutrition Research Center, 430West Health Sciences Drive, Davis, CA 95616, USA

Daniela Hampel and Lindsay H. Allen
USDA/ARS Western Human Nutrition Research Center, 430West Health Sciences Drive, Davis, CA 95616, USA
Department of Nutrition, University of California, One Shields Ave, Davis, CA 95616, USA

Muttaquina Hossain, M. Munirul Islam and Tahmeed Ahmed
Nutrition and Clinical Services Division, International Centre for Diarrhoeal Disease Research, 68 Shaheed Tajuddin Ahmed Sarani, Mohakhali, Dhaka 1212, Bangladesh

Anna Hepworth
School of Molecular Sciences, Faculty of Science, The University of Western Australia, Perth, WA 6009, Australia

Donna Geddes
School of Molecular Sciences, Faculty of Science, The University of Western Australia, Perth, WA 6009, Australia
School of Molecular Sciences, University of Western Australia, 35 Stirling Highway, Crawley, 6009 WA, Australia

Chooi Kok, Kathryn Nancarrow and Karen Simmer
Centre for Neonatal Research and Education, School of Medicine, Faculty of Health and Medical Sciences, The University of Western Australia, Perth, WA 6009, Australia
The Neonatal Directorate, King Edward Memorial Hospital, Perth, WA 6008, Australia

M. Teresa Cabezuelo
Department of Physiology, Universitat de València, Avda. Blasco Ibañez, 15, 46010 Valencia, Spain
University Hospital Doctor Peset, Gaspar Aguilar, 90, 46017 Valencia, Spain

Rosa Zaragozá
Department of Human Anatomy and Embryology-INCLIVA Biomedical Research Institute, Universitat de València, 46010 Valencia, Spain

Teresa Barber and Juan R. Viña
Department of Biochemistry and Molecular Biology-INCLIVA Biomedical Research Institute, Universitat de València, 46010 Valencia, Spain

Malgorzata Witkowska-Zimny, Ewa Kamińska-El-Hassan and Edyta Wróbel
Department of Biophysics and Human Physiology, Medical University of Warsaw, Chalubinskiego 5, 02-004 Warsaw, Poland

Amal Nasser, Fadumo Omer, Fatima Al-Lenqawi, Rehab Al-awwa, Tamam Khan, Asmaa El-Heneidy, Rana kurdi and Ghadir Al-Jayyousi
Department of Public Health, College of Health Sciences, Qatar University, 2713 Doha, Qatar

Wan Jun Tie
School of Molecular Sciences, M310, The University of Western Australia, Crawley, Perth, WA 6009, Australia

Magalie Sabatier, Clara L. Garcia-Rodenas, Peter Kastenmayer, Mario Vigo, Stéphane Dubascoux, Daniel Andrey, Marine Nicolas, Janique Richoz Payot and Valentine Bordier
Nestlé Research, Société des Produits Nestlé SA, 1000 Lausanne, Switzerland

Carlos A. De Castro
Nestle Research Singapore Hub, Société des Produits Nestlé SA, 29 Quality Road, Singapore 618802, Singapore
Clinical Development Unit, Nestlé Research Asia, Singapore 138567, Singapore

Ching Tat Lai
School of Molecular Sciences, University of Western Australia, 35 Stirling Highway, Crawley, 6009 WA, Australia
School of Molecular Sciences, M310, The University of Western Australia, Crawley, Perth, WA 6009, Australia

Emily E. Little and Leslie J. Carver
Department of Psychology, University of California, San Diego, CA 92093, USA

Cristine H. Legare
Department of Psychology, The University of Texas at Austin, TX 78712, USA

Sara Moukarzel
Larsson-Rosenquist Foundation Mother-Milk-Infant Center of Research Excellence, University of California, San Diego, CA 92093, USA

Alejandra M. Wiedeman, Roger A. Dyer and Sheila M. Innis
British Columbia Children's Hospital Research Institute, Vancouver, BC V5Z 4H4, Canada
Department of Pediatrics, Faculty of Medicine, The University of British Columbia, Vancouver, BC V5Z 4H4, Canada

Lynda S. Soberanes and Yvonne Lamers
British Columbia Children's Hospital Research Institute, Vancouver, BC V5Z 4H4, Canada
Food, Nutrition, and Health Program, Faculty of Land and Food Systems, The University of British Columbia, Vancouver, BC V6T 1Z4, Canada

Alexandra D. George and Melvin C. L. Gay
School of Molecular Sciences, M310, The University of Western Australia, Crawley, Perth, WA 6009, Australia

Peter E. Hartmann
School of Molecular Sciences, M310, The University of Western Australia, Crawley, Perth, WA 6009, Australia
School of Molecular Sciences, The University of Western Australia, 35 Stirling Hwy, Crawley, WA 6009, Australia

Sambavi Kugananthan
School of Molecular Sciences, M310, The University of Western Australia, Crawley, Perth, WA 6009, Australia
School of Human Sciences, The University of Western Australia, Crawley, Perth, WA 6009, Australia

Index

www.ingramcontent.com/pod-product-compliance
Lightning Source LLC
LaVergne TN
LVHW060538210926
848485LV00005B/1222